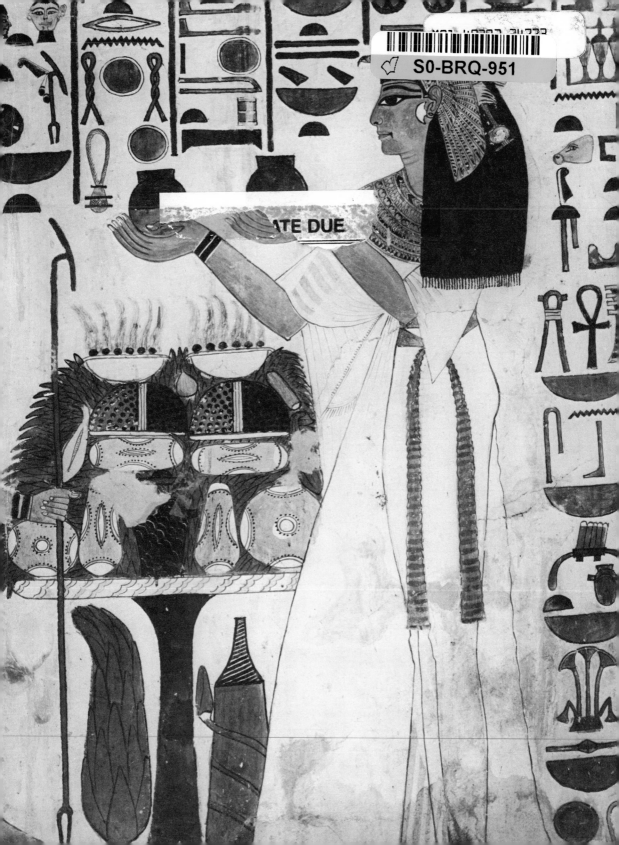

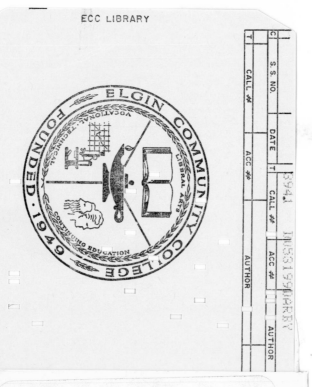

Food:
The Gift of Osiris

VOLUME 1

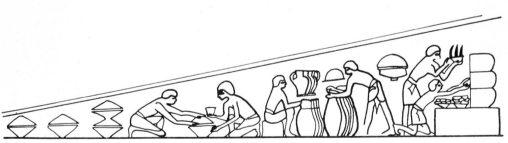

handling of honey

Frontispiece: The God Osiris. Tomb of Sennutem (number 1) at Thebes. (Deir el Medina); New Kingdom, Ramessid Period, date uncertain. Photographed 1967

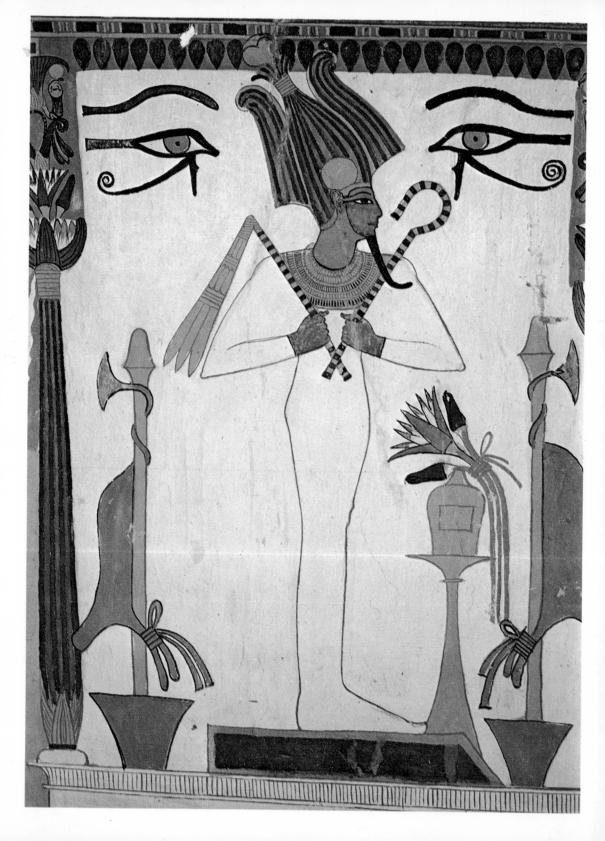

Food:
The Gift of Osiris

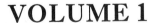

WILLIAM J. DARBY

Vanderbilt University, Nashville,
Tennessee, U.S.A. and
The Nutrition Foundation,
New York, U.S.A.

PAUL GHALIOUNGUI

Cairo, Egypt

LOUIS GRIVETTI

University of California,
Davis, California, U.S.A.

VOLUME 1

ACADEMIC PRESS

1977

London New York San Francisco

A Subsidiary of Harcourt Brace Jovanovich, Publishers

ACADEMIC PRESS INC. (LONDON) LTD.
24/28 Oval Road, London NW1

United States Edition published by
ACADEMIC PRESS INC.
111 Fifth Avenue, New York, New York 10003

Library of Congress Catalog Card Number: 75-19630
ISBN: 0-12-203401-5

Text set 11/12pt Monotype Baskerville, printed by photolithography and
bound in Great Britain at The Pitman Press, Bath

For

Elva Darby
Hugette Ghalioungui
Georgette Grivetti

Preface

The cultural significance of given items of food, in a given society, and at a given time, is widely, though often only subconsciously, recognized. Less generally is it appreciated that the social implications of eating particular foods vary from one period to another or from culture to culture. Conversely, some attitudes persist for exceedingly long periods of time and through diverse social eras, and all the while the current explanations or interpretations of the conditions that gave rise to them may differ considerably from earlier explanations or from their factual origin.

These concepts are particularly well illustrated, retrospectively, by the unparalleled wealth of evidence pertaining to foods over the 7,000 or more years of history recorded in that relatively small geographic area commonly referred to as "the Middle East". Inasmuch as many modern food attitudes are associated with the religious or ethical concepts of the three dominant religions, Christianity, Islam and Judaism, which all originated there, an understanding of the genesis of food habits in this region should be of especial interest to the major cultures of the Western world.

However, these religions and the associated cultural attitudes toward food did not develop *de novo*; they were based upon practices and codes of earlier, highly developed social structures and civilizations, partial records of which are available. These records (or fragments of them) are so scattered through the storehouses of knowledge that they are inaccessible to scholars except within the inventories of their particular scholarly disciplines. We have, therefore, attempted to assemble as much as possible of the evidence that is interpretable in terms of food use and changing attitudes towards foods, as those occurred in courses of the history of the regions studied. Where feasible, we have also tried to relate these concepts to the position of certain foods today.

The constant concern of the ancient physician for diet is a recurrent theme in the writings of the classical physician-scholars Hippocrates, Celsus, Avicenna, and others. The use of foodstuffs in prescriptions from the records of Egyptian physicians from the time of Imhotep onwards, and their instructions, reveal much concerning the "art of food" at a given time, or the availability of food items. Hence, we judge that our account would be incomplete without reference to food in medicine.

The broad understanding thus obtained should provide a useful perspective to our own changing habits and attitudes, as well as to foreign habits that might seem to us strange or incomprehensible. Hopefully, it may afford a greater appreciation of that neglected area of history, namely, the cultural role that food plays in societies. Accordingly, the present work should be of interest to readers of widely diverse backgrounds: agriculturalists, anthropologists, archaeologists, classicists, ecclesiasticists, Egyptologists, food scientists, historians, nutritionists, medical historians, sociologists and others. It should appeal also to that inquisitive general reader who is intrigued with the origin and evolution of his own value judgements and living practices, and who experiences the thrill of romance in the magnificent and colourful fragments of knowledge of earlier civilizations from which the roots of his culture and traditions have been so richly nurtured.

We recognized the enormity of our undertaking and the diversity of sources and disciplines that had to be drawn upon. We have sought, therefore, the counsel and guidance of a wise circle of competent colleagues. We have appreciated the role of food in mythological, mystic, and religious beliefs in determining attitudes and, conversely, the influence of these beliefs upon food acceptability, and have, therefore, sought cues from diverse sources in order that others with deeper knowledge and insight may extend our understanding of food and its cultural significance.

The numerous illustrations have been carefully selected as documentary evidence supplied to allow the reader to appreciate both the wealth and the limitations of this knowledge base. Their inherent beauty may add to the attractiveness of the work, but the reader is urged to study them for their remarkable content.

Due to the richness of the associations, it has been difficult to limit the text, but the focus is on Egypt and the Nile valley, with emphasis on the social and cultural concepts relative to foods through the ages. The diversity of the evidence utilized and the weight given by the thoughtful, critical scholar to particular types of evidence made it desirable to document the sources drawn upon. It is hoped that by so doing others in specialized disciplines may be stimulated to pursue the contribution that their field can offer to improve knowledge of the cultural role and position of foods in society.

Volume 1, after a short survey of the state of nutrition in Ancient Egypt, considers the available information on the major food articles of animal origin—protein rich meats, ranging from the sumptuous beef to the popular and often deprecated fish and seafoods. Reflection on the evidence presented indicates that these food stuffs, then as now, were more accessible to the ruling class, the wealthy, the priesthood, the affluent. Much of the evidence is gleaned from scenes depicting the life-style of the nobility, the leisure class, the pharaohs, or the scholarly traveler. Permanent records of practices by the common man are few, except as seen through the eyes of the élite. Hence, inferences must be drawn from sources of other kinds in order to synthesize a picture of the food culture of the majority of the people of an historical period.

The animal world, however, played more than a nutritive role in Egyptian thought. It did inspire realistic scenes of husbandry and sport, but it was also an inexhaustible source of inspiration that fed the need of symbolic expression, in literature and art, of the powers and virtues of gods and kings who were called bulls or hawks or were given their shape.

A further step was taken when animals were illustrated, not in solemn divine or royal functions, but in plainly human activities. The general tone was humoristic, animals cooking, brewing, plucking the harp or blowing the oboe. More often it was a burlesque caricature of the ceremonious decoration of tombs and temples, a parody that reached at times a philosophy of the absurd, comparable to the contemporary literature of despair: birds using ladders to climb a tree while a hippopotamus is already seated in its foliage and eating its fruits, humans led by goats, cats serving mice, an army of rats storming a fortress manned by surrendering cats, and the like (Curto, no date). It behoves the student, therefore, in examining this symbolic art or the graphic heralds of Aesop, Muqaffah, and other fabulists of old, to bear in mind such artistic motivations.

The items discussed in Volume 2—cereals, vegetables, fruits and alcoholic beverages, especially beer, are better representatives, however, of the staple diet and of the bulk of caloric intake of the majority of the people in antiquity. Rather than the "meat and wine" of the affluent society, "bread and beer" in Ancient Egypt, "bread and salt" in Biblical and Arabian traditions, "bread and butter" in modern Western usage, are the usual synecdoques for daily food.

The East has always been fond of expressing its wisdom in aphoristic metaphors and parables which springing as they do from the common experience of the people, tersely betray the ecological conditions of their birth. A proverb like "What could the Fellah know of apples" expresses better than a lengthy statistical study the relative scarcity of that expensive fruit and its high "social status" in rural Egypt. "Goose chicks can swim", could have been conceived only in a well-watered countryside. Conversely, the ritual use of sand as a cleansing agent, is borne out by the adage "When water comes, cleaning with sand (*tayammum*) is excluded" and the religious injunction to cleanse with sand cooking vessels defiled by dogs could have been born only in a waterless desert: in these two examples, the Arabian peninsula.

Accordingly, since ages immemorial, street-cries and popular maxims express the meaning of food to the Egyptian people. We have tagged some of these to various food items, drawing from our personal experience and from several publications, more especially from the voluminous collection of proverbs by Mrs F. A. Ragheb (1939), many of which re-appear among the over 800 maxims and street-cries that Miss C. Wissa Wassef recorded in her thesis on the rural and alimentary traditions of the Copts (1971). These traditions are mostly general to all ethnic groups in Egypt, underscoring autochthonous practice as distinct from the ostentatious Turkish and Persian Court cuisines imported during the last five centuries. Her work is invaluable to students of food culture and customs in their relation to seasons, fasts, agricultural cycles and milestones of life (birth, baptism, wedding, delivery, mourning).

William J. Darby   *November 1976*
Paul E. Ghalioungui
Louis Grivetti

Acknowledgements

This investigation was supported in part by Public Health Service Research Grant No. AM 08317 from the National Institute of Arthritis and Metabolic Diseases. Dr Karl Mason of that Institute has been most helpful throughout our researches.

Research facilities and support granted in part by US Naval Medical Research Unit No. 3 (NAMRU-3), Cairo, ARE—supported by Bureau of Medicine and Surgery, United States Navy Work Unit No. MR005.20–0150, and the National Institutes of Health Grant No. 112501.

The opinions and assertions contained herein are private ones of the authors and are not to be construed as official or reflecting the views of the United States Public Health Service, the Navy Department, the Naval Service at large, or the ARE Ministry of Agriculture, Ministry of Culture and National Orientation, or the Ministry of Health.

We wish to thank the several officials of the Arab Republic of Egypt whose skills and assistance, cooperation, and cordial relationships made possible this study.

Our special gratitude is expressed to Dr Gamal Mokhtar, Under Secretary of State, Department of Antiquities, ARE, from whose experience, guidance, and skill we greatly benefited.

Throughout his tenure as Director General of Antiquities, Dr Mokhtar's schedule has been one of accelerated organization, especially during the intense activities of the past few years. He maintains a calm and friendly professional ease, an unhurried cordiality that he extends to all investigators. Dr Mokhtar's field is Egypt, past and present. His goal is to share the accumulated knowledge with all inquiring scholars. For his friendship, hospitality and scholarly assistance, and for the free access he allowed us to the unique collections and holdings of the Department of Antiquities of the ARE, we are most grateful.

The authors acknowledge their special indebtedness to Mrs Gloria Martin, who skillfully rendered the large number of excellent, accurate, informative pen and ink drawings made from photographs and other documented sources. These add immeasurably to the clarity of the text, the documentation of sources of information and impart a uniformity of illustrative material that could not otherwise have been obtained.

To each of the several hundred persons who helped with this work we are grateful. We wish, however, to recognize especially the interest and assistance of the following persons:

Ministry of Agriculture, ARE:
    Dr Abbas El-Itriby, Under-Secretary of State
    Dr Mahmoud Helmy El-Kawas, Director-General, Agriculture Museum, Dokki
    Mr Edward Riskalla, Deputy Director-General, Agriculture Museum, Dokki
    Mr Hussein Kamel El Monayar, Administrative Assistant, Antiquities Division, Agriculture Museum, Dokki
    Mr William Nazir, Specialist in Ancient Agriculture, Antiquities Division, Agriculture Museum, Dokki
    Mr Hassan Khattab, Specialist in Ancient Agriculture, Antiquities Division, Agriculture Museum, Dokki
    Mr Ramzy Higazi, Director, Training Division, Department of Foreign Relations, Ministry of Agriculture, Dokki
    Mr Medhat Abu Shahba, Engineer, Department of Foreign Relations, Ministry of Agriculture, Dokki

Ministry of Culture and National Orientation, ARE:
    Dr Henri Riad, Director General, Egyptian Museum, Department of Antiquities
    Dr Abdel Hamid Youssef, Director, Centre for Documentation, Department of Antiquities
    Dr Abdel Hamid el Dahly, Archaeological Inspector, Luxor, Department of Antiquities
    Mrs Zeinab el Dawakhly, Librarian, Centre for Documentation, Department of Antiquities
    Mr Mohamed Salah, Archaeological Inspector, Necropolis of Thebes, Department of Antiquities
    Mr Ramadan Saad, Archaeological Inspector, Karnak, Department of Antiquities
    Mr Ali el-Khouli, Archaeological Inspector, Saqqara, Department of Antiquities
    Mr Magdi Abdel Maboud Abdalla, Chief Guard, Necropolis of Thebes, Department of Antiquities

To Dr Serge Sauneron, Director, Institut Français d'Archéologie Orientale, Cairo, we offer our great appreciation for use of the vast archives and library materials of this unique Egyptological institution, for valuable information on many Egyptological details, and for the hieroglyphs used in the book that were provided by the presses of the Institut.

To Professor Charles Kuentz, the distinguished Egyptologist and former Director of the Institut Français d'Archéologie Orientale in Cairo, we are indebted for highly valuable help and information on historical and philological details.

Members of the Division of Nutrition of Vanderbilt University have long cooperated with the United States Naval Medical Research Unit No. 3 (NAMRU-3) in Cairo, ARE. We particularly wish to acknowledge this support. To both past and present colleagues at NAMRU-3 we are especially grateful,

Dr John R. Seal, M.C., USN, Director, NAMRU-3 (1958–61)
Dr James Boyers, M.C., USN, Director, NAMRU-3 (1962–63)
Dr Lloyd F. Miller, M.C., USN, Director, NAMRU-3 (1964–67)
Dr Donald C. Kent, M.C., USN, Director, NAMRU-3 (1967–70)
Dr Henry Sparks, M.C., USN, Director, NAMRU-3 (1970–73)
Dr Walter Miner, M.C., USN, Director, NAMRU-3 (1973–present)
Dr Imam Zaghloul El Sayed, Director-General, Ministry of Health Laboratories, ARE.
Dr Vinayak Narayan Patwardhan, Assistant Director for Nutrition and Biochemistry
Dr Harry Hoogstraal, Department Head, Department of Medical Zoology
Dr Dale Osborn, Mammalogist, Department of Medical Zoology
Mr Kenneth Otto Horner, Ornithologist, Department of Medical Zoology
Mr Abdel Aziz Salah, Administrative Assistant
Mr Ibrahim Helmi, Technician, Department of Medical Zoology
Mr Samir Araman, Technician, Department of Medical Zoology
Mr Abdalla Diab, Technician, Department of Bacteriology
Mr Sobhy Gaber, Research Associate, Department of Medical Zoology
Mr Hassan Touhami, Laboratory Aide, Department of Medical Zoology
Mr Abdou Hosny Aly, Nurse, Department of Tropical Medicine

With permission of the ARE Department of Antiquities, Mr Ward Patterson has prepared stone rubbings of selected nutrition reliefs from Old Kingdom tombs at Saqqara. Photographs from his unique collection are used with his permission. Mr A. Bergère, Cultural Attaché, French Embassy, formerly in Kuwait, now in Libya, offered friendly assistance and placed at our disposal texts from his fine Egyptological library.

The staff of the library of University of Chicago, particularly Mr Stanley Gwynn, Miss Shirley Lyon, and Mrs Alexandria Denny of the Breasted Library, assisted the authors during early phases of research. Of distinct help in the translation and organization of archaeological texts were Dr Aida Nureddin and Mrs Georgette Stylianos Mayerakis Grivetti.

Miss Juanita Frazor, Executive Secretary, Department of Biochemistry, Vanderbilt School of Medicine, endured our tempers, illegible handwriting and endless revisions. Her tenacity, skill, and cheerfulness are attributes greatly to be admired.

Although the organization and final content are the sole responsibility of the authors, the text benefits from the review by and encouragement and criticism from professional colleagues from several fields:

> Dr Paul E. Johnson, Executive Secretary, Committee on Food Protection, National Research Council, National Academy of Sciences, Washington, D.C.
>
> Dr E. Neige Todhunter, Visiting Professor of Nutrition, Department of Biochemistry, Vanderbilt University School of Medicine, Nashville, Tennessee
>
> Dr Dale Osborn, Mammalogist, Department of Medical Zoology, NAMRU-3, Cairo, ARE.
>
> Dr Kent Weeks, Medical Historian/Egyptologist, Metropolitan Museum, New York
>
> Professor V. Täckholm, Faculty of Science, Cairo University
>
> Dr James S. Dinning, Associate Director, Rockefeller Foundation, Bangkok, Thailand
>
> Dr Wallace Aykroyd, Oxford, England
>
> Dr Frederick J. Simoons, Professor of Geography, University of California, Davis
>
> Mr Kenneth Otto Horner, Ornithologist, Department of Medical Zoology, NAMRU-3, Cairo, ARE.

Dr Richard Hall, Vice President, McCormick and Co. Inc., Hunt Valley, Maryland

Dr Maynard Amerine, Professor of Enology, University of California at Davis

To all Egyptologists, from Champollion to present, whose research and insight provided the keys to the mysteries of Egyptian civilization, we are humbly grateful.

Finally, the authors sincerely appreciate the warm understanding, the interest and patience that has characterized our pleasant relationship with the Academic Press Inc. (London) Ltd. during the production of this book. The encouragement, creativity in design and unstinting cooperation of all of the staff, but especially of Jane Duncan, have made this a remarkably happy author–publisher relationship.

William J. Darby   *November 1976*
Paul E. Ghalioungui
Louis Grivetti

Abbreviations

The following abbreviations to references appear throughout the text.

A.R.   *Ancient Records of Egypt*: see Breasted, J. H. (1906).

ASAE   *Annales du Service des Antiquités de l'Egypte.*

Ber.   The Berlin Papyrus: see Wreszinski, W. (1909). *Der grosse medizinische Papyrus des Berliner Museums*, Leipzig: Hinrichs.

B.I.E.   *Bulletin de l'Institut d'Egypte*, Cairo.

B.I.F.A.O.   *Bulletin de l'Institut Français d'Archéologie Orientale*, Cairo.

Carlsb.   *The Carlsberg Papyrus*, Det Kgl. Videnskabernes Selskab histor.-philologische Meddelelser XXVI, E. Iversen, Copenhagen (1939).

Ch.B.   *The Chester Beatty Papyrus*, Hieratic papyri in the British Museum, 3rd series, Translated by Jonckheere, F. (1947). Brussels: Fondation Egyptologique Reine Elisabeth.

Deipnos.   see Athenaeus, *The Deipnosophists.*

Diod.   see Diodorus Siculus.

Eb.   see Ebbell B., *The Papyrus Ebers*, The Ebbell classification is noted in Roman characters; the Wreszinski in Arabic numerals.

F.   Faulkner, R. O. (1962). *A Concise Dictionary of Middle Egyptian*, Oxford University Press.

Fl.   see Loret, V. (1892b). *La Flore Pharaonique.*

G.   Gardiner, A. H. (1950). *Egyptian Grammar*, 2nd Ed. Oxford: Oxford University Press.

Geo.   see Strabo, *Geography.*

Gpfl.   see Keimer (1924a). *Die Gartenpflanze.*

H.   see Wreszinski (1912). *Der Londoner medizinische Papyrus . . . und der Papyrus Hearst . . .* Leipzig: Hinrichs.

Her.   see *Herodotus.*

I. and O.   see Plutarch, *Isis and Osiris.*

J.E.A.   *Journal of Egyptian Archaeology.*

JNEAS   *Journal of Near Eastern Studies.*

K.   *Hieratic Papyri from Kahun and Gurob*, Griffith, F. Ll., London (1898).

L. London Medical Papyrus: see Wreszinski, W. (1912). *Der Londoner medizinische Papyrus . . . und der Papyrus Hearst . . .*, Leipzig: Hinrichs.

MAE see Hayes, W. C. (1964). *Most Ancient Egypt.*

N.H. see Pliny, *Natural History.*

Pyr. *The Pyramid Texts in Translation and Commentary*, by Mercer, S. A. B. (1952). 4 vols. London: Longmans, Green and Co.

Ram III Gardiner, A. H. (1955). *Five Ramasseum Papyri.* Oxford: Oxford University Press; and Barns, J. W. B. (1956). *Five Ramasseum Papyri*, Oxford: Oxford University Press.

S. *The Edwin Smith Surgical Papyrus.* Translated by Breasted, J. H. (1930). Vol. I. Hieroglyphic transliteration, Translatic and Commentary. Vol. II. Facsimile plates and line for line hieroglyphic transliteration. Chicago: The University of Chicago Press.

S.P. *Select Papyri*, see Hunt, A. S. and Edgar, C. C. (1932–34).

Wb. see Erman, A. and Grapow, H. (1957). *Wörterbuch der aegyptischen Sprache.*

Wb.Dr. see von Deines, H. and Grapow, H. (1959). *Wörterbuch der aegyptische Drogennamen*, Berlin: Akademie-Verlag (Grundriss der Medizin der Alten Aegypter, Vol. 6).

Z.A.S. *Zeitschr. für Aegyptische Sprache und Altertumskunde.*

Zaub. Zaubersprüche für Kind und Mutter, Berlin Papyrus 3027 Erman, A. (1901), Abhandlungen der königlichen Preussicher Akademie der Wissenschaften zu Berlin.

T. see Täckholm, V. L. (1941–69). *The Flora of Egypt.*

Note on Vocalization of Symbols used in Transliterating Hieroglyphic Sounds

ʾ the glottal stop heard at the commencement of German words beginning with a vowel, ex. *der Adler* (Arabic *alif hamzatun*)

i̯ Consonantal *Y*

ʿ a guttural sound unknown in English, corresponds to Hebrew *avin*, Arabic *ain*

ḥ emphatic *h*, corresponds to Arabic *ha*

ḫ like *ch* in Scottish *loch*

h perhaps like *ch* in German *ich*

š *sh*

ḳ backward *k*; rather like our *q* in *queen*, corresponds to Hebrew *qoph* Arabic *kaf*

ṯ *tsh*

ḏ *dj*

Conventionally an *e* is intercalated between consonants in pronouncing Ancient Egyptian words except when an ʾ or an ʿ which are read *a*, are present.

Adapted from Gardiner (1950), p. 27.

Contents

Contents   xxi

Chapter 5   Other Mammals: Ovines, Wild Species, Equids, Cervinae, Canidae, Miscellaneous **211**

Contents   *xxiii*

Contents of Volume 2

List of Illustrations Volume I

Endpapers:
Front left. Ptahhetep. Saqqara.
Front right. Nefertari. Thebes.
Back left. Mereruka's tomb. Saqqara.
Back right. Tomb of Ptahhetep. Saqqara.

Half-title page. Handling of honey (Fig. 9.2).
Title page. Youth devouring a duck (Fig. 6.25).
Frontispiece (Colour plate) The god Osiris.

Chapter 1 Introduction

All photographs taken by authors except when specifically acknowledged otherwise.

Chapter 4 Meat: Pork

Chapter 5 Other Mammals: Ovines, Wild Species, Equids, Cervinae, Caridae

Chapter 7 Fish

Chapter 8 Reptiles, Shellfish, Molluscs and Arthropods

Chapter 9 Sweetening Agents

Chapter I   Introduction, Evaluation of Data, Special Discussions

Introduction

Conceptual Organization of the Text

History and archaeology rise above mere chronicle, whenever they aim at fulfilling the teaching of Socrates inscribed on the temple of Apollo, at Delphi, "know thyself".[1] To know man's food, whether in the twentieth century or in antiquity, is to know and understand a host of interrelated knowledge derived from archaeology, art, climatology, geography, history, medicine, mythology and religion.

The present text is a study of foods through a period extending from the time of the prehistoric nomadic hunters who roamed along the Nile Valley, through the agricultural revolution, to the era of greatest expansion of Ancient Egypt.

It concerns their use, their cultural significance, the varied attitudes towards each of them, and the impact of these attitudes upon modern beliefs and usage.

The information gained from such a study is manifold. Thus, to the historical anthropologist the identification of genera or species foreign to the site of discovery may afford evidence of prehistoric trading, migrations or cultural relations. For example, the finding of marine shells in inland Pre-Columbian sites confirmed the existence of certain suggested trade routes, and similar conclusions might perhaps be derived from the finding of Red Sea shells at Jericho (see Biggs, 1969). This is an aspect that we shall hardly touch. We are more concerned here with nutrition.

Today's accelerated race of scientific and technical change has not yet erased the repeated famines that recur in many parts of the globe.

1

To combat under-nutrition, scientists of all nations work toward the development of new and better strains of plants, cheaper fertilizers, better storage techniques, improved animal husbandry, new sources of protein, and formulation of new foods.

But the cultural heritage of patterns of behaviour that obstructs change is seldom the object of inquiry and understanding. New foods and dietary products may be rejected by needy populations for reasons of taste, palatability, colour, texture or cost. On the other hand, rejection often occurs because of fears, superstitions and ingrained attitudes understandable only through broad knowledge of a culture and its past. Small wonder that problems reflecting the inevitable *status quo* should persist, that educational efforts fail, population increments continue to outstrip economic gains, logical efforts to change food habits be foiled, and that scientifically indefensible fads gain widespread credence.

Because the historical focus of this text is upon Egypt and the neighbouring geographic region, it is useful to review some background of concepts related to Egypt in antiquity.

Ancient Egypt: Definition of Area and Boundaries

The present well-defined political boundaries of Egypt are the result of nineteenth- and twentieth-century politics. No such fixed boundaries were recognized by Ancient Egyptians, Greeks or Romans and, throughout antiquity, the boundaries remained vague. Strabo* noted that

"... neither can we tell the boundaries either of Aethiopia or of Libya, nor yet accurately even those of the country next to Aegypt ..." (17, 3, 23)[2]

It is appropriate for the perspective of this work, therefore, to regard Egypt as a sphere of reciprocal influence rather than an area or nation with well-delineated boundaries.

The western limit of Egypt has always been ill defined because of the sparsely inhabited desert. Herodotus (II, 17–19) described Libya as

---

* The Appendix (p. 809) contains an alphabetical list of the Greek and Roman authors cited within this text.

encompassing most of the land that today lies within the modern state of Libya, in addition to the western desertic regions of Egypt. This ambiguous Egypto-Libyan entity included the northern coast, a fertile agricultural region extending west along the Mediterranean from Alexandria to Solloum, in addition to the lush western oases of Siwa, Qara, Bahriyah, Farafra, Dakhla and Kharga, which all lie within the frontiers of modern Egypt.

Cultural contacts between Egypt and "Libya" in antiquity were sporadic and usually of military nature. At the close of the Old Kingdom,* *c.*2200 B.C., the Libyans harassed the northwestern positions of Egypt, and exerted their political control for a limited period of time. Again, in 950 B.C. Egypt was conquered by "Libyan" kings and was under their rule for nearly 150 years. Hence, the retrospective Egyptian sphere embraces materials that can be dated to a period of "Libyan" supremacy in Egypt, and that geographically can be assigned to the western desert of modern Egypt, primarily, the oases and the northern coastal region.

Throughout recorded history Egypt has been linked with its southern neighbours[3] and, earlier, the Nile Valley was a natural funnel directing nomads out of East Africa and into the eastern Mediterranean and Europe. Similarly, the Nile Valley was a major corridor for the southward retreat of early man from Europe back into Africa as he fled the advance of cold in the Glacial Period. These indistinct migrations of ancient hunters left traces of their passage in the crudely chipped flint tools abandoned at camp sites adjacent to the Nile.

It is not clear to what extent early migrants from the south influenced or, in turn, were influenced by religious ideas and technology developed within the Nile Valley. Several traditions commonly described as "Ancient Egyptian" were probably imported from the South.[4] There is little doubt, likewise, that the earliest settlers in the southern Nile Valley derived portions of their heritage from East Africa and the savannah cultures south of the Sahara Desert.

Ethiopia or *Aethiopia*, as it was known to the Ancient Greeks and Romans, represented a vast unexplored land with vague northern boundaries. These fluctuated at different periods of history, but usually approximated the Ancient Egyptian city of *abw*,[5] the modern city of Aswan.

This "Ethiopia" included large tracts of land lying within the

---

* The Appendix (p. 818) contains chronologic tables and lists of kings.

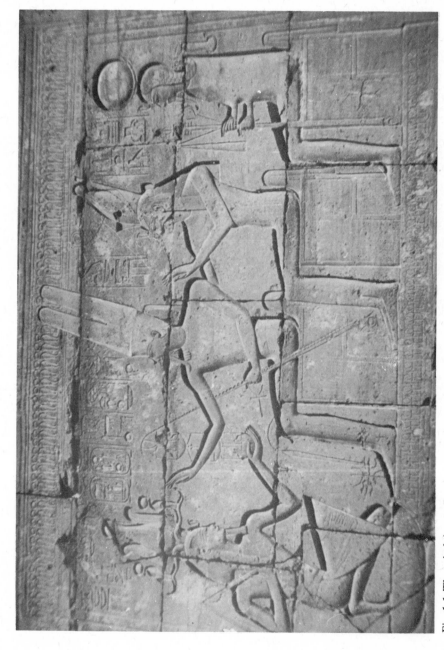

Fig. 1.1. The triad Amon-Ra, Mut and Khonsu at Karnak; temple of Amon-Ra, New Kingdom, nineteenth dynasty, *c.* 1250 B.C. Photographed 1969. Note the ram's horn in the composite crown worn by kneeling Pharaoh.

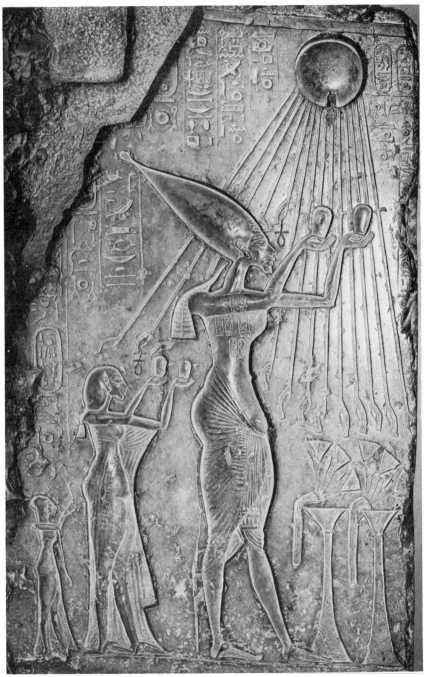

Fig. 1.2. Aten as a radiating sun disc. New Kingdom, eighteenth dynasty, reign of King Amenhotep IV (Akhenaten), *c.* 1360 B.C. Photographed with permission of the Ministry of Culture and the officials of the Egyptian Museum, Cairo, ARE (1969).

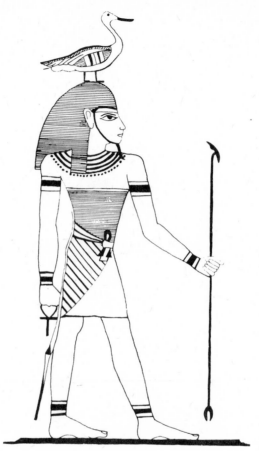

Fig. 1.3. Geb, god of earth. Redrawn from Wilkinson (1878), Vol 3, p. 60, Fig. 516.

present states of Sudan, Ethiopia, Somalia, as well as undefined portions
of Uganda, Kenya, and central Africa. The different cultural entities
that these represented figure prominently in Egyptian history and
tradition—for example, Nubia,[6] Kush[7] and Punt.[8] The populations
that inhabited them, some real, others imaginary, were discussed in
Greek and Roman texts, and the names given them by ancient traveller-
historians reflect their reputed dietary practices—e.g. the "root
eaters", "ostrich eaters", "locust eaters", and "fish eaters".
   About 750 B.C., the whole of Egypt was conquered by "Ethiopian"
monarchs whose capital was situated at Gebel Barkel in the modern

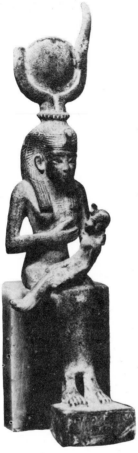

Fig. 1.4. Bronze statuette of Isis suckling the infant Horus. Cairo Museum.

Sudan. Because of the cultural links and continued contacts with "Ethiopia" the dietary heritage of Egypt cannot be divorced from this southern area (Huffman, 1931; Butt, 1952; Murdock, 1959). But, regardless of geographical or political frontiers, the exchange with Africa as a whole, including "black" Africa, as far as the Sahara, the Fezzan, Katanga, Ghana, the Tchad, the Ivory Coast and even Madagascar, has been extensive (Forde-Johnson, 1959; Davidson, 1965; Meyerovitz, 1960; Wainwright, 1951).

Similarly, no sharp boundary between Egypt and Asia can be defined. Periodic migrations between them have occurred throughout

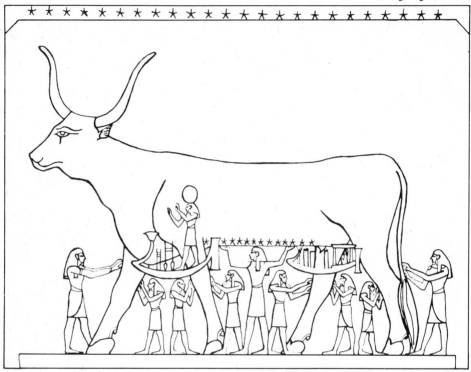

Fig. 1.5. The goddess Hathor/Nut. Tomb of Seti I at Thebes (Valley of the Kings) New Kingdom, nineteenth dynasty, *c.* 1298 B.C. Redrawn from Budge (1904), (1969 edition, Vol. 1 p. 368).

history. Such contacts, *c.* 5000 B.C., may have brought agriculture to Egypt from Southwest Asia (compare Flannery, 1965 and Hugot, 1968). On the other hand, new evidence from Upper Egypt suggests the initiation of agricultural development there several thousand years earlier (Wendorf *et al.,* 1970). Whatever its origin, it is this development that provided a constant and reliable food source, and permitted the indigenous hunting-gathering nomads of Egypt to settle and follow other pursuits that eventually led to the full blooming of that remarkable entity of "Ancient Egypt".

Politically, Egypt has to a varying degree occupied or, at least, exerted a direct influence over nearby Asia. Byblos entertained relations as far back as the legendary times when Isis landed there in her search for Osiris. At the height of the New Kingdom, the sphere controlled by Thutmose III almost reached the southern borders of modern Turkey.

Conversely, periods of Asiatic power saw the eastern boundary of Egypt recede to the region of north-central Sinai.[9] At various times,

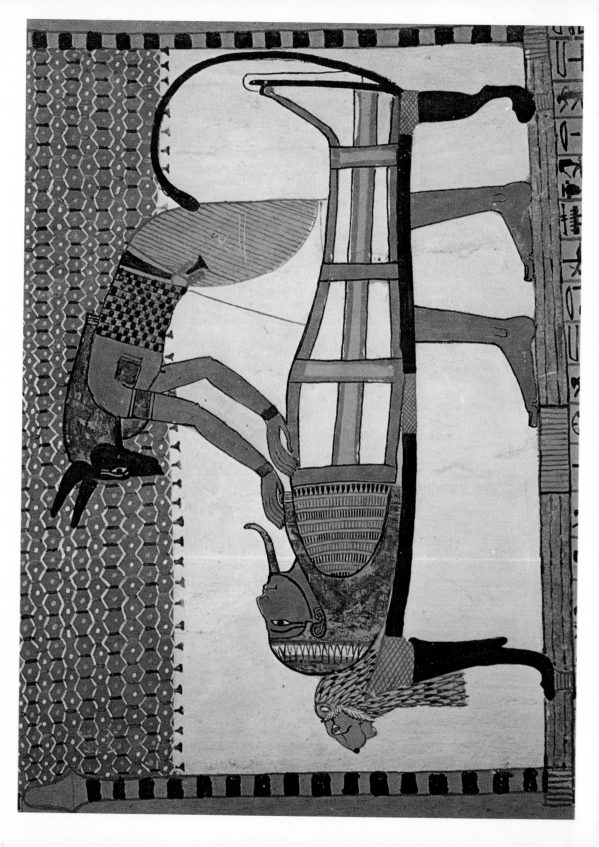

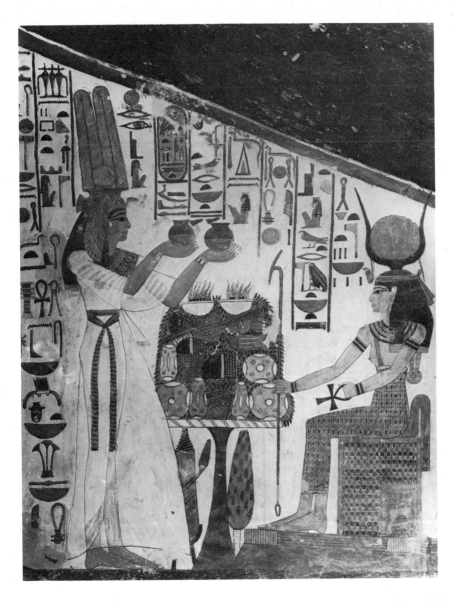

Fig. 1.6 a. (Facing page) The god Anubis. Tomb of Sennutem (number 1) at Thebes (Deir el Medina); New Kingdom, Ramessid Period, date uncertain. Photographed 1969.

Fig. 1.6. b (Above) Isis (right) and Queen Nefertari (left). Tomb of Queen Nefertari at Thebes (Valley of the Queens); New Kingdom, nineteenth dynasty, *c.* 1232 B.C. Centre of Documentation, Cairo, ARE (1969).

two Asiatic peoples conquered Egypt wholly or in part. From 1730 B.C. the Hyksos[10] ruled the Delta and north-central Egypt until they were expelled by Ahmose I in 1580 B.C. Twice the Persians were conquerors, first under Cambyses in 525 B.C. and then under Artaxerxes II (Ochus) in 341 B.C. All these periods were no doubt marked by the introduction of new varieties of food, including certain seeds, nuts, fruits and vegetables, that became regular components of the Egyptian diet.

With the Hebrews, apart from direct Biblical evidence, foreign words in the Old Testament are clear evidence of the process of cross-fertilization. Ellenbogen (1962) in a statistical study of these "Fremd-wörter" found that 22% were of Egyptian origin and apparently all Pre-Exilic. Conversely, Erman (1927) found almost all foreign words in New Kingdom Egyptian to be borrowed from the inhabitants of Palestine; while, together with Humbert (1929) and Weill (1950) he found in Hebrew literature a number of features that strikingly remind one of the Egyptian writings.

In the north, the Mediterranean which forms the geographic limit of Egypt did not prevent cultural exchange, trade, commerce, or conquest, no more than the western or eastern deserts. The Minoans,[11] who created one of the early great European civilizations, sailed from their island home of Crete in the sixteenth to fifteenth century B.C. to establish trade relationships with Egypt. Later, Greek colonies at Naucratis and elsewhere prospered in the Egyptian Delta. In 332 B.C., Alexander the Great invaded Egypt, expelled the Persians and founded the city which bears his name. His successors, the Ptolemies were to blend Greek attitudes into Egyptian thought, and this combination was reflected in new dietary attitudes and traditions. The subsequent conquest of Egypt by the Romans led by Augustus (Octavianus) in 30 B.C., further modified the established Graeco-Egyptian conventions. Even today one finds appreciable Greek traces in language and customs in the northern areas.

Even earlier, ever since the dawn of history, the interchange of visitors, slaves, foreign wives and traders, also brought their share to the homogenization of food customs and prejudices. It is difficult to minimize the mimetic influence of foreign groups, or of conquered peoples on the conquerors. To quote a few examples, this is what made England a tea-drinking country before it became a coffee-drinking country; introduced tobacco into Europe and Mexican food, Italian pizza, Chinese delicacies, Kosher-type delicatessen foods and many other delicacies to North American tables.

It would be a great error, therefore, to ignore Greek or Roman contributions to the Egyptian diet on the grounds that they represented beliefs lying outside the sphere of Egyptian thought. The peoples of the whole of the present-day Arab Middle East were, in fact, influenced to a greater or lesser extent, but permanently, by these major historical periods. This is attested by magnificent Greek and Roman vestiges, notably at Jarash, Palmyra, Baalbek or Alexandria, by linguistic remains, and by the multilingual inscriptions found everywhere, the most revealing of which are those left by successive invaders on the shores of the Dog River, near Beirut. In the same way, the records of Greek and Latin writers must be considered a valuable background in understanding the development of attitudes to foodstuffs in Egypt and the Middle East.

Religion

The gods of Ancient Egypt were as many as its cities before their union. There is no evidence, however, that at that momentous point of her history, any group forced compliance to its beliefs. Indeed, throughout its history, Egypt has been known for its remarkable absorptive tolerance and philosophical elaboration of the most varied concepts, out of which its theologians eventually grouped gods into families of eight, *Ogdoads*, or nine, *Enneads*.

At Hermopolis Magna, today Ashmunein, the Ogdoad consisted of four couples, Nun/Nunet, Heh/Hehet, Kek/Keket, and Amon/Amonet. The most ancient Ennead, created at Heliopolis to account for the Creation, taught that Ra-Atum had created the couple Shu (Air and Vacuum) and Tefnis (Humidity). These engendered Earth (Geb) and Heaven (Nut) who brought forth two couples: Osiris/Isis and Seth/Nephthys. Horus, Thot, Anubis, Maat, and other lesser gods were later combined into an additional Lesser Ennead.

Such groupings, however, were not stable. Gods were interchangeable and numbers varied, as in Karnak where Amon-Ra headed an Ennead that accommodated fifteen gods.

On the whole, beliefs were strongly influenced by the vivid contrast between the black fertile earth of the Nile Valley, and the sterile red desert. The stark opposites of flood and emergence, and

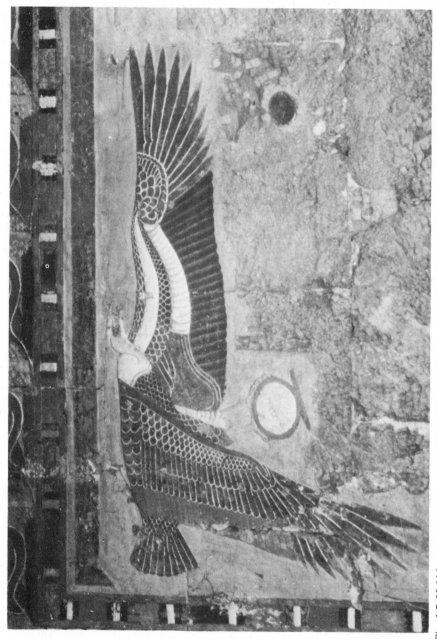

Fig. 1.7. Nekhbet, protective goddess of Upper Egypt. Funerary temple of Queen Hatshepsut at Thebes (Deir el Bahari); New Kingdom, eighteenth dynasty, *c.* 1500 B.C. Photographed 1969.

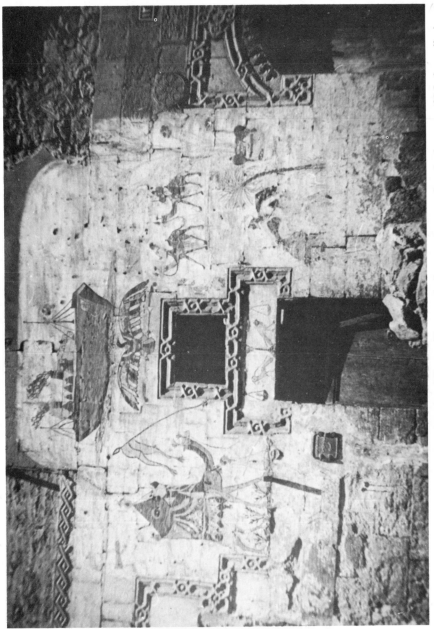

Fig. 1.8. Nekhbet as a motif in modern Egyptian folk art. House painting commemorating the journey of Moslem pilgrims to Mecca. Photographed 1966; Cairo (Darb El Ahmar).

birth and death, deeply coloured the themes that underlay literature, legend and religion alike.

On the other hand, the myth of Osiris that perhaps embodied a veiled remembrance of the conquest *c.* 3200 B.C. of the North by the South, was the loom on which many aspects of Egyptian culture were woven. As told by Plutarch (*I. and O.*, 355, 12, D-358, 19, E) it may be summarized thus:

The sun god, Ra, was in love with the beautiful Nut, goddess of the sky. But having found that she had mated with her brother, Geb, the earth, he placed a curse upon her pregnancy, prohibiting birth on any day, in any month of any year. At that time the calendar consisted of 360 days. Thot, god of secret science and knowledge, being asked for help, gambled with the moon, asking, if he won, for only 1/70 part of her daily illumination. The moon agreed and lost. Thot then assembled the illumination he had gained into five new days, on each of which Nut gave birth to one of her quintuplets, Osiris, Horus-the-Elder, Seth, Isisi and Nephthys.

Osiris took Isis as his mate, and Seth took Nephthys; Horus-the-Elder remained alone and went to live in the northern Delta.

Osiris brought civilization to the Egyptians and taught them cultivation, law, and how to honour the divinities. After having accomplished this, he travelled abroad to bring his teachings to the rest of the world and, while away, he placed Isis on the throne of Egypt.

When Osiris returned to the Nile Valley after civilizing the world, Seth, who coveted the throne, had built a sumptuous chest to the specific body measurements of Osiris, and he invited him to a banquet where he offered the magnificent hand-built chest to whomever should lie down inside, and fit in it. All attempted, but no one fitted until Osiris lay inside, whereupon Seth and his associates nailed on the lid, sealed the chest with lead, and cast it in the Nile, where it floated to the sea.

Isis, having learned of the murder, started a long journey seeking everywhere information about her husband and the whereabouts of the chest. She was joined in the search by Anubis, offspring of an illicit meeting between Osiris and his sister, Nephthys. Children told her that they had seen the chest float by on its way northward. Isis then travelled north and east towards the city of Byblos, where she learned that the chest had finally come ashore.

The chest had indeed been caught in a bushy tree along the shore

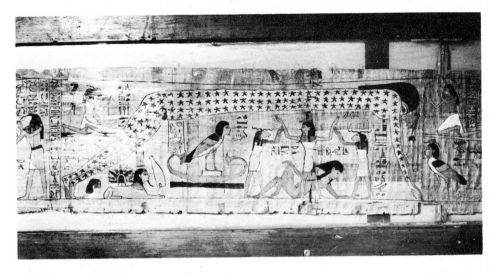

Fig. 1.9. Nut, goddess of the sky. New Kingdom funerary papyrus; date uncertain. Photographed with permission of the Ministry of Culture and the officials of the Egyptian Museum, Cairo, ARE (1969).

that grew about it, protecting the god from harm. The king of Byblos admired the tree, cut it down, and made from it a pillar for his palace, the chest unknowingly being held captive beneath the bark.

At Byblos, Isis did not at first reveal her identity, nor her purpose. But after she succeeded in becoming an intimate of the queen and the nurse of her baby, she made herself known, and asked for the pillar containing the chest, which was gladly given by the king. Thereupon, she transported it back to Egypt and hid it, while she visited her brother, Horus-the-Elder, to rest.

Seth, while hunting wild boars during the full moon, found the chest, and immediately cut the body of Osiris into fourteen parts which he scattered the length and breadth of the Valley of the Nile. Isis, returning from her visit, failed to find her husband's body, and thus began her more difficult second search for its fragments.

After great hardship she recovered all parts except the phallus, which Seth had dismembered and thrown into the Nile, where it was lost forever, devoured by three fish, the *Lepidotus*, the *Phagrus* and the *Oxyrhynchus*. But the lamentations of Isis came to the attention of Thot, who provided her with a magic spell whereby Osiris was

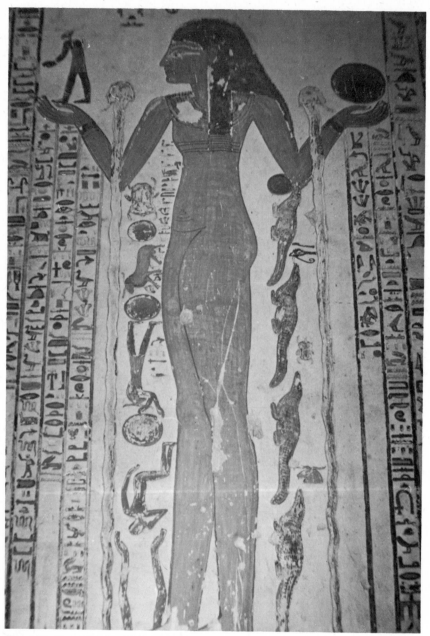

Fig. 1.10. Nut. Tomb of King Rameses VI at Thebes (Valley of the Kings); New Kingdom, twentieth dynasty, *c.* 1130 B.C. Photographed 1969. Note beetle under the right arm.

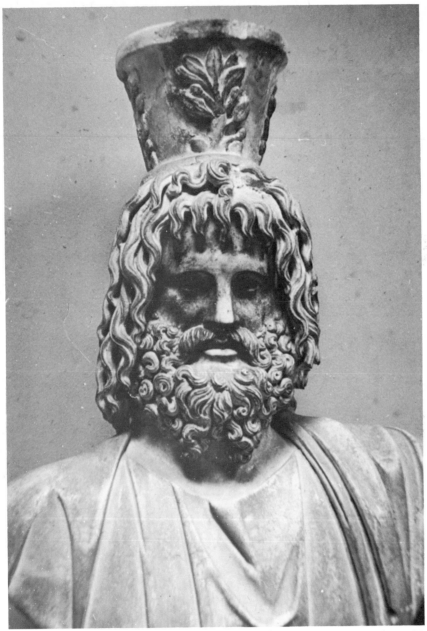

Fig. 1.11. Serapis. Ptolemaic Period; date uncertain. Photographed 1967 with permission of the Ministry of Culture and the officials of the Graeco-Roman Museum, Alexandria, ARE.

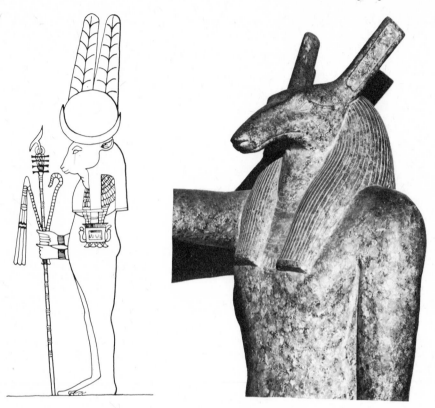

Fig. 1.12. (left) The god Oser-Apis. Redrawn from Budge (1904), (1969 edition, Vol. 2, p. 198).

Fig. 1.13. (right) Seth. Medinet Habu; New Kingdom, twentieth dynasty, reign of King Rameses III, *c.* 1198 B.C. Photographed with permission of the officials of the Egyptian Museum, Cairo, ARE (1969).

resurrected and his missing member recreated, whereupon he mated with Isis, and conceived Horus the avenger (Horus-son-of-Isis-and-Osiris).

Horus grew in knowledge, spirit, and strength. During his childhood his father Osiris reappeared on several occasions, and instructed him in the methods of justice, nobility, and honour. After being trained in the use of arms, he set out to avenge the death and mutilation of his father. He clashed with Seth in terrible battle,

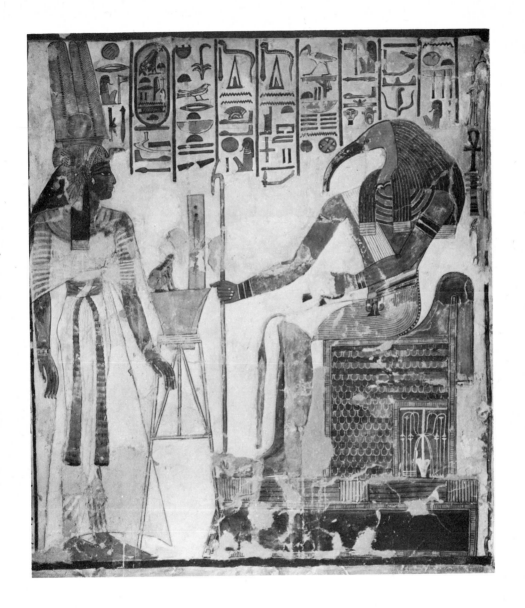

Fig. 1.14. Thot. Tomb of Queen Nefertari at Thebes (Valley of the Queens); New Kingdom, nineteenth dynasty, *c.* 1232 B.C. Photograph used with permission of the Ministry of Culture and the officials of the Centre of Documentation, Cairo, ARE (1969).

each horribly mutilating the other. In the end, however, he prevailed, spared the life of his uncle, was upheld as the true ruler of Egypt, and ascended the throne.

There is no evidence, however, that the conquering worshippers of Osiris imposed their beliefs on the conquered or entirely abolished their religion. The "evil" Seth was continuously worshipped in certain communities, as in Ombos in the South, and in Tanis in the Delta. The Sethan inclinations of kings Peribsen and Seti I, and similar ideas that Rameses II inherited from his father Seti I, were, at times or in certain places, regarded as righteous, while at other times or places, they were considered abominable!

Concepts of good and evil as attached to particular beliefs or practices must, therefore, be approached cautiously. Inasmuch as food is connected with the Osirian cycle, the presence or absence of a foodstuff in a tomb thus reflects how the deceased viewed this food at that particular locality and time, and this view might have differed radically under other circumstances. Thus comparisons and contrasts should be correlated with time and place.

Evaluation of Data

Chronologic Scope

We are concerned primarily with the period from 5000 B.C. through A.D. 305, which spans the Pre-Dynastic, Dynastic, Ptolemaic (Greek), and Roman Egyptian Periods (Appendix, pp. 816–828). Nevertheless, our text deals necessarily at greater length with the so-called historic period, since this is the period that has left most vestiges and records. Civilization, however, as a living phenomenon, is as incapable of spontaneous generation as any living being. Here and there, we shall be referring to what we know of the obscure prehistoric times that set the basis on which "historic" civilization grew. These were the periods where many novelties that affected the alimentary field appeared, of which the expansion of agriculture and cattle-breeding, the manufacture of leavened bread, of beer and, possibly, of wine, and the organization and control on a substantial scale of artificial irrigation, a development that was a necessary prerequisite of the expansion and regularity of agricultural production.

It is at that period that Nile and, possibly, maritime navigation, developed and played their parts. For if the latter could not, at that stage, significantly influence the economics of food, fluvial navigation helped in securing a better distribution of food materials and in alleviating the consequences of poor harvests.

Above all, the Pre-Dynastic era, possibly more in Egypt than elsewhere, was the start of the gradual transformation of the Eneolithic, that led its economy from mere hunting and gathering to near total reliance on agriculture and pasture.

Hunting counted no longer as a main source of food, although fishing did so because of the favourable hydrologic conditions.

By the end of the Pre-Dynastic, alimentation mainly relied, as later in historic times, on cereals. This was not entirely a progress, but because the diet was complemented by fruits, vegetables and dairy and fishing products, the late Pre-Dynastic Egyptian was not likely to have been malnourished. In fact, we cannot agree with Saffirio's statement that the difficulty of keeping pace with the rapid demographic and social development may have meant a deficiency in quantity if not in quality except, of course, when the yearly flood was inadequate or in periods of political or social turmoil.

The challenge of increasing demands was met through unremitting toil, and Egyptian production succeeded in sustaining the progress of an expanding population in spite of the rigid limits of the arable land.

Unfortunately, the available information pertains mostly to Upper Egypt and the Fayoum. It would be helpful if we could complete it with some evidence on the resources north of the Delta, a region that enjoyed a noteworthy cultural development. Our knowledge of that area is very limited, however, owing to the bad state of preservation of most Delta sites, as a result of the repeated storm of wars and the yearly floods.

Organization of Source Materials

The continued work by scholars in fields related to nutrition makes it repeatedly necessary to revise or change one's hypotheses or deductions. Of the several texts published in the past two centuries that include sections on diet and food attitudes in Egyptian antiquity most are now out of date. New archaeological material is yearly excavated in Egypt and elsewhere, and publication is sometimes delayed up to 50 years after first discovery.[12]

To facilitate taking appropriate account of these factors, the present material has been arranged within an accepted chronology based on Engelbach (1961) and Ehrich (1965), with complete citation, geographical location within or outside Egypt, data relative to status and social divisions, and religious implications if known. Subsequent evidence may be fitted into this framework later to permit additional analysis.

The available sources that allow one to identify with a high degree of probability the primary foods of the Ancient Egyptians during various periods of history, are listed below in Table 1.

Certain precautions in utilizing this material are, however, mandatory. When reconstructing history, the modern scholar must beware of his tendency to interpret ancient traditions, thoughts and attitudes in terms of twentieth century motivations, social values and training. Interpretation of written history 51 centuries removed from the present, with roots extending even centuries further back into time, is at least tenuous.

In addition, many modern texts dealing with antiquity make generalized conclusions regarding ancient attitudes and beliefs, without giving due regard to their variation in time, or to the different levels of culture existing in the same area.

As an example, merely labelling the years 3200–332 B.C. the "Dynastic Period" misleads the uninitiated to visualize this long span of time as a discrete historical era, to be contrasted or compared to the Pre-Dynastic, Ptolemaic (Greek), Roman, Byzantine, Arabic, Turkish and Modern Periods.

But the technology and ideas prevalent in the Dynastic Period under King Narmer (first dynasty, *c.* 3200 B.C.) and those current during the reign of King Nectanebo II (thirtieth dynasty, *c.* 350 B.C.) probably differed as much as Stonehenge and the England of today. Conversely, the reigns of King Nectanebo II, of Artaxerxes II, and of Alexander the Great, are commonly treated as three distinct periods (Dynastic, Persian and Ptolemaic), despite the fact that, chronologically, they are separated by a mere twelve years.

Other sweeping generalizations on artistic, nutritional, or religious concepts in Ancient Egypt neglect differences in social strata. The statement found in many nineteenth- and twentieth-century texts, that

Table 1

Nature of material cited in this text

Egyptian archaeological material

1. Preserved animal and plant remains
   a. Food found in the stomach and intestines of human mummies
   b. Animal and plant foods found inside tombs
      1. sealed tombs (i.e. uncontaminated materials)
      2. opened or pilfered tombs (i.e. the possibility of a more recently introduced food being found in an earlier tomb)
   c. Plant materials identified from stems and seeds preserved in ancient mud bricks

2. Religious, funerary and domestic art
   a. Reliefs or paintings from temples and tombs that depict foods, offerings, sacrifice, or methods of food preparation and preservation
   b. Statues, models, or dioramas that depict foods and their preparation
   c. Reliefs or paintings from temples and tombs which depict the domestication, care, and feeding of Egyptian animals

3. Literary sources (papyri, tomb, or temple texts)
   a. Lists of daily food allowances (or diets) provided for the soldiers, workmen and servants
   b. Lists of food offerings made to the temples or gods
   c. Foodstuffs utilized in medical prescriptions
   d. Cosmological and mythological texts

Material relatively foreign to Egypt

1. Greek, Roman and Arabic mythology
2. Religious texts: Bible, Talmud and Koran
3. Descriptive accounts by Greek, Roman, Arab and modern travellers, historians and naturalists

Contemporary Egyptian material

1. Personal experience and interviews on dietary traditions with persons representing the various ethnic divisions within Egypt today
2. Analysis of modern methods and traditions of agriculture, marketing (from field to consumer) and food attitudes

Egyptians ate beef, fish and fowl, is true only in part, for the pre-
ponderance of evidence is directly associated with the nobility, priesthood, or royalty, to the near exclusion of information about the peasantry (Table 1), and it is unlikely that the diet and food attitudes of the
poor farmers near Memphis in Lower Egypt would have been identical
to those of High Priests of the New Kingdom of Thebes in Upper
Egypt.

One may even argue that the diet of the lower classes in Egyptian
antiquity was not greatly different from that of the farmers of Egypt
today, without of course the benefit of the many varieties introduced
later. Primarily, the subsistence diet of the farmer is determined by
availability, ease of preparation and storage, and bulk. Thus a farmer
may eat a vegetable from his field during one season, whereas he eats an
entirely different kind at other periods. Furthermore, when both men
and women work in the fields, the time spent in preparing food must
not be excessive. In addition, satiety is in part determined by the bulk
of the food and, among a labouring society, there is a preference for
filling, bulky, foods. It is likely that the foods used by the peasantry in
Egyptian antiquity were determined to a greater degree by similar
considerations than by the religious dictates depicted in tombs and
temples; and it is unlikely that the acceptance–avoidance patterns
adopted by the nobility and priests greatly influenced the eating habits
of the peasantry.

Factors that Affect Evidence on the Presence or Absence of a Food Substance in Antiquity

When we come to evaluate archaeological and literary evidence, we
have to consider this from several viewpoints.

Selective Preservation of Materials

Desiccation by sand and heat has preserved innumerable food vestiges.
But which materials are preserved and which are lost through decomposition is not a random matter. Bone, teeth and horny chitinous parts are

more likely to survive than soft structures. This could result in erroneous conclusions inasmuch as excavations might reveal more material of animal than of vegetable origin. At the same time, the presence of animal or plant material at a site does not prove its use as food, and several possibilities must be considered before including them in a food list.

Interpretation from Incomplete Data

Two of these possibilities are seasonal variations and regional preference.

An observer accustomed to luscious, tasty, fresh fruit, who ate dried dates out of season, might cast disparaging remarks on the quality of fruits produced in the region: thus Pliny's remark

> "... all over the Thebaid [Upper Egypt] and Arabia the dates are dry and small with a shriveled body, and as they are scorched by the continual heat their covering is more truly a rind than a skin ..." (*N.H.*, 13, 9, 47)

This remark might have followed a meal of dates dried and preserved during summer when, on the other hand, a visit during winter would have familiarized the author with the tender, plump, fresh dates.

On the other hand, deductions that appear valid when viewed against modern or known historical models, may be quite inaccurate.

Assume, for example, that a future archaeologist unearthed at various sites in North America, the following items:

1. three menus—a 1925 Boston dinner, a 1945 Waco, Texas dinner, and a 1969 Seattle breakfast;
2. a meagre, well preserved pot-luck supper;
3. checklist of animals caged in the zoo at San Diego, California;
4. a fragmentary book concerning local folklore of Biloxi, Mississippi;
5. two menus in diaries, one belonging to a New York banker; the other, attributed to an Apache Indian;
6. a bronze sculpture of an American Bison.

What may be deduced from this information? Do bean dishes listed on the menus indicate regional preference, seasonal distribution, or both? Might the absence of beans at Seattle indicate a local avoidance, or simply regional distribution? To what extent is the pot-luck food representative of the dinners of the majority of American citizens?

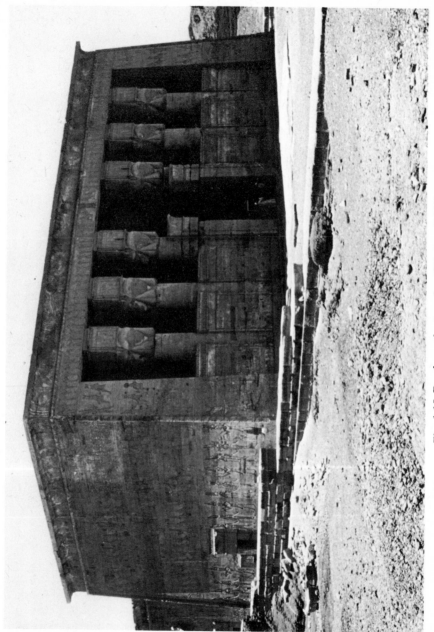

Fig. 1.15. Dendera; the temple of Hathor (1969).

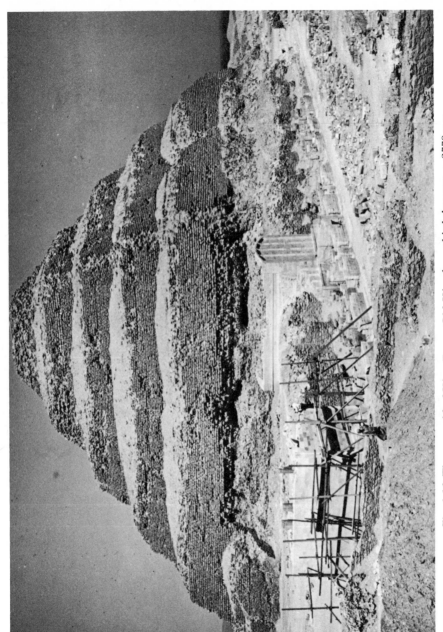

Fig. 1.16. The pyramid of King Zoser; Old Kingdom, third dynasty, *c.* 2770 B.C.

Might items included in this dinner be indicators of religious acceptability and, conversely, might foods not included be indicators of
religious avoidance? Does the presence of wild cattle, sheep, goats, and
swine in the zoo indicate that these animals were eaten by the citizens
of San Diego? Do dietary traditions mentioned in southern folklore (fried
chicken, grits, chitterlings, turnip greens) apply to all levels of southern
society? Did the Apache Indian prefer cheap wine, flat cakes of corn-
bread, and chicken, and reject champagne, dinner rolls, and steak
in order to remain culturally distinct from the New Yorker? Was
the bison statue indicative of religious worship? If so, was bison ever
eaten? Did eating bison flesh reflect religious conflict with those who
avoided it?

Such questions appear ludicrous in the light of complete knowledge,
but the materials discussed are American parallels to the data available
from different periods of Egyptian history.

On the other hand, survival of archaeological evidence is obviously
in part determined by relative abundance, but the validity of deducing
regional variations from modern distribution is questionable. Theophrastus (4, 2, 9), for example, wrote that olives grew in Upper Egypt.
Strabo (17, 1, 35) denied this, stating that Egypt had no olive trees
except those at the Fayoum oasis and Alexandria. Could this discrepancy represent regional variation in crops? Might it reflect the
extent of travel by each within the country? Or is one of the two writers
in error?

Oversight of the Informant

In literary records a specific food may be omitted because the item was
so common or obvious to the Ancient Egyptian that he neglected to
mention it during discussions with Greek or Roman visitors. A modern
example of omission of the commonplace may be cited.

Until recently, a high percentage of farmers in the Delta of northern
Egypt were affected with Schistosomiasis (Bilharziasis).[13] One clinical
sign of this disease is haematuria or the presence of blood in the urine,
which is so common that not passing blood has in the past been considered unusual. If asked non-leading questions concerning health, the
villager rarely volunteered information relative to haematuria. He
viewed the sign lightly and considered it a usual part of his way of life.

On the other hand, the first appearance of this sign in an urban citizen would elicit immediate concern.

Table 2

Selective oversight and interpretation of data

Excavations at archaeological site "X" revealed no information relative to plant or animal "Y", a food commonly eaten now. Greek and Roman literary descriptions do not mention the plant or animal. What is the interpretation?

Plant present or absent	Interpretation
1. Absent	Was never present in the region or country
2. Absent	Present in the region and country but avoided at site "X" a. Not used as food throughout the country, though used as food today b. Not used as food at site "X" because of religious or other avoidance, but eaten elsewhere in the country
3. Present	Not evident during excavation because it was perishable (selective preservation)
4. Present	Missing because of selective preservation; not mentioned by recorder because: a. informant neglected to mention its presence or use, because he considered it unimportant or of no interest (informants' selective oversight) b. informant neglected to mention it because of religious attitudes (information not volunteered) c. informant did mention its use and occurrence, but recorder omitted it from descriptions through neglect, error or cultural bias (recorder's selective oversight)

Oversight of the Recorder

Travellers always experience a marked attraction towards unfamiliar elements of another culture, and are apt to emphasize these elements in their descriptions. A Greek or Roman traveller might likewise fail to note an important food in Egypt because it was too familiar in his own country to be considered worthy of recording.

The tourist from New York does not take photographs of an average street in San Francisco, but rather of Fisherman's Wharf, the Golden Gate Bridge, Haight-Ashbury, and the nearby Sequoia forests. Persons who view the photographs several thousand years hence could erroneously conclude that San Francisco in 1976 consisted only of "fishermen and hippies who together built a metal bridge in order to utilize the northern forests of giant trees!".

The "Silent Voice"

The absence of refuting data—the "silent voice"—is sometimes used to support a thesis, but writers seldom use the same criteria in their descriptions of the different lands they visited. A food might have been described by one writer as common to Libya and Phoenicia; another writer might describe the same food in Syria; and both might omit direct reference to Egypt. Is it correct to assume the presence of the food in Egypt from factors of physical geography, ecology? Or does the negative evidence indicate a religious or cultural difference. This negative argument is the weakest of analytical methods, and but few steps removed from pure speculation, since further investigation may bring forth invalidating evidence.

Social Position and Experience of Chronicler

In antiquity, as today, persons without financial means could little afford to travel. Hence, the descriptions of the ancient historians and naturalists were written by members of the upper level of Greek and Roman society, and reflected the attitudes, interests and bias of the wealthy.

In addition, one may assume that ancient travellers, as today, visited with their peers—priests with priests, wealthy nobles with the ruling group, and foreigners with resident citizens of Greek or Roman descent. Ancient writers, moreover, like those of today, were conscious of their audience, that consisted primarily of the upper class citizenry of their home city and country. Would this audience find pleasure in descriptions of pastoral Egyptian life and commonplace foods, or would they expect exciting reports of unusual customs?

Thus occurs "selective oversight" especially in relation to foods of the poorer classes.

The Egyptian, on the other hand, may not have regarded the Greek traveller as his peer and may have introduced thereby bias in his information. There is evidence that the Egyptian priests with whom Greeks and Romans associated might not have been the most knowledgeable, literate, or accurate.

Uppishness is indicated by the remark attributed to an unknown Egyptian priest who told Solon of Salamis (seventh century B.C.), one of the seven philosopher sages of Ancient Greece

> ". . . Solon, Solon, you Greeks are always children; an old [knowledgeable] Greek does not exist . . ." (Plato, *Timaeus*, 22, B)

The writings of Carneades of Cyrene (third to second century B.C.), preserved as references in the works of Porphyry of Tyre (third century A.D.), recorded the aloofness of the Egyptian "high clergy"

> ". . . they do not associate with any one who was not a religious character . . . they also led a solitary life, as they only mingled with other men in solemn sacrifices and festivals. But at other times the priests were almost inaccessible to any one who wished to converse with them. For it was requisite that he who approached to them should be first purified, and abstain from many things [foods] . . ." (Porphyry, 4, 6)

But, although the Ancient Greek and Roman writers generally observed through the eyes of an elite alien traveller, and recorded their observations for a select audience, some were more observant than others, and possessed a curiosity that, despite bias, resulted in accurate descriptions of everyday events in Egyptian life and food, descriptions that often have been supported by archaeological data.

Errors of Information from the Informer

It is also plausible that some of the Egyptian priests and informers filled the eager ears of visitors with flights of inventive or superstitious fantasy which were dutifully recorded as "Egyptian truths".

It is an easy delight to fabricate extemporaneous tales that ring true to uninformed ears preconditioned for reception of the exotic and unusual. The early Greek or Roman visitor likely encountered the equivalent of today's Egyptian *dragoman* (guide) with his unique flowing style and vast, almost depthless reservoir of tales that may change from day to day.[14] These errors are not readily assessable. But errors could have been introduced, likewise, during interviews with supposedly knowledgeable but still gullible Greek or Roman residents in Egypt who were interviewed about Egyptian culture. These resident aliens most probably were never able to grasp the complexities and dynamics of Egyptian culture (Badawi and Khafaga, 1966). Thus, the fantasy of his informants may well account for the mixed reputation acquired by Herodotus.

Plagiarism

Too often the uninitiated consider the classical writings of the Greeks and Romans as representing original personal opinion. In some instances, however, the writers were guilty of gross plagiarism. Hence, the recurrence of a statement does not necessarily reinforce its validity.

Thus, most ancient authors were eager to quote passages from *The Iliad* and *The Odyssey* and, through this device, to assume acceptability, authenticity, and status. For example

> ". . . even the poet [Homer], we are told has mentioned it when he says: 'nay, not for all the wealth of Thebes in Egypt, where in ev'ry hall there lieth treasure vast; a hundred are her gates, and warriors by each issue forth two hundred, each of them with car and steeds' . . ."
>
> (*Diod.*, 1, 45, 6)

Homer was always credited by later historians, for to omit him as the source would have cancelled the reason for inclusion of the reference. One wonders, therefore, why the ancient authors were less careful about acknowledging other sources. Herodotus is commonly given as the originator of the phrase, "Egypt is the gift of the Nile" (II, 5). Herodotus, however, did not coin this phrase; present research attributes it to Hecataes of Mileteus who travelled in Egypt nearly 100 years prior to Herodotus! (Bury, 1958, pp. 49–50).

The extent of that kind of plagiarism is difficult to assess unless one is steeped in Greek and Roman classics and philology. The more flagrant examples can be detected, however, by comparison of texts arranged by author in chronologic sequence.

1. "... this is like millet ... these heads the Egyptians heap together and leave to decay, and when the pod has decayed, they wash the head in the river and take out the fruit, and having dried and pounded it, they make loaves of it which they use for food ..."

(Theophrastus, 374–285 B.C.)

2. "... it contains grains like millet seeds. The natives pile these heads in heaps to rot, and then separate the seeds by washing, and dry them and crush them, and use them to make bread ..."

(Pliny, A.D. 23–79)

If the earlier description contained one inadvertent error the later copy would perpetuate the mistake. Likewise, if through the course of cursory reading the earlier were not consulted, the secondary source would be given prime authorship!

Difficulties of Language, Transliteration and Translation

"... O Egypt, only fables will remain from your cults, and even your children will no longer believe in them; nothing will survive but the words engraved in stone, that tell of your exploits ..."[15]

(Hermes Trismegistus, Fustigière translation, 1945, p. 327)

The cryptic language of Ancient Egypt challenged all understanding until the beginning of the nineteenth century. Many of the translational difficulties stem not only from the complex and variable analysis of individual ancient words, but from ideas ingrained in the mind of the translator which may be quite different from those of the original author.

The Ancient Egyptian writing and its later derivatives took several forms, hieroglyphic, hieratic, demotic; and the language persisted into Coptic. The artistic religious form of Ancient Egyptian was called by the Greeks hieroglyphic, a name that stems from Greek (sacred carvings) rather than from Egyptian. The cursive form of Ancient Egyptian, likewise religious in nature, was termed hieratic (sacred) by the Greek visitors, and was basically a non-ornamental script. Demotic, on the other hand, was a late development that eventually became the style used in everyday writing.

Coptic, a term derived from the Greek, was the language in use after the third century A.D. It represents the evolved form of Ancient Egyptian, and it substituted Greek alphabetical signs for Egyptian

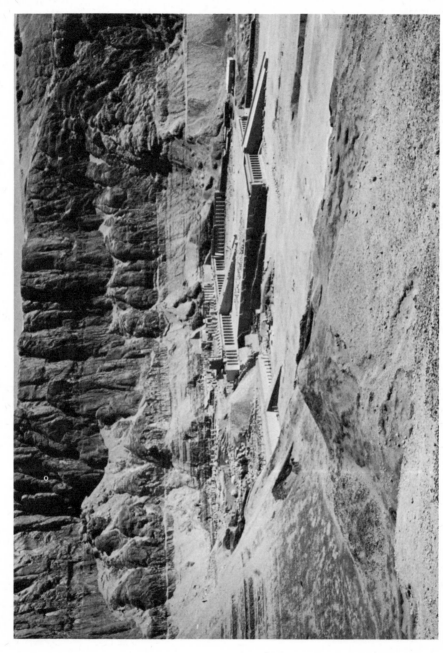

Fig. 1.17. The funerary temple of Queen Hatshepsut at Deir El Bahari (1969). New Kingdom, eighteenth dynasty, *c.* 1500 B.C

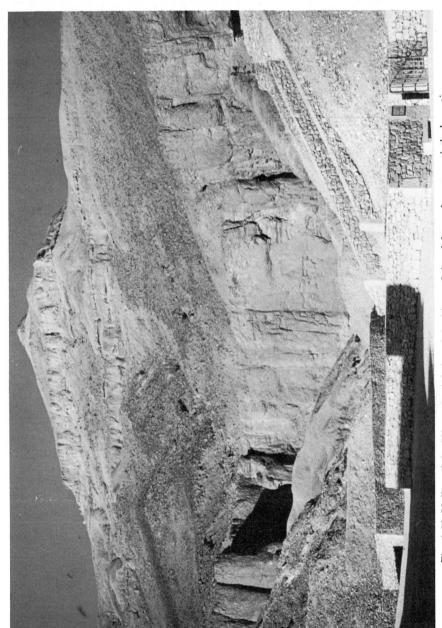

Fig. 1.18. Valley of the Kings. Burial site of the kings of the eighteenth to twentieth dynasties.

symbols, with the addition of seven signs, ultimately derived from hieroglyphic, for sounds unknown to Greek. During the Christian era, it split
into three distinct dialects: Akhmimic, Bohairic and Sahidic. Bohairic
eventually became the written form for all Coptic.

Ancient Egyptian writing was based on more than 500 individual
signs. Those that stood for one or several consonants are called phonetic
signs, and those that represented an object or an idea are called ideo-
graphic characters. Others follow the word to determine the meaning
of the foregoing sound signs, and are called determinatives.

Like its related affiliates of Aramaic, Arabic and Hebrew, Ancient
Egyptian was written using only the consonantic skeleton of words, i.e.
the vowels were omitted. Such a written structure presented innumerable difficulties for early translators. It is as if one wrote in English
"bat", "bet", "bit", and "but" by the single word "bt" followed
by the respective determinative sign. Translation was further compli-
cated by the fact that the consonantal order might follow no set rule. It
could be a function of artistic style and ornamentation. Texts could be
written from left to right, right to left, down, or up, depending upon the
scribe, the context, and decorative details. Fortunately, some rules
usually permit one to find the order in which they were to be read.

Early translators were somewhat disinclined simply to transcribe
consonants, and began the regrettable practice of inserting "missing"
vowels. This has led to much confusion and to problems of synonymy,
for example, regarding the word for "barley" (*Hordeum* spp.); *'it*
(Gardiner, 1950, p. 555), *iait* (Maspero, 1901, p. 66) and *iot* (Kees,
1961, p. 74).

One would like to pronounce this Ancient Egyptian word *'it* correctly,
but any vocalization using twentieth century linguistic models would be
a guess of low reliability. Now the practice of "random" insertion of
vowels has been suppressed, but occasionally is still encountered.
This will explain to the reader occasional differences in spelling the
same word in our text, according to the source quoted or to various
schools of Egyptology.

In addition to difficulties of reading and pronunciation, Ancient
Egyptian words for foods, plants, and animals are difficult to identify
and evaluate. Translation constantly undergoes re-evaluation. Recent
studies have reaffirmed some, but altered other translations made by
the earlier Egyptologists such as Breasted, Budge and Erman.

Similar difficulties beset readers of the works of the early Egyptological botanists and zoologists. The pioneering work of Loret, and

Schweinfurth has, in the past, been outdated by modern botanists, zoologists and chemists such as Greiss, Keimer, Lucas, Moustapha, the Täckholms, Drar and others. No doubt, these translations will be further refined by new generations of workers.

Classification of Food Materials, Identification of Sites and Problems of Synonymy

Differences between mediaeval and modern English reflect but 900 years of history.[16] What, then, of the 5000 years of linguistic change from Ancient Egyptian into Coptic? The language of the Middle Kingdom is considered by Egyptologists to be the classic form of Ancient Egyptian (Gardiner, 1950, pp. 1–2), but it widely differed from that of the Old and New Kingdoms and from that of the Post-Dynastic era.

Some Greek and Roman visitors referred to Egyptian words in their writings, but these were transcribed in alphabetical characters that did not cover all sounds native to Ancient Egyptian; hence, the resemblance to true Ancient Egyptian written forms is unreliable. Moreover, Greek and Latin vocalization was not constant at a given time in the different districts where they were spoken. Hence, even if transliterations were accurate, they might be obscure when comparing foreign writers.

One problem faced by the food historian is the identification of Ancient Egyptian words with terms used by the Greeks and Romans. As an illustration, was barley (*Hordeum* spp.) grown in Egypt? To answer, one must find whether the Latin word, *Hordeum*, was in fact equal to barley. Once this equivalence is established it must be decided whether *Hordeum*, as discussed by Pliny (*N.H.* 18, 14, 72–74), is identical to *Krithi* described in Egypt by Theophrastus (8, 2, 7). In turn are both *Hordeum* and *Krithi* identical to Coptic *Beti* (Crum, 1962, p. 45) and to '*it* of Ancient Egyptian as written during the Middle Kingdom?

In addition, early man saw little reason to concoct specific words to define fine taxonomic divisions of plant and animal species; hence the deeper one delves into history the more general become the groupings.

Such vague divisions plague many purists of scientific taxonomy who desire more sharply defined terms, to place them conveniently within specific boundaries. Classification, however, is but a product of modern methodology, and thus the ancients cannot be faulted.

Thus, ancient descriptive groupings may mask the presence of an animal, plant, or food, because they placed it in a general category rather than specifically naming it. The term "gazelle" in the description of one traveller might have specifically applied to *Gazella dorcus*. Yet "gazelle", as used by another traveller, might also include other desert game, such as the addax, hartebeest, or oryx, whose only link is that they all possessed "horns".

Adherence to strict descriptive, taxonomic, or classificatory detail at the expense of "general knowledge" may, likewise, cause problems. Few present-day Egyptians would recognize the Ancient Egyptian word for their country, *kmt*,[17] "The Black Land," but all would recognize "Egypt". The word "Egypt", however, stems from *Hikuptah*, "The House of the Ka of Ptah". Foreigners used this name for the whole land, and the Greeks invented the legend of Aigyptos who fled his home in the Nile Valley and settled in the Argive region of the Peloponnesus. If one strives for historical accuracy and ignores tradition, consider the difficulty of changing all texts on "Egypt" to "*kmt*"!

(a)

niwt

(b)

w3st

(c)

Iwnw šm'w

Most Egyptian sites are now designated by names derived from Ancient Egyptian, Coptic, Greek, Biblical, Latin, Arabic, even European linguistic tradition. The site of Luxor, for example, represents a classic example of this complexity. The modern name, Luxor, is a linguistic corruption resulting from the inability of European visitors to pronounce the plural Arabic noun *el Qusur*, a word translated as "castles". Yet none of the ancient names for this site resemble the modern term. The Romans called Luxor the "Great-City-of-God" (*Diospolis Magna*), taken from the Greek, *Diospolis Megale*. But the Greeks also knew the site as Thebes, as recorded first by Homer and copied by a host of other authors. Ancient Egyptians themselves had several names for the site, among them: (a) (The City),[18] (b)[19] and (c)[20] (The Southern Town).

Today, even the term Luxor is not all inclusive. It is applied specifically only to the main village, and to archaeological sites situated on the southern east bank of the Nile, whereas the northern portion of the east bank, with its associated archaeological sites, is termed Karnak. Thebes, on the other hand, is the name commonly applied in general to the archaeological sites on the west bank wherein are intermingled the villages of Drah abu el Naga, Sheik abu Gurna, Murrai, and several others.

Food Patterns

Scholars involved in food research have long realized that the acceptance or avoidance of foods can be assessed from several different viewpoints, and that the reasons for food acceptance or rejection are diverse and cover a variety of social and physiological parameters. For example, a food that is normally forbidden by religious or social dictate may, at specific intervals, be consumed with approval. Furthermore, foods may be avoided, not only for adverse reasons such as disgust or religious hatred, but also out of respect for the food itself or to associated deities. Table 3 summarizes the possible positive and negative

Table 3

Basic attitudes towards individual foodstuffs

Accepted or rejected	Positive attitude	Negative attitude
Food eaten	Out of respect for, or to honour a god Pleasing with good taste no economic restrictions	Revenge Ritualistic reinforcement of a past event
Food avoided	Out of respect for, or to honour a god Partial avoidance (fasting)	To avoid offence to a god Observable health effect Economic restrictions

attitudes towards specific foods as reflected in both consumption and avoidance. These may be classed into two major categories: factors relative to the food itself and factors stemming from cultural and human interactions. Table 4 summarizes this duality.

Finally, the archaeological and literary references to food and diet in Ancient Egypt should be arranged within a chronologic sequence and according to their geographic distribution within the Nile Valley. Whenever possible we have tried such a correlation. It may, therefore, be pertinent to discuss here the bases of Egyptological dating.

Table 4

Patterns of food avoidance

Considerations relative to the substance itself

Effect on consumer's health: assumed cause-effect relationship: discomfort, pain, vomiting, diarrhoea, death, either immediate, or happening before next meal. *Examples:* toxic plants, seasonal shellfish avoidance
Esthetics: unpleasing appearance, taste, or smell. *Example:* Carrion
Religious patterns[a]

1. Avoidance believed to be directly dictated by revelation. *Examples:* Biblical bans
2. Avoidance codified by Clergy

   a. direct association with a god: i. avoided out of respect or to honour the god. *Example:* Ibis and hawk in Osiris worship; ii. avoided not to offend a god. *Examples:* pork, oxyrhynchus, and fish, in Osiris worship
   b. indirect association with a god; because of impurity. *Examples:* salt and beans in Osiris worship

Relative availability

1. Foodstuff uncommon or inexistent
2. Threatened extinction of foodstuff (see p. 142)
3. Females avoided to assure perpetuation of the species. *Example:* possibly cow flesh in Osiris worship. Palm wine production restricted to old male date trees

Considerations due to human interaction

Voluntary patterns

1. Individual, familial or tribal differentiation

   a. related to growth, maturation, or sexual differentiation. *Examples:* crocodile flesh not allowed to pre-pubescent males, but allowed to hunters; crocodile eggs denied to women
   b. resulting from cultural contact or conflict

Table 4—*continued*

1. Dietary differentiation from traditional enemy. *Examples:* dietary codes relative to pork, and different attitudes in Egypt towards same food
2. Avoiding mixing two foods, although each eaten separately, possibly because of their conflicting significance. *Examples:* Israelite separation of meat and dairy products; present day avoidance of fish with milk

Involuntary patterns

1. Mimetic or complimentary towards conqueror who avoids the food Overt pressure not exerted, but avoidance assimilated as subjects are brought into the new culture. *Examples:* pork avoidance among worshippers of Seth, diffused from Horus worshipping conquerors Fish discouraged by attitude of Ethiopian kings
2. Economic avoidance. Desired but denied because of relative expense, or because its production is no longer economic in an abstainer community.

---

[a] It is difficult to separate 1 and 2 under this heading.

Egyptological Dating

". . . the number of years from Osiris and Isis, they say, to the reign of Alexander, who founded the city which bears his name in Egypt, is over ten thousand, but according to other writers, a little less than twenty-three thousand . . ."

(*Diod.*, 1, 23, 1–2)

Time relationships of Egyptian history are assessed by a variety of methods. Early assessments were based upon the relative thickness and position of archaeological layers or strata (stratigraphic techniques), but archaeologists soon recognized that stratigraphy, superposition, and relative thickness were slender points upon which to base an estimate of time, and permitted only very speculative guesses. Floods, draught, fire or war are but a few of the forces that affect the formation and thickness of strata and deposits of dirt or human refuse on various locations of the same site form different thicknesses (Fig. 1.20).

Fortunately, there are five major documents that provide the chronology of Ancient Egyptian rulers, with additional information,

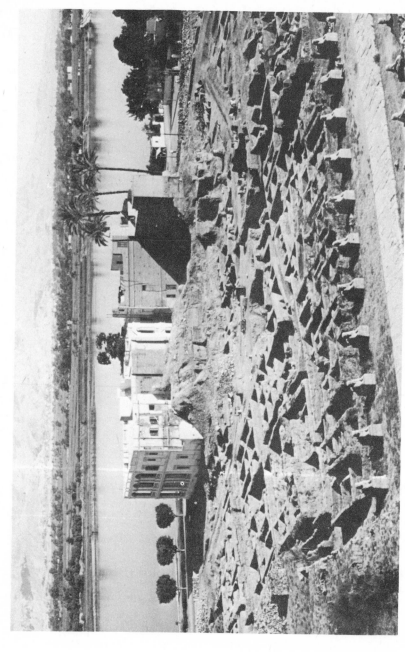

Fig. 1.19. Stratigraphy and archaeology. Over 3,000 years of history are depicted in this illustration of the area just north of the temple of Luxor. The stone road and the sphinxes (bottom) date from the New Kingdom. Ancient Egyptian buildings straddled this road, and were later overlain by remains of buildings of Greek, Roman and Byzantine construction. The sequence is crowned by a twentieth century home with television. Photographed 1969.

such as years of reign and the major historical occurrence during each year. Comparison of these royal lists with excavated sequences and materials supports their basic credibility. These documents are:

the Abydos list: a wall inscription found inside the temple of King Seti I at Abydos, that lists in chronologic order 76 "ancestor" kings between Menes and Seti I;

the Karnak tablet: from the temple of Amon at Karnak. It was inscribed during the reign of King Thutmose III, and originally contained 61 names of earlier Egyptian kings—but not in chronologic order. Only 48 names are presently legible;

the Palermo stone: the major fragment from one or many slabs on which were inscribed the royal Egyptian annals. The portion in the Museum at Palermo, deals only with the fifth dynasty and earlier kings, but gives additional interesting information (Figs 1.20, 1.21);

the Saqqara tablet: a wall inscription from the tomb of Tjunersy, at Saqqara, containing a list of 57 kings who reigned before Rameses II. Only 50 are legible at present;

the Turin papyrus: this document, written during the reign of King Rameses II, contains the annals and names of kings with their length of rule. Unfortunately, it is in a very fragmentary condition and chronologic placement of several portions of the papyrus is still hypothetical. See Gardiner (1961, pp. 47–51, 62–64) Engelbach, (1961, pp. 15–16).

These Ancient Egyptian lists fit fairly well with a document written by an Egyptian priest, Manetho of Sebennytus, who was selected by King Ptolemy II (Philadelphus) to compile a list of all kings of Egypt, including the length of each reign and specific notes of importance. This study, entitled *Aegyptiaca*, divides Egyptian history into thirty periods called dynasties, a concept basically unchanged today. Manetho's list of kings is no longer extant and is known only by quotations in the works of secondary or tertiary authors: originally he was quoted by two writers of the third century A.D., Eusebius of Caesarea and Sextius Julius (Africanus). Their works, too, are lost. But these were in turn quoted, in regard to Manetho, by Syncellus Georgius, a Byzantine historian also known as George the Monk, whose text has survived.

Manetho (fragment 4 *Excerpta Latina Barbari*, pp. 17–19) described the "demigods" who lived to great lengths of time

". . . some say that the god Hephaestus reigned in Egypt for 680 years; after him Sol, son of Hephaestus, for 77 years; next, Sosinosiris, for 320 years; then Orus the Ruler, for 28 years; and after him, Typhon, for 45 years. Total for the reigns of the Gods, 1550 years . . ."

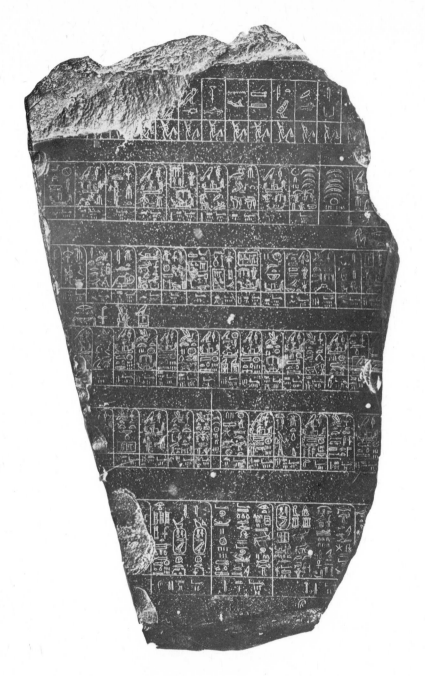

Fig. 1.20. The Palermo stone with the names of the Pharaohs. (Cairo Museum)

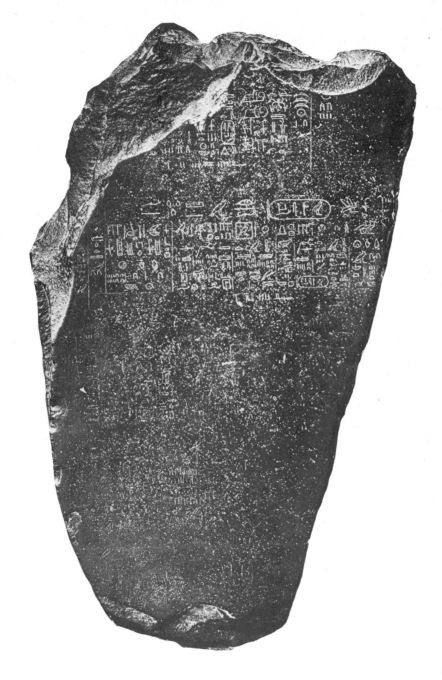

Fig. 1.21. The Palermo stone, Back view. (Cairo Museum)

An interesting explanation for such lengthy spans of life was made during the first century B.C.

> ". . . but since this great number of years surpasses belief, some men would maintain that in early times, before the movement of the sun had as yet been recognized, it was customary to reckon the year by the lunar cycle. Consequently, since the year consisted of thirty days, it was not impossible that some men lived twelve hundred years . . ." (*Diod.*, 1, 26, 1–6)

These surviving lists of Egyptian kings and the important quotations attributed to Manetho can establish only *relative* dates of reign. Egyptologists, however, use the observable regularity of the Nile flood in association with astronomic constants to fix points in Egyptian history. This regularity of the Nile flood,[21] that is such that fifty observations on the day of peak flood passing the same position can be averaged to the *same day* of the year (Childe, 1953, pp. 4–5), may have been the original impetus for setting the 365-day solar calendar used in Ancient Egypt.

(d)

ꜣḥt

This calendar was based on observations carried out on the star Sirius. The star was known as *spdt*[22] to the Ancient Egyptians but, in later writings, the Greeks called it both Sothis and the "Dog star".[23] The peculiarity of this star is that it rises and sets on the horizon, that for a certain period of its yearly shift it lies within the sun's halo and thus disappears from vision, and that its emergence heralds the Nile flood. The last coincidence re-inforced Egyptian faith in cosmological regularity.

(e)

prt

The coincidence between the peak day of flood and the heliacal rising of Sirius profoundly influenced Egyptian religion and chronology. The 365-day or observable calendar year, was introduced early in Egyptian history, by linking the Nile flood with the emergence of Sirius (*A.R.*, I, 38–46; Engelbach, 1961, pp. 65–71). This Egyptian year of 365 days consisted of twelve months of thirty days each grouped into three seasons of 120 days; (d) flood,[24] (e) winter (or planting),[25] and (f) summer (or harvest).[26] At the end of the three seasons, a five-day intercalary period (g)[27] was inserted, completing the 365-day calendar. These are the five days gained by Thot on the moon, as previously related on page 14.

(f)

šmw

(g)

hrw 5 hrym rnpt

As the 365-day year passed, the lag of 1/4 day between the calendar year and the astronomic year was not at first noticeable, and day 1 of the actual flood season would correspond with the first day of the flood calendar. Accumulation of the 1/4 day difference over a long period, however, revealed the instability of the calendrical system; thus over a

480-year period the actual peak day of the flood would occur 120 days earlier, and the cycle was realigned only every 1,460 years. When such a shift had been completed it was cause for rejoicing. This return to regularity every 1,460 years is called a Sothic cycle.

In the third century A.D., Censorinus, a Roman grammarian and chronologist, wrote that the 365-day and astronomic calendars of Egypt coincided at a date that could be placed between the years A.D. 160–144. This four-year margin is not due to an error by Censorinus, but to modern uncertainty as to the placement of his date within the framework of the modern Julian calendar. But, despite this ±2-year deviation, a ratio can be calculated in order to set Ancient Egyptian dates within the Julian calendar system.

With the help of these sources and of additional data from geneologies of long-lived officials who served several kings, historical records, business documents, temple calendars, records of the lives of sacred animals, synchronysms with other peoples and other miscellaneous data, a fair chronology can be deduced. Thus, the earliest known record of flood-Sirius divergence enabled archaeologists to establish the onset of the Middle Kingdom (twelfth dynasty) at 2000 B.C. (±9 years).

No mention has been made of the results derived from the use of C^{14} In the words of Parker (1971), this is

"because, for dynastic Egypt, we are in most cases already well within the range of accuracy of the method. For the periods of predynastic Egypt . . . Carbon-14 dating has considerable value, and eliminates quite decisively the 'long' chronologies favoured by some older scholars, which would place the First Dynasty and Menes in the 5th and 6th Millenia B.C. . . ."

Notes: Chapter 1

1. According to Pausanias (10, 24, 1). Others variously attribute the saying to Socrates, Solon, Plato or Pythagoras.
2. Translations of Greek and Roman texts are quoted by book, chapter, or paragraph of the ancient work, not of the modern translation.

3. This link was noted by visiting foreigners as early as the first century B.C. "... they say, also, that the Egyptians are colonists sent out by the Ethiopians, Osiris having been the leader of the colony ..." (*Diod.*, 3, 3, 1–2).

4. The Egyptian *hb-sd* festival, sometimes called the *hb-sd* jubilee, was a religious ceremony periodically performed to enact the ritualistic death (or murder) and subsequent re-birth of the king. During this ceremony, the sovereign, supposedly dead for a few days, succeeded himself as a young king reborn with fresh vigour and virility. The whole rite was probably a vestige of the custom of the ritual murder of the king that was, until very recently, current among certain African tribes, like the Shilluk, who live along the White Nile.

5. *F.*, 2; *G.*, 549.

6. Nubia is the region south of Aswan, down to Dongola in the Sudan. The word is derived from *nbw*, the Ancient Egyptian term for gold (*F.*, 129).

(h)

7. Kush: (h) in Nubia (*F.*, 284).

kȝš

8. Punt, the *Pwenet* of the Ancient Egyptians (*F.*, 88), was a southern land of vast riches with which Egypt traded since the earliest dynasties. It is especially known for the visit of Queen Hatshepsut's ships *c.* 1504 B.C. recorded in the temple of Deir al-Bahari at Thebes in a series of reliefs detailing the vast amount of goods brought from thither. It was situated in the region of Ethiopia, Somalia or Yemen, but its exact location has not been ascertained.

(i)

9. The Ancient Egyptian city of *Snw*: (i) (*F.*, 231), known to the Greeks as Pelusium the "gate to Egypt". Its ruins are found on the north coast of Sinai, between Port-Said and El-Arish.

snw

10. A little known Semite group, sometimes called the "Shepherd Kings".

11. Named after the legendary King Minos, ruler of Knossos in Crete.

12. Although several thousand tombs are known, those published to date are numbered in mere hundreds.

13. Bilharziasis, named for Theodor Bilharz who discovered in Cairo the worm that causes the disease. There are two species of the worm, *Schistosoma mansoni* that affects mainly the colon and causes dysenteric symptoms and hepatic fibrosis, and *S. haematobium* that affects principally the urinary tract. Before the recent massive therapeutic campaigns, 95% of the population in certain parts of the Delta were affected, and the complications of the disease were a major cause of mortality. The reader who might consider the attitude towards Bilharziasis unusual, might recall that not many decades ago gonorrhoea was considered in many European countries a sign of virility and tacitly accepted as a sign of manhood. Another parallel would be the acceptance in the USA of "athlete's foot", an infection caused by *Tinea pedis*, as something to be ignored, unless specifically asked about.

14. How often have we listened to the wealth of tales of such guides!
15. A similar prophesy concerned the Spartan city of Lacedaemon: ". . . for if the city of the Lacedaemonians should be deserted, and nothing should be left of it but its temples and the foundations of its buildings, posterity would, I think, after a long lapse of time, be very loath to believe that their power was as great as their renown . . ." (Thucydides, 1, 10, 2).
16. Modern English, likewise, varies. When one hears Americans, Britishers, Australians and South Africans speak the "mother tongue", one recalls a familiar wit's apt quip: "America and England, two sister countries separated by a common language".
17. *F.*, 286; *G.*, 611.
18. *F.*, 125; *G.*, 572, The Southern City.
19. *F.*, 54; *G.*, 559.
20. *F.*, 13; *G.*, 552.
21. This struck all ancient travellers: ". . . nor does the Nile ever deceive; it is a river that keeps its appointments both in the times of its increase and the amount of water that it brings, a river that never allows itself to be convicted of being unpunctual . . ." (Achilles Tatius, 4, 12, 2). An attempt to explain the flood appeared in the writings of nearly all ancient writers, like Herodotus (II, 19–27) who also quoted the opinions of Hecataeus, Thales of Miletus and Anaxagoras.
22. *F.*, 224; *G.*, 625.
23. Plutarch wrote, on the authority of Eudoxus ". . . the soul of Isis is called by the Greeks the Dog star, but by the Egyptians Sothis . . ." (*I. and O.*, 359, 21 D). Elsewhere, he also wrote that Sothis meant in Egyptian "pregnant" or "to be pregnant" (*I. and O.*, 376, 61, A). Other myths and beliefs were also linked to this star, among which that the antelope was the first creature to know when the Dog star arises, and manifests the fact by sneezing (Aelian, 7, 8)!
24. *F.*, 4.
25. *F.*, 91.
26. *F.*, 267.
27. *F.*, 150.

Chapter 2

The Nutritional State of the Ancient Egyptians

*"O ye, who preside over food, who are
      attached to plentifulness,
Commend him to the cup-bearer of Rê,
that he may commend him to Rê himself,
That they may seize and give him, that
they may take and give him barley, spelt,
      bread and beer,
That which Rê bites, he gives to him, that
which he nibbles, he gives to him."*

(*Pyr.*, 120a *et seq.*)

The accurate assessment of the nutritional position of a country requires data on such interrelated matters as the extent of the arable area, the efficiency of prevailing techniques, the animal and industrial resources, the density of the population in country and town, the extent and nature of foreign trade, the social structure, and the existence of infections and diseases likely to interfere with nutrition or to affect human productivity. All these factors affect the cost of living and ultimately the purchasing power of the individual. The difficulty of gathering such extensive information is great even in contemporary society; it is a near impossibility in retrospective studies covering the ever-changing face of a culture that spanned over thirty centuries, from the Neolithic to the plenitude of Egyptian splendour.

The Cultivated Area

Butzer (1960) estimated the cultivated area of the Egyptian land at the end of the Pre-Dynastic era at 16,000 sq. km (roughly 6,000 sq. miles), and he calculated that this could nourish some 100,000 to 200,000 inhabitants.

Daumas gave a terse account of later periods, while, at the same time, underscoring the fragmentary nature of documentation (1965, pp. 218, 219). One would like, he said, to know the size of the population throughout the centuries. Unfortunately, there are no accurate estimates. Nevertheless, we do not have the impression—and we emphasize the word impression—that Egypt was overpopulated. A rough estimate may be made from later historians' reports. Herodotus reckoned that the number of towns under Amasis was 20,000, but he could not vouch for the accuracy of his statement. He preferred to introduce it by "They say . . .". Diodorus evaluated them at 18,000 before Ptolemy Soter under whom, he said, they increased to 30,000; and he estimated the population at 7 million. As it is certain that the Greeks carried out periodic censuses, these figures may have solid bases.

Daumas further said that one must be content with impressions. The population must have been dense under the twelfth dynasty and grown even denser under the eighteenth when, at Thebes, it appears to have been considerable. Under the nineteenth dynasty the Delta, especially in its eastern part, was the seat of a great demographic expansion. If we admit that under Amenophis III Egypt, then at the peak of its greatness, nourished nine to ten million souls, it is evident that it was well populated, but not beyond what its rich soil and its unceasing relations with Nubia, the Fertile Crescent, and the Aegean could support. Under the Saitic rule, the population reached, according to some estimates, 20 million; but this number, which has been deducted from modern data, does not rest on any positive information.

Now, these figures compare fairly well with more recently documented ones. Before the High Dam was built the cultivable area constituted by the long green ribbon along the Nile, which opens up in the Delta like a blossoming Nile lily, totalled about 23,000 sq. km (about 9,000 sq. miles). The population was 7 million in 1882 and 12,751,000 in 1917 (L'Egypte, p. 160). It now exceeds 36 million.

The exceptional fertility of the "black land" that gave the country its name, *kmt*, need not be dwelt upon. The peasants could not have starved in a land that nourished in a single princely domain at El-Kab 122 oxen, 100 sheep, 1,200 goats, and 1,500 swine; or that could provide Rameses III with the 514,698 large cattle and 680,764 geese that he offered to the temples in 31 years (Erman and Ranke, 1952, p. 506).

Nevertheless, a text that seems a stylistic exercise meant to extol the merits of the scribe's profession over those of other crafts draws a gloomy picture of the peasant's lot

"Remember you not the condition of the cultivator faced with the registering of the harvest-tax, when the snake has carried off the corn and the hippopotamus has devoured the rest. The mice abound in the field. The locusts descend. The cattle devour. The sparrows bring disaster upon the cultivator. The remainder that is on the threshing-floor is at an end, it falls to the thieves. The yoke of oxen has died while threshing and ploughing. And now the scribe lands on the river-bank and is about to register the harvest-tax. The janitors carry staves and the Nubians rods of palm, and they say 'Hand over the corn' though there is none. The cultivator is beaten all over, he is bound and thrown into the well, soused and dipped head downwards. His wife has been bound in his presence, his children are in fetters. His neighbours abandon them and they are fled. So their corn flies away. But the scribe is ahead of everyone . . . Mark it well." (Gardiner, 1961, p. 33)

The Cost of Living

Data on the cost of living contains even greater gaps. To quote again Daumas (1965, p. 228), without having known money in its proper sense, Egypt not only invented an abstract monetary standard, but actually utilized fixed weights of metal as exchange media. In rare cases, before the custom of striking money appeared in the eastern Mediterranean in the sixth century B.C., some of the great temples stamped ingots, and just before Alexander's conquest, some Pharaohs stamped metallic pieces with hieroglyphic inscriptions. There was, however, no generally used official currency. Nevertheless, no financial document written in proper legal form dispenses with metallic evaluations. Thus, a house would be estimated say at 10 *chats*, and payment could consist of a piece of cloth worth 3 *chats*, in addition to a bed worth 4 *chats*, and another piece of cloth worth 3 *chats*.

A *chat* probably weighed 7·5 g, and a *dbn* was worth 12 *chats*. The nineteenth dynasty introduced a new standard, the *qite* which was worth 1/10 of a silver *dbn*. Ten bronze *dbn* equalled 1 silver *qite*. The price of silver relative to bronze was thus 100:1 under Rameses III. Later, it fell to 60:1.

By the end of the eighteenth dynasty, a cow was worth 8 silver *chats*, and a goat 1/2 *chat*. In the Fayoum, an *aroure* (2,756 sq. m) fetched 2 silver *chats*, i.e. 1/6 of a *dbn*. Four hundred years later, it cost 11 *qites* (1·1 *dbn*) which represented a considerable increase. Slaves were very expensive: 4 *dbn* and 1 *qite* for a small girl, and 7 *dbn* for a man. The cost of labour seems equally exorbitant: 2 *chats* a day for a girl, no doubt a weaver, which equalled 1/4 of the price of a cow, and 1 *chat* for an unqualified male labourer.

However, when we read that a gown cost the equivalent of $18, a shroud of finer cloth, $23, and a pot of scent $53 (Daumas, 1965) we are left with the questions: of what kind was the cloth, of what fineness the shroud, and of what quality the scent? Unless we discover some day a show window with price tabs, there is no answer!

According to Baer (1962) cattle cost up to 130 *dbn* of copper, corresponding to 65 sacks of grain or the yearly income of a craftsman at Deir el-Medineh. Under Amenophis IV, a cow could be bought for 0·5 *dbn* and a bull for 0·67 *dbn* of silver. Much later, under Sheshonq (twenty-first dynasty), the price of an ox was 0·2 *dbn*, of a cow 1·08 *dbn*, and of slaves from 1–5 *dbn* of silver.

Daily Allowances and Diets

Rations changed, similarly. As an example, Reekmans (1966) cites the rapid change of conditions before and after year 38 of Ptolemy Philadelphus (248–247 B.C.) due no doubt to changing economic conditions. Whereas the grain issued to workers, in a certain area, provided before that year an adequate caloric intake estimated as 3,780 for men and 2,520 for women and children, after that date the provision was hardly adequate for any kind of work, providing 2,840 and 1,820 respectively. His calculations, however, took into account only grain.

The importance of food at all periods in Egypt is reflected in present day proverbs that perpetuate attitudes related to eating as metaphors. Some comment on overeating and greed

"If God hates somebody, he drives his belly against him."

Others stress the necessity of foresight

"Yesterday's lunch does not silence today's hunger."

Still others make fun of pretence and incompetence

"If his cook is a beetle, what sort of meal does he expect?"

All this implies that food in Egypt was abundant and varied. As we shall see in the following chapters, cereals, vegetables, fruit, birds and fish, were within arm's reach of the poorest; while the rich had, in addition, abundant cattle and more costly or sophisticated items. Herodotus (II, 77), describing the way of life of the average Egyptian, wrote

"They live on bread made of spelt which they form into loaves called in their own tongue *cyllestis*. Their drink is a wine which they obtain from barley ... Many kinds of fish they eat raw, either salted, or dried in the sun. Quails also, and ducks, and small birds, they eat uncooked, merely firstly salting them. All other birds, excepting those which are set apart as sacred, are eaten either roasted or broiled."

Seventeen centuries earlier, a stele of the Silsileh quarries mentioned the daily allowances for a thousand men sent by Pharaoh Seti I to transport the monument of Amon-Ra-Osiris and his divine Ennead

"20 *deben* [1,820 gm] of bread, two bundles of vegetables, and a roast of flesh."

The "King's Messenger and Standard-Bearer" fared better

"... Good bread, ox flesh, wine, sweet oil, olive oil, fat, honey, figs, fish, and vegetables, every day ..." (*A.R.*, III, 207, 208)

As was befitting, kings had even richer menus. King Unas' bill of fare, which is not the richest, but definitely the oldest Royal list to be preserved complete (sixth dynasty, *c.* 2600 B.C.), mentions

"... milk, three kinds of beer, five kinds of wine, ten kinds of loaves, four of bread, ten of cakes, fruit cakes, four meats, different cuts, joints, roast, spleen, limb, breast, tail, goose, pigeon, figs, ten other fruit, three kinds of corn [wheat], barley, spelt, five kinds of oil, and fresh plants ..." (*Pyr.* 16*d*–115*c*)

Later, better commercial communications with neighbouring or conquered countries added delicacies from Cyprus, Babylonia, Naharin and the lands of the Hittites.

These were, of course, rations for the gods. For whereas King Cheops, in appreciation of the tales of magic that diverted him, offered a thousand loaves of bread, one hundred jugs of beer, and a whole ox to the memory of the king under whom the miraculous events had happened, he rewarded the author of the prodigee with only one cake, one jug of beer, and one portion of meat (Lefebvre, 1949, pp. 74–80).

Nor should we think that all Egyptians had the gastric capacity of the hero of one of these tales. Djedi the magician no doubt owed to his magic the capacity to consume daily five hundred loaves of bread, a haunch of beef, and one hundred jugs of beer. Such tall tales were common among the Ancient Egyptians. Plutarch related that a certain Heraclides, unable to find a drinking companion, was in the habit of inviting people in for rounds of drink, some before luncheon, others for luncheon, still others for dinner and finally new people for an afternoon bout. Without any let-up, he was a match for them all and fully carried his part of the four sessions of drinking (Plutarch, *Table Talk*, 1, 6, 624).

In spite of such obvious embellishments, of the different epochs in which they were written, of the tattered state of some of them, and of the stereotyped character of some expressions, Egyptian popular tales, the "Oriental Nights" of antiquity, offer a faithful picture of daily life, abounding in carefully noted details. Table 1 shows the frequency with which items of diet appear in the tales collected by Lefebvre (1949), and indicates that, in order of frequency, the commonest were bread, beer, meats, fruits and vegetables.

Child Feeding

Children were breast-fed for three years, a rather long period by Western standards, but not unusual in other countries. Mothers who could not or would not feed their children resorted to wet nurses, whose profession was strictly regulated by law in Ptolemaic times.

There exists no statement that cows or other animals were ever used as wet nurses. There are, however, texts that intimate such usage, and numerous representations of young boys at a cow's udders (Fig. 2.1). In a curious inscription of *The Pyramid Texts* (Utterance 267; Erman, 1927, p. 9), a mother goddess says

> "... My son, O king, take to thee my breast and suck it. How is it that thou hast not come on every one of thy days ... He has come to these his two mothers, the two vultures, they of the long hair and the pendulous breast ... They draw their breasts to his mouth and nevermore do they wean him ..."

This is indeed an interesting text, for after a jump of over four thousand years the vulture motif is now recognized by psychoanalysts as a symbol of motherhood (Freud, 1947, p. 45). Through such utterances and pictures, princes and kings asserted their divine filiation.

Table 1

Frequency with which different articles of food are mentioned in Egyptian tales (calculated from Lefebvre, 1949)

Cereals and bread		Meats	
Barley	6	Just "meat"	3
Wheat	4	Boiled meat	1
Bread	15	Beef, ox	6
Cakes	5	Ox liver	1
	—	Cattle (bovines?)	2
Total	30	Mutton	1
		Pig	1
Vegetables		Small animals	2
Just "vegetables"	2	Wild game	1
Lentils	2		—
Lettuce	1	Total	18
Cucumber	1		
	—	Fowl	
Total	6	Birds	4
		Water game	1
Fruit		Roast fowl	1
Just "fruit"	2		—
Figs	2	Total	6
Grapes	2		
Sycamore, 2 kinds (each)	1		
Cyperus esculentus	1	Fish	
	—	Fish	1
Total	9		
Miscellaneous		Beverages	
Milk	4	Beer	16
Honey	1	Wine	5
Olive oil	1		—
(from Syria, Palestine)	—	Total	21
Total	6		

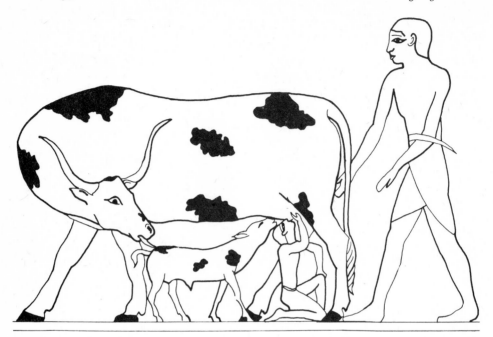

Fig. 2.1. Young boy sharing with a calf, a cow's milk (Rosellini, I., 1834, MCXXVII).

The theme of the suckling prince is also the subject of a chapter of *The Book of the Dead* illustrated by statuary groups, where the dead Prince, painted black (the colour of death), meets Hathor in her marshy kingdom of the West. The goddess offers him her milk; he drinks the divine beverage that restores him to life (the second life); and is thereafter painted red, the colour of life, at the udder (Fig. 3.3).

Otherwise, cow milk was fed to infants and instructions were given on how to distinguish by smell good from bad milk (*Eb.*, XCIII, 788; XCIV, 796) (see also Chapter 19, Vol. 2).

Diseases of Overeating

Generally speaking, therefore, the average Egyptians were well nourished. Even the poorest took enough nutriment before the introduction of maize (and the subsequent appearance of pellagra), and the

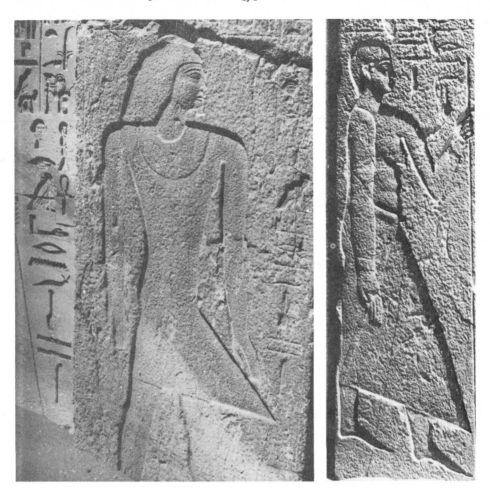

Fig. 2.2. Ankh-ma-Hor's tomb. Saqqara. Old Kingdom. The owner of the tomb is shown, aged and obese as he was in real life (right) on the outer face of the gate of the tomb; and thin and young on the inner face of the same gate (left). Photographed 1969.

diversion of agricultural lands to production of cash crops such as cotton and sugar cane. Herodotus wrote that they were the healthiest people after the Libyans (II, 77). Their portraits are superb examples of athletic manhood. However, there is reason to believe that the models of these portraits, that bear a remarkable resemblance to modern Fellaheen, were the common people who toiled hard and ate a much more frugal diet than the wealthy. The latter were probably much heavier. One reason for our doubt is that, especially under the Old Kingdom which is known for the realism of its artists, one may meet, in the same person and on the same panel, an admirably lean and muscular portrait beside the big belly, double chin, and hanging breasts reflecting years of gracious living (Fig. 2.2).

This could only mean that the beauty of their portraits stemmed less from a universal perfection of their physique than from the belief that, by drawing their portraits in that way, their souls would be re-incarnated and live forever after death in these idealized bodies.

Obesity

Obesity, however, was regarded as objectionable. Plutarch wrote of the Egyptian priests that they did not want the bull Apis to be fat

> "... nor themselves, either; but rather they desire that their bodies, the encasement of their souls, shall be well adjusted and light, and shall not oppress the divine element by the predominance and preponderance of the mortal" (*I. and O.*, 353, 6)

The few obese portraits we know were usually artists' charges against their better-fed patrons, the wealthy, and the class of foremen or supervisors who had finally acceded to sedentary positions after years of hard toil: a doorkeeper in the temple of Amon-Ra Khor-en-Khonsu (Winlock, 1942); a cook in Ankh-ma-Hor's tomb; a fat man quietly enjoying food presented to him by his lean servants in Mereruka's tomb (Fig. 2.3); or the local yeoman, the famed Sheikh el Balad, but never a Pharaoh.

When dealing with foreigners, however, the artists' verve was freed. No fear of sanction prevented them from reproducing the phenomenal corpulence of the Ethiopians Harwa[1] and Agrigadiganen,[2] or from accurately copying the lipodystrophy of the Queen of Punt (Fig. 2.4).

Overdrinking

The affluent were, as always and everywhere, much given to overeating and drinking. Priests were said to avoid superfluity, but the "bons

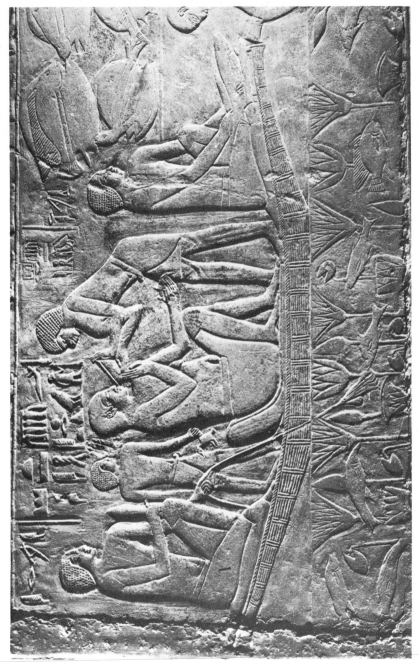

Fig. 2.3. From Mereruka's tomb. Saqqara. Old Kingdom. The fat man in the barge. Photographed 1969.

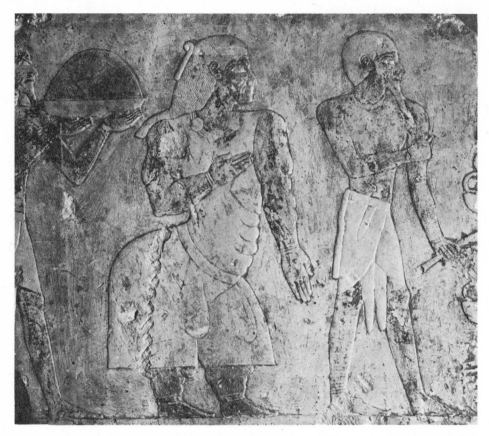

Fig. 2.4. The Queen of Punt. Cairo Museum. *c.* 1500 B.C. Used with permission.

vivants" at the conclusion of banquets, had a servant go round with a wooden image of a dead body and saying

". . . Drink and be merry for when you die such you will be . . ." (*Her.*, II, 78)

Herodotus further relates that King Amasis, when he was chided by his friends because of his drinking during his leisure time, answered that

". . . bowmen bend their bows when they wish to shoot, and unbrace them when the shooting is over. Were they always strung they would break and fail the archer in time of need." (II, 173)

The native production of beer and wine was very large. We may see representations in museums and tombs of buxom lasses preparing the dough to be fermented and of the jolly vintners, intoxicated by the fumes of fermenting grapes, holding fast to hanging ropes, to keep their balance in the vats. About 1200 B.C., a group of vintners delivered 1200 jars of good wine and 50 of medium quality (Posener, 1962, p. 300). Their clients were very particular about the quality of their beverage. Jars were marked with the year, the variety, the vine, the vineyard, the owner, and the person responsible (see Chapter 14).

Numerous moralizing poems described the dubious joys of drinking

> ". . . You trail from street to street smelling of beer
> You are like a broken rudder . . .
> You are performing acrobatics on a wall
> Here you are learning to play the flute and to pluck the lyre
> Look at yourself beside a pretty girl, drenched in perfume,
> a garland of flowers round your neck, beating on
>   your stomach, reeling and rolling about on the ground
>   covered with filth."

(Posener, 1962, p. 69)

In Paheri's tomb, a lady orders the butler

"Give me eighteen cups of wine, I want to drink to ebriety; my throat is as parched as straw."

Elsewhere, in the middle of another banquet, an elegant lady is relieving her overfilled stomach (Fig. 14.13). In a humorous drawing, the butler, too partial to his master's wine, hardly responds to the knocks at the door of the cellar of a man who says: "He is asleep", while another comments: "He is drunk with wine". Still irresponsive, the butler answers in a sleepy drawl one might well imagine "No, I am not at all asleep" (Fig. 2.5).

Atheroma

Atheroma, widely associated with rich living, has been reviewed by Buchheim (1956). It was found in several mummies of the historic period (Ruffer, 1921), including those of Rameses II (Elliot Smith and

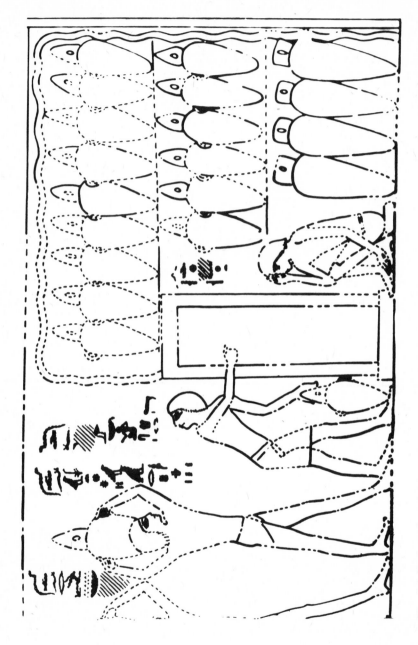

Fig. 2.5. Butler asleep behind the cellar door. The persons knocking at the door are commenting "He is drunk with wine" (Tomb of Antef, Säve-Söderbergh, 1957, plate XV).

Dawson, 1924, p. 156), of a Lady Teye of the twenty-first dynasty (Long, 1931), and of pharaoh Meneptah (Shattock, 1909). The recent development of mummy radiography has disclosed even more strikingly its frequency (Gray, 1966; Harris and Weeks, 1973) in Pre-Dynastic mummies (Moodie, 1931). Histological examination revealed its conformity to usual types: vascular narrowing, lipid deposition, reduplication of the internal elastic lamina and medial calcification (Sandison, 1962).

Diabetes Mellitus

Evidence of other metabolic diseases that may be precipitated or caused by dietary excess include polyuria, possibly of diabetic origin, which is the object of many medical prescriptions (*Eb.*, XLIX, 264; *L.*, 274, 280), in one of which it is treated with honey. The Egyptians did not appear to know the sweet taste of diabetic urine; otherwise, one would be tempted to look at this as a substitutive therapy.

Gall-stones

Multiple gall-stones were found in a twenty-first dynasty Priestess of Amon, and gout, in a body of the Early Christian Period (Elliot Smith and Dawson, 1924, p. 156).

Renal Calculi

Renal calculi may result from metabolic derangements as well as from Bilharziasis or dehydration. Both of the latter conditions were common in Egypt, and renal and vesical calculi were also found in mummies, although they were extremely rare: only two cases with vesical calculi, and three of renal stones among 30,000 Ancient Egyptian and Nubian bodies examined (Elliot Smith and Dawson, 1924, p. 156; Ruffer, 1921).

Underfeeding and Famine

On the opposite extreme of the scale, excessive thinness is illustrated in a tomb at Meir by a skinny shepherd (Cledat, 1901) who probably belonged to a Beja population living in the desolate fringes of the desert (Fig. 3.16).

The occurrence of famine is documented by many texts of various periods that Vandier collected in his classical monograph (1936). Drioton compared them to an account of famine due to a low Nile flood, written by Abdal-Latif al-Baghdady in 1229 (1965), noting that some of the most odious details of the mediaeval account, those that related incidents of cannibalism, had their parallel in two of the Egyptian accounts, one of the tenth, the other the eleventh dynasty (Drioton, 1943a). Indeed, they had their counterpart only some time ago among the victims of an air crash in the Andes, and the eaters were absolved by men of religion because they ate already dead bodies (*St Louis Globe*, December 28, 1972).

Drought

Egypt is utterly dependent on the periodic Nile flood for its subsistence. Rulers to this day have repeatedly tried to equalize its flow, ever since Menes attempted in the fourth millenium B.C., according to Herodotus, to dam it south of Memphis (II, 99), through the legendary Moeris [probably Amenemhat] who was credited by the same Herodotus with diverting its excess into Lake Moeris (II, 101) and the successive building and raising of dams in modern times.

Various Ancient Egyptian offices connected with irrigation are known: intendants of the lakes, managers of dams or locks; supervisors of drainage; and controllers of the inundation, of the growth of the land brought by the Nile, and of the filling up of ponds (Petrie, 1925, p. 110). Any whim of the Nile god Hapi (Fig. 2.6), whose generous corpulence equalled only the abundance of his gifts, brought disaster and famine. This was graphically told in a rock inscription that recalls the Biblical story of Joseph.

"The eighteenth year of King Zoser, the following information was sent to the governor of Aswan, Medari: '. . . I am overwhelmed with sorrow for the

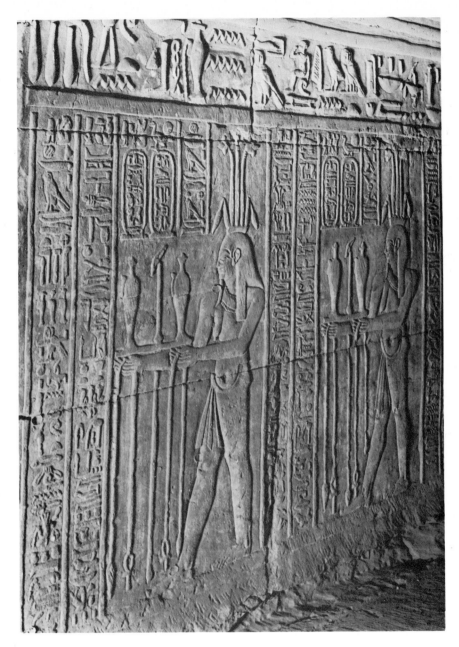

Fig. 2.6. The Nile god, Hapi, shown as a fat man with hanging breasts, as symbols of his bounties. His head is crowned with lotus plants, and he holds a tray from which hang lotus buds. Temple of Edfu. Ptolemaic period. Documentation Centre, Cairo.

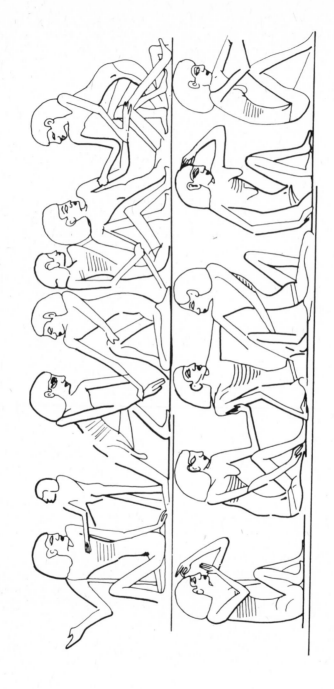

Fig. 2.7a. Scene of Famine. Unas ramp. Redrawn from Drioton (1943a).

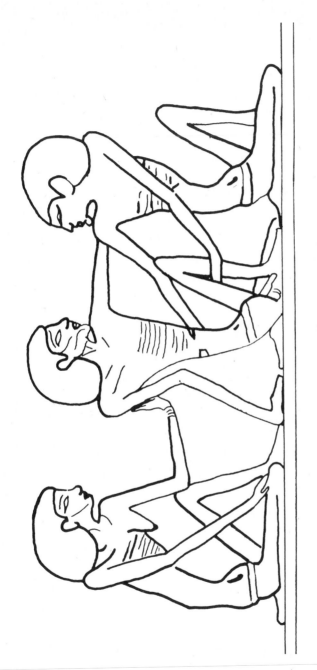

Fig. 2.7b. Enlargement of part of scene depicted in Fig. 2.7a.

Throne and the inmates of the Palace; my heart is filled with immense affliction, for the Nile has not been full in my time for seven years. Grain is lacking; fodder is dry, there is a dearth of edible things. If one calls for help, people turn aside, not to answer. Children cry, young people waste, men's hearts fail them, their legs give way. Squatting on the ground, they stretch their hands forth towards us'."

The strikingly realistic bas-relief on the Unas ramp in Saqqara (2600 B.C.) could illustrate this text (Drioton, 1943a). The artist caught the sticking out ribs, hollow flanks, bony limbs and drooping breasts of his characters (Fig. 2.7). Some sway on their legs, on the point of fainting. Others devour their fleas and suck their thumb. In Drioton's opinion these bas-reliefs are a graphic representation of popular sayings.

Excessive Floods

An excessive flood could be equally disastrous. This was recorded twice: under Nesubenebded of the twenty-first dynasty (*A.R.*, IV, 627–628); and again under Osorkon II (twenty-second dynasty, ninth century B.C.), when the water rose over two feet above the pavement of the temple. In descriptions of the time the temples of Thebes were said to be like marshes, and the people like water-birds. The great Amon Festival could not be held and to abate the flood this god's statue was brought forth from the temple in his sacred barge to be prayed to (*A.R.*, IV, 742–743).

As a safeguard against these meagre years, the authorities, like the Biblical Joseph, stocked grain in silos (Fig. 2.8); (see also Chapter 12); and distributions were occasions for royal ceremonies and recorded on special stelae.

Apart from such cataclysms how did malnutrition exist, and how could it arise in the middle of plenty? The answer is that the mere lists of available foods may be most misleading. The foods listed may be available only in limited amounts or to a favoured few; many nourishing articles may be rejected out of ignorance, of early conditioning, or in compliance with religious bans.

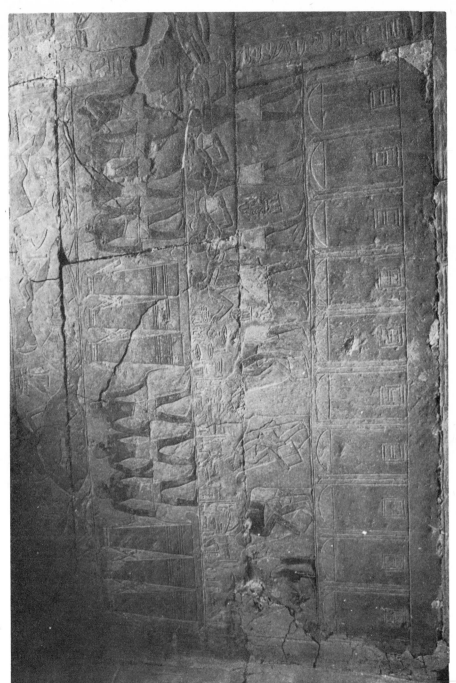

Fig. 2.8. Silos. Each silo had an opening in its lower part to allow the withdrawal of grain poured in it from above. Tomb of Mereruka. Saqqara. Old Kingdom. Photographed 1969.

Taboos

As we shall see in the following chapters, the evidence shows beyond doubt that taboos in Egypt—in spite of the tales, told and retold in Greek chronicles—involved only a few meats, and were limited to certain districts, to certain holy periods of the year, to discrete historical periods, or to restricted classes of people. The Clergy and Nobility, who had a vested interest in religion, might have abided by them; not the commoner who, traditionally, disbelieved, challenged, or was just disinterested and could not afford to be too choosy. Who would believe that fish was defiling on listening to a maid *deshabillé* enticing her lover with a fretting red fish in her hand

> ". . . My brother, it is pleasant to go to the [pond] in order to bathe me in thy presence, that I may let thee see my beauty in my tunic of finest royal linen when it is wet . . . I go down with thee into the water and come forth again to thee with a red fish, which lieth beautiful on my fingers . . . Come and look at me . . ." (Erman, 1927, p. 243)

Intestinal Malabsorption

Another cause of malnutrition in the midst of plenty or, at least, of an adequate nutritional intake, is the "conditioning" effect of intestinal disease, helminths, or other abnormalities that alter intestinal absorption or increase nutrient losses. In hot countries, the main agents of such "conditioned deficiences" are intestinal helminths and diarrhoeas. This long recognized or suspected notion has been recently proved in the laboratory by Waslien *et al.* (1973) who showed considerable depletion of iron, zinc and protein, and diminished concentrations of vitamins in Egyptian patients harbouring intestinal parasites (Table 2).

Intestinal Parasites

The Egyptian papyri mentioned many intestinal worms by name: *ḥft, pnd* (*Eb.*, XVI–XXIII, 50–85), *betju* (*Eb.*, XLI, 205); *ḥrrw* (*Eb.*, XIX, 62), equated by Ebbel with *Ascaris, Taenia*, hookworm and *Schistosomia* respectively. But these identifications are, to say the least, problematical.

Schistosoma haematobium ova, however, because of the resistance

Table 2

Percentage incidences of low serum values for nutrients

	Fe <80 mg%	Zn <100 μg%	Alb. <2.8 g%	vit. A <20 μg%	Carotene <40 μg%	Folate <3 μg%	B12 <100 pg%	vit. E <.5 mg%
Hookworm and Schistosomiasis	100	100	—	15	—	—	18	—
Hookworm	—	—	26	—	—	0	4	—
Schistosomiasis	80	—	20	25	25	0	0	25
S. mansoni uncomplicated	100	—	0	14	7	13	0	25
Polyposis	100	—	53	50	43	19	0	40

From Waslien *et al.*, 1973.

of their chitinous egg-shells, were found in the urinary tracts of many mummies by Ruffer (1921, pp. 17, 18) and their most obvious manifestation, haematuria, is often mentioned in the medical papyri.

Nothing is known of the ancient incidence of the intestinal variety due to *S. mansoni* which, on account of its dysenteric and hepatic complications, is especially likely to cause malnutrition. At present, its connection with the perennial irrigation lately introduced in Lower Egypt has restricted its spread to that part of the country. It has spared Upper Egypt where the practice, since Pharaonic times, of alternating irrigation with drying of the land, did not allow the survival of its intermediate host. With the extension of continuous irrigation, made possible by the erection of the High Aswan dam, its future spread to Upper Egypt is now one of the main concerns of the Health Authorities. It is possible that Ancient Egypt remained free of that scourge, except in the marshy, continuously wet areas of the Delta.

Bilharziasis: Cirrhosis of the Liver

Hepatic cirrhosis was not unknown. Ruffer (1921, p. 78) described dense connective tissue around a few bile ducts in the liver of a mummy. He called these appearances cirrhosis, without further details. Some illustrations in Old Kingdom tombs at Saqqara, the necropolis of Memphis, show abdominal distension, scrotal and umbilical herniae (Fig. 2.9) such as may be caused by ascites. The exhibition of gynaecomastia (Fig. 2.10) in the same tomb suggests hepatic cirrhosis as a

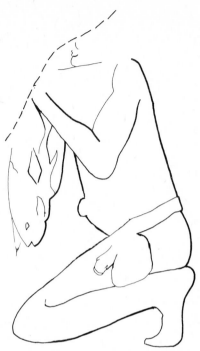

Fig. 2.9. Tomb of Mehu. Saqqara. Old Kingdom. A fisherman with abdominal distension umbilical hernia and scrotal distension. (?hydrocele? hernia) Redrawn from authors' photograph 1965.

cause (Ghalioungui, 1962). Whether this was nutritional, post-infective, or bilharzial is debatable. But the genital hyperplasia in other individuals of the same tomb (Fig. 2.11) is a strong indication that Memphis was then, as it is today, an area of bilharzial endemicity. It is of course well known that, in the affected field hands, malnutrition often adds its harm to those of bilharziasis.

Âaâ

One of the few diseases given a name of its own in the medical papyri is the mysterious *âaâ*. Its symptoms include abdominal distension and pain, palpitation, cardiac "stitches" and "escape", probably meaning extrasystoles. Jonckheere (1944) and Scheuthauer (1881) added to these symptoms blood-stained evacuations on the flimsy grounds that the word *âaâ* (see a) was determined by a phallic sign, and that, in a

(a)

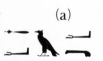

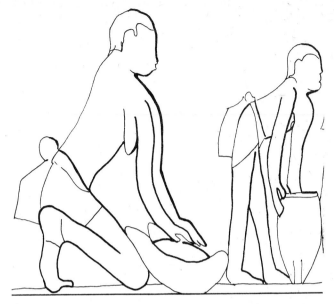

Fig. 2.10. Gynaecomastia. Mehu's tomb, Saqqara. Old Kingdom.

magical papyrus, a formula to treat it is inserted between a prescription for anal bleeding, and another for uterine haemorrhage.

It was also argued, both because of the phallic determinative and because one of the fifty prescriptions that mention it says

". . . to be taken by a man in whose belly there are worms; it is *âaâ* that caused them to appear . . ." (*Eb.*, XIX, 62)

that Egyptian physicians had discovered the *Schistosoma* worm. It was, accordingly, boldly stated that *âaâ* was identical with urinary bilharziasis.

Nevertheless, the minuteness of the *Schistosoma* worm, its hidden location in the portal tributaries whereas the invoked text places it in the "belly", the non-mentioning of *âaâ* in any of the numerous passages concerned with haematuria (e.g. *Eb.*, 49; *Ber.*, 165, 187, 188 etc.), the attribution in the texts of the worms to *âaâ* rather than of *âaâ* to worms, and the current interpretation by Egyptologists of the phallus as meaning "poison" or "seed", are all arguments against the consideration of *âaâ* as schistosomiasis. An alternative interpretation explains *âaâ* as the occult poison of an evil causative spirit or demon (von Deines and Grapow, 1958, Vol. IV, p. 111).

Âaâ has also more plausibly been identified with "Egyptian chlorosis", equally stated without serious reasons, to be due to schistosomiasis. Its symptoms are, in fact, consistent with this diagnosis, and
the presence of this parasite and hookworm could well cause blood-loss
and iron deficiency. In Egypt, "chlorosis", an obsolete term for hypo-
chromic anaemia, is still a serious problem. Its causes are partly dietary
but, to a larger extent, parasitic.

The relation of anaemia to parasitism has been accepted for a
long time as a fact, and recent scientific evidence establishes beyond
doubt the role of parasites in its causation in Egypt (Waslien *et al.*, 1972).
This has been extensively reviewed by Patwardhan and Darby (1972).
According to Rifat and Nagaty (1961), 50% of dermatology out-
patients in Cairo and 76% of out-patients in the countryside carry
protozoal or helminthic infections. In other areas, they found infection
rates of 84% after a single examination of urine and faeces (Nagaty *et al.*,
1961). Other investigators confirmed these results.

If the association of *âaâ* with worms is one day substantiated, then the
hardly visible *Schistosoma* that Egyptian physicians credited with
the disease will not alone be held responsible, but, rather hookworm,
ascaris, and the other intestinal worms, that certainly they had seen
wriggling in the stools of their patients.

There is, moreover, no inconsistency in accepting *âaâ*, as suggested
by von Deines and Grapow, as a demoniac entity and, at the same time,
connecting it with visible worms, since worms, in Egyptian thought,
could be the executive agents of the disease-causing spirits.

Vitamin Deficiencies

Pellagra

A vitamin deficiency, often, though not always, associated with
parasitism is pellagra. The earliest mention of that condition in connection with Egypt was made by Sonnini (1799) who observed in
Upper Egypt persons covered with boils that the local people called
Habe Nili, and wondered whether these were cases of "peleagra".
In his statement, however, he was obviously led astray by his ignorance
of the language and lack of experience, for *hab el Nil* (Nile boils) is the
local name of the very common sudamina that prevails during the hot
and humid flood season.

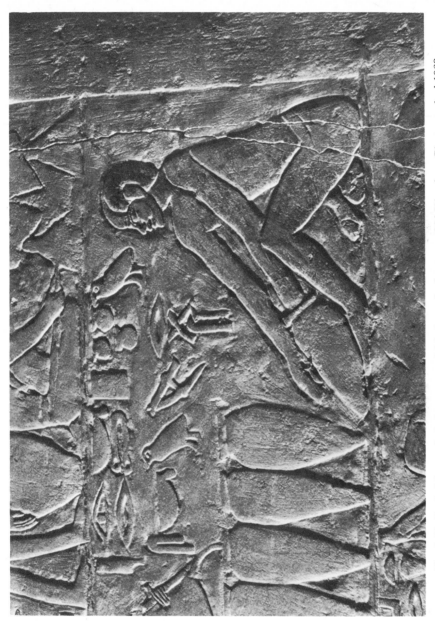

Fig. 2.11. Genital hyperplasia in a potter. Mehu's tomb. Saqqara. Old Kingdom. Photographed 1969.

The history of pellagra in Egypt has been discussed in detail by Patwardhan and Darby (1972). The first to describe it in that country was Pruner (1847a, b). His diagnosis was rejected by Hirsch (1885); but Pruner's previous familiarity with the disease in Italy, and the subsequent confirmation by Sandwith (1898, 1905) and others (Marie, 1910; White, 1910) strongly support Pruner's conclusions.

Today, pellagra is much commoner in Lower than in Upper Egypt (Patwardhan and Darby, 1972). This is presumably related to the greater reliance there on maize rather than on sorghum, and to the higher incidence of parasitism. The association with maize has been repeatedly stressed by various authors and this was early attributed to the absence of tryptophane from zein, the chief protein of this cereal (Sandwith, 1913). The discovery that tryptophane is converted into nicotinic acid in the body brought this theory in line with modern concepts.

Maize, however, was unknown in Ancient Egypt. The statement by Abdou (1965) that it was introduced only in 1840, would place it only seven years before Pruner's report, but this statement is surely erroneous. Patwardhan and Darby (1972) have argued that it must have been established much earlier, since in 1833 the production of that cereal was estimated to be 13,382 metric tons, occupying the fifth most important place as a good crop. The Täckholms (Vol. I, p. 546) quoted writers who mentioned it still earlier, Forskaal in 1761–1762 and Delile in 1798–1801, and they concluded that it must have been introduced in Egypt some time in the sixteenth century. This left ample time for the appearance of pellagra.

But there is also a sorghum pellagra (Patwardhan, 1961) and, even in the absence of maize, undernutrition and parasitism may certainly render its appearance possible.

Night-blindness

The available ancient medical texts do not specifically mention other nutritional deficiencies, but they describe some syndromes that are very suggestive of avitaminosis. To treat an eye disease called *shaw* (*Eb.*, LVII, 351) or *sharw* (*L.*, 35), local applications of pressed roasted beef liver, or of beef liver juice, were recommended. Ebbell noted that Dioscorides (II, 45) advised the same treatment for night-blindness and concluded that *shaw/sharw* was identical with it. Considering the richness of liver in vitamin A, this is a plausible suggestion.

Scurvy

Another disease, called *wnm-n-snf* (the blood-eater), was said to affect the limbs (*Eb.*, LXXXVII, 724, 725; *H.*, 129), the cardia (*Eb.*, XLIII, 211), the inside of the body (*Eb.*, LXXXVII, 722) and, in one case, the gums (*Eb.*, LXXXIX, 749). Ebbell (1937) interpreted it as scurvy. As a treatment, onions mashed in fat, or local applications were recommended.

Rickets

Rickets is not mentioned although it probably existed. Neither Ruffer (1921) nor Elliot Smith and Dawson (1924, p. 157) ever found rickety changes in the bones they examined; but Ruffer published pictures of deformed statues (Fig. 2.12) whose malformations he attributed to that disease (1921, pp. 43, 47, plate IX). In addition, one of the attendants on the alabaster barge of Tut-ankh-Amon's treasure may have suffered from rickets (Fig. 2.13).

Dental Caries

Insofar as dental caries is an index of the nutrient intake, or of the type and consistency of food, it is of paramount importance to the historian of nutrition, in view of the abundant evidence that correlates it with the carbohydrate content and physical character of food. Caries has an antique history. It has been found in the early hominids *Paranthropus crassidens* (Robinson, 1952), the Java *Pithecanthropus* (Brodrick, 1948), and Palestinian Neanderthal forms (Sognnaes, 1956). The most surprising specimen was a Rhodesian Neanderthaloid skull in which 15 cavities were found in 11 out of 13 teeth. Fermentation of food debris would seem to have been a cause since most of the caries did not form occlusively. Brothwell made the gratuitous suggestion that this individual, like the modern Bushman, was inordinately fond of honey (1958). He also concluded that caries really started to be common with the swing of a hunting–collecting economy to an agricultural one of high cereal consumption, and that the

"last straw was the introduction of sugar in the twelfth century [A.D.]."

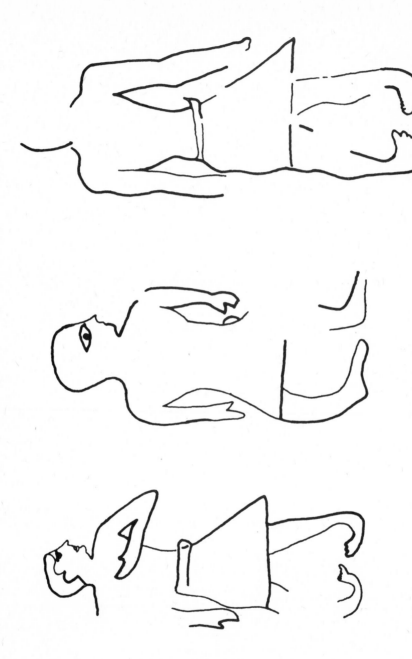

Fig. 2.12. Evidence of rickets. Redrawn from Ruffer (1921) plate IX, Figs 10 and 11.

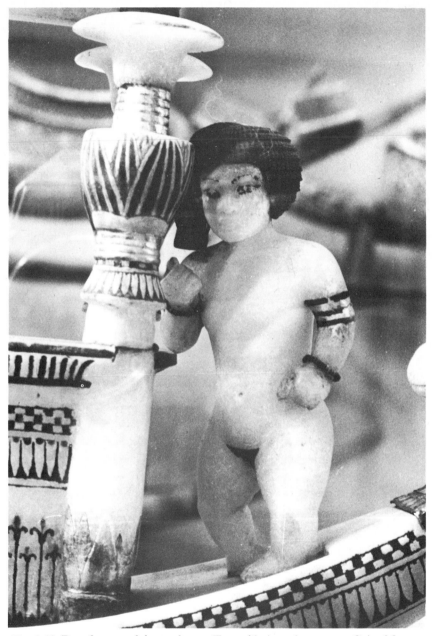

Fig. 2.13. Dwarf on an alabaster barge. Tut-ankh-Amon's treasure, Cairo Museum. Used with permission. Photographed 1969.

More historical documentation is required before accepting this broad generalization.

Current evidence of the infectious nature of dental caries, as reviewed by Russell (1974, p. 635), might make it more to the point to relate this rising incidence to the increased contact with Europeans affected with the condition that was occurring from approximately that period.

In Ancient Egyptian papyri, a prescription (*Eb.*, LXXXIX, 743) that recommends filling the teeth with a resinous composition suggests that caries was not unknown, but it is the general opinion of all those who investigated dental remains that, although pyorrhea, attrition, alveolar abscesses, and periodontitis were frequent and severe, caries were distinctly rare in the early periods (Ruffer, 1921, p. 315). Elliot Smith (1924, p. 158) who studied large numbers of teeth from different epochs, sites, and social classes, concluded that in the Pre-Dynastic and Proto-Dynastic periods the condition was quite rare among the poor, in whom it never became common until modern times, but, as soon as people learned to live in luxury, it became as common among the well-to-do as in Europe in his time. He found in 500 skeletons of the Pyramid age, unearthed at Giza and, at every subsequent period, that the disease was widely prevalent among the wealthy, while the poorer, who lived mainly on a coarse, uncooked vegetable diet were relatively free of the defect. One asks whether this reflected an increased contact of the wealthy with other peoples—encounters that permitted them the introduction and spread of cariogenic organisms.

By Christian times, Ruffer (1921, p. 144) found that caries had spread in severe fashion to all classes. Early comments on possible etiological factors were limited to the extreme roughness of the food, as confirmed by examination of the intestinal contents. The higher incidence in the wealthy and in later epochs was referred, therefore, to retention and fermentation, rather than to any nutritional deficiency. The relative roles of gradual changes in oral microflora and of the food cannot yet be deciphered.

Iodine Deficiency

Iodine deficiency is now widespread throughout many regions of Africa, and goitre is common throughout the Lebanon, Syria, Iraq and the Sudan. In fact, goitre is found in this region wherever it is looked for. In Egypt, its incidence was reviewed by Ghalioungui (1964b) and

Pathwardhan and Darby (1972). It increases the farther one goes inland. There is no evidence of its existence in Ancient Egypt but this does not exclude its existence. It is even doubtful whether the thyroid had a name in Egyptian (Lefebvre, 1952). But the carving in the round that was fashionable with Ptolemaic artists gave most of their productions swollen necks, a fact that accounts for the error of calling Cleopatra goitrous (Iason, 1946). The first reference to goitre in Egypt was actually made by Dolbey and Omar (1924), and to its endemicity, by Ali Ibrahim (1932). It was not mentioned by the medical members of the French Expedition under Bonaparte or by any ancient traveller. The only indication of thyroid disease at that period is the exophthalmos of a few Old Kingdom statuettes discovered at Giza (Ghalioungui, 1964a).

The reader may wonder at our apparent inconsistency in describing the Ancient Egyptian's diet as adequate, and yet presenting evidence of malnutrition, but, especially in the last two centuries, considerable changes have modified the peasant's diet. The introduction of maize; the intensive cultivation of cash crops, like cotton and sugar cane, that has deprived the small farmer from the products of his small plot of land; the extensive draining of lakes that yielded abundant fish; the inundation of fertile land by the successive elevations of the Aswan dam, have made the peasant rely on purchased food (Vilter *et al.*, 1954), of which maize flour is the cheapest, until resettlement policies of the government fully bear their fruits.

Conclusions

In conclusion, and prejudging in part the content of subsequent chapters, one may state the following points.

1. The available evidence indicates that the poorest could obtain, either by barter, or as governmental rations, or by fishing, fowling hunting, or gathering, adequate if not abundant nourishment.

2. Taboos were restricted to a few foods: some species of fish, pork, beans, onions. They were observed by a limited section of the population belonging to the clergy and nobility. These varied in different areas. Generally, commoners did not abide by them.

3. Among the rich, obesity and certain metabolic disorders that

may be related to excessive food intake, especially arteriosclerosis, gall-stones, and, possibly, gout and diabetes, were not unknown.

4. Evidence is available of alcoholic excess, although this was regarded as reprehensible.

5. Worm infestation was common, and must have exacted a toll from the nutriture. When nutritional intake was barely adequate, malnutrition must have resulted.

6. References to specific nutritional deficiencies in Ancient Egyptian general literature are limited to accounts of famine due to vagaries of the Nile flood.

7. There is in the medical papyri evidence consistent with a few other deficiency diseases: iron deficiency anaemia probably conditioned by parasitism, and possibly scurvy, avitaminosis A, but the evidence is thin. Rickets is suggested by a few artifacts.

8. An obscure syndrome, called *áaâ* was probably a combination of undernourishment and polyparasitism, and similar to chlorosis of the European and American physicians of the last century.

9. Hepatic cirrhosis was probably existent, but it is not possible currently to establish its etiology.

10. There is no evidence of goitre or pellagra, which seem to be diseases of more recent eras.

11. Dental caries existed early but increased in extent and frequency first among the well-to-do, then spread throughout the population.

All of this, despite a wide variety of foods! Hence, problems of distribution of foods must have plagued that civilization, as they do ours. The interpretation of disease characteristics and changes throughout long periods of history must recognize the complex, often subtle, socio-economic and environmental alterations and must not be made in an over-simplistic expectation of direct, obvious relationships.

Notes: Chapter 2

1. See Ghalioungui and Dawakhly (1965), Fig. 29.
2. See Ghalioungui and Dawakhly (1965), Fig. 28.

Chapter 3   Meat: Beef

If you miss the meat, get the broth
(Egyptian proverb)

Introduction

One of the most significant of man's achievements has undoubtedly
been the domestication of several varieties of cattle, and their utilization
as draught, meat and dairy animals. Our knowledge of the domestic
species of Egypt indicates familiarity with antelopes, gazelle, sheep,
goats and ibex; but, as in many agricultural societies, preference was
given to bovines. It seems, however, that man succeeded with domestication only after trial and failure with many kinds and species, and it
speaks both for his industry and for the adaptability of the animals
with which he worked that he could develop peaceful varieties from
their fierce ancestors.

Although it is difficult to judge the correctness of the opinion that the
art of domestication sprang from the similarity of its methods to those
used in keeping cult or totem animals in temples or sacred precincts and
that, therefore, domestic animals were originally cult animals (Kees,
1956), there are certain indications that slaughter and eating had
peculiar meanings in primitive man's thought.

The Meaning of Eating

From what we know of very early man, his mind was already harbouring the germs of notions that later developed into the abstruse concepts
of microcosm–macrocosm affinities, and of the possibility of resolving
the Universe into a few elements, forces, or qualities. In that respect,
both the humoral theory and its rival, iatrochemistry, and cure by both
"contrary" and "like" substances, in spite of their opposition were
constructed on similar conceptual bases.

Until the eighteenth century, physicians prescribed drugs, not on account of their pharmaco-dynamic properties, but because of the elements (sulphur, mercury and salt, according to the iatrochemists; water, earth, fire and air, according to the humoralists) which supposedly entered into their composition, and which, added to those in the body, corrected its composition.

According to this mode of thinking, eating was not the mere taking in of a nutrient. It was the means of replenishing the body with the forces or essences of which it had run out.

Cannibalism

Similarly, the underlying motive of cannibalism, excluding conditions of extreme necessity, as in the 1972 Andes air crash (*St Louis Globe*, December 28, 1972), was and still is the acquisition of the forces and essence of the eaten individual with its results: identification, especially if this was a god, and the continuation of the dead person's life in the eater. An early example of both these incentives is that of the Massagetes who, according to Herodotus (I, 216) sacrificed their kinfolk when they grew very old, and feasted upon them. The latter, they reckoned, were the happiest of people, and they wailed over the fate of those who had not had that dubious privilege.

At the antipodes of the Massagetes' country, in Pre-Columbian Mexico, cannibalism was a religious ritual. It still is so in portions of central Africa, where members of secret cannibal sects, after partaking of human flesh, have to undergo ritual purification before returning to society.

The so-called "Cannibal Hymn" of *The Pyramid Texts*, that dates to the sixth dynasty, but is a relic of extremely older customs and concepts, explains the development of the thought process involved. The theme is the arrival of Pharaoh Wenis (Unas) in the other world as a conqueror, and his subsequent deification

397a :   Wenis is the bull of the sky . . . who lives on the being of every god
397b :   Who eats their entrails (?) who comes when their belly is filled with magic
397c :   From the Island of Fire
400a :   It is Wenis who eats men and lives on gods
403c :   It is Wenis who eats their magic and swallows their spirits

Having eaten the gods, absorbed their magic and spirits, Unas now becomes their master. He commands, and is served

405a: It is the great ones who are in the North of the sky who place for him the fire

405b: To the kettles containing them with the thighs of their eldest ones

406a: Those who are in the sky serve Wenis

406b: The cooking pots are wiped out for him with the legs of their women

407a: Wenis is the Great Mighty One who has power over the Mighty Ones.

He is even in the position to create gods

407b: Wenis is the figure of a god who endows with divinity (?) the great figures of the gods

And the hymn ends by rehearsing the whole process of assimilation

411b: Wenis flourishes, their magic is in his belly

411d: He has swallowed the intelligence of every god

412a: The lifetime of Wenis is eternity, his limit is everlastingness

It is curious that Biblical literature should offer a parallel in Ezekiel (39, 18)

"Ye shall eat the flesh of the mighty and drink the blood of the Princes of the Earth."

Though these utterings had become mere metaphors, it is nevertheless to such vestigeal beliefs that we owe organotherapy, the precursor of endocrinology.

Apart from these relics of a common past, anthropophagy does not appear to have flourished in Egypt, at least in historic times. The subject has been discussed by many authors who often failed, however, to distinguish between cannibalism, ritual sacrifices and the slaughter of prisoners of war.

A frequently quoted story is that of King Busiris who complied to the revelation of a seer from Cyprus that the famine which had ravaged Egypt for nine years would cease if every year a stranger were slaughtered (Apollodorus, *The Library*, 2, 5, 11). However, this tale, which actually places human sacrifices in the class of agricultural rites has been doubted even by the Greeks, because the names of all the characters it mentions are Greek, except Busiris which is the name of a town, not of a king.

Griffiths (1948), on the basis of the above story of questionable historicity, and on the alleged sacrifice of "Typhonian" men, wrote, however

"The evidence suggests that human sacrifices were not frequent in Egypt in the period of the Egyptian dynasties, but that in a later era, they became common in certain areas and cults."

After discussing whether the increase was the result of Hyksos, Greek or Persian influences, he concluded

"The reasons for their increasing prevalence in later times are at present unknown, and will probably remain so; for to approach them requires much more detailed knowledge of the mental and spiritual processes of the Egyptians than is available through their literature and monuments."

Most references to cannibalism among Egyptians are tragic descriptions of famine, when all laws break down, as was fully discussed in the section on "Famine" in Chapter 2. Diodorus, who cited such an example, expressed his astonishment that under these circumstances

". . . not a single man was even accused of having partaken of the sacred animals . . ." (1, 83, 8–9)

Herodotus mentioned only two examples of cannibalism. One is his account of how the Greek and Carian mercenaries of Egypt punished a Carian deserter who had helped the enemy, by cutting his sons' throats and drinking their blood before the battle (III, 11). The second is his description of the Ethiopian ordeal suffered by the Persian troops (III, 25). In neither were Egyptians involved.

The few examples of cannibalism we know were initiated by mob hatred rather than by need. Juvenal, exiled in Egypt, and probably ill-disposed towards the inhabitants of his exilic prison, related

". . . near Tentyra, they [the enemies] retreat in panic confusion. One of them goes too fast, goes down in his terror, is captured, cut into bits . . . a banquet eaten up, bones and all, by the victorious rabble . . . (Satire, 15)

One cannot refrain from relating here, the melodramatic, but delightful, adventure of Leucippe, kidnapped in the marshes south of Alexandria by brigands who ripped her abdomen, roasted her bowels and ate them up. In fact, she had been saved by one of the officiating priests, a friend in disguise, who had filled a sheep skin with its entrails and fitted her with it. Then, using a sham dagger with a blade retracting into the handle, he had slit the sheep skin. The tale ended happily with the beautiful Leucippe falling into the arms of her lover, Clitophon (Achilles Tatius, 3, 15–22).

Suetonus told another tale, that was adduced as evidence of cannibalism (*De vitae Caesarum*, VI, 37). He said fo Nero that he wished

> ". . . to make an Egyptian who was accustomed to eat raw flesh . . . have living men thrown to him . . ."

But there is nothing in that wish of Nero to suggest cannibalism.

The situation is only partly different with regard to eating vegetable matter. Because plants do not readily appear endowed with life, man did not generally concede them any religious status, but when he learned to cultivate a few staple crops and to rely on regular harvests he translated the successive cycles of sowing, growing and harvesting, into divine myths. Thus it came about that maize was a god in Central America (Netzahualpili) as was wheat in Greece and the Near East.

On the other hand, some vegetables were credited with occult associations, either because they possessed hallucinogenic properties, or for some other reason, such as the alleged resemblance of the mandrake to the human body.

Among edible plants, beans were said by Herodotus (II, 37) and other Greeks to be avoided by Egyptian priests. It has been suggested that the reason was the impurity of their emanations. This may be no joke, however, as it was recorded that Pythagoras forbade them to his disciples because they were generated by the same putrefactive material that generates human beings, or because he thought that the souls of the dead dwell in them (Pliny, *H.N.*, XVIII, XXX, 18).

By a remarkable coincidence, the Egyptian word for beans *iwryt*, is so close to *iwr*, to conceive, or to generate, as to suggest a similar association; and it has been stated that Orphics and Pythagoreans, whose master Pythagoras studied in Egypt, called eggs "beans" (*kuamoi*), by a pun on the word (*kuesis*), conception (Plutarch, *Table Talk*, II, 3, 365).

It seems of course, unthinkable that the first hominids could have elaborated such concepts, but one thinks of the cave men who thought that they could ensure rich hunts by drawing their quarries on the walls of their caves. In their ignorance of the details of digestion and assimilation, they quite naturally believed that the flesh they ate was incorporated as such in their bodies, with all the qualities of its previous owner. This is why, according to Apollodorus (*The Library*, 3, 13, 6), the centaur Chiron raised the infant Achilles on the intestines of lions and the marrows of bears.

The Significance of Slaughter

Furthermore, from the attribution of higher meanings to animals, there arose the notion that taking life was as sacred as giving it. Killing was a divine privilege of the gods or of their incarnation, the kings or priests, and it had to be performed according to a proper ritual, usually stated to have been revealed. Any other way of obtaining flesh was sinful. And it also followed that permitting an animal's flesh or forbidding it, depended on the significance attached to it.

This helps to understand why every civilization imposed some food restriction, applying to the whole animal or only parts of it, usually directed at the totemic animal of the tribe or of its rival. (See Chapter 1.)

Distribution of Bovines During the Pre-Dynastic Period

That bovines ranged in Egypt during the Pleistocene, long before man appeared in the Nile Valley, is indicated by fossil evidence. Bones of *Bos primigenius* have been found in sequences of that period in the Fayoum (Benedite, 1918, p. 8). By the Late Palaeolithic Sebilian in Upper Egypt, two new forms of early bovines had appeared: *Bos africanus* (Sandford, 1934, p. 86; *MAE*, 1964, pp. 67–68), and *Bos brachyceros*, in addition to the ancestral *Bos primigenius* (Gaillard, 1934, p. 29).

Bovines were certainly hunted by the early settlers living in the Fayoum (Caton-Thompson and Gardiner, 1934, p. 34), at Merimda Beni Salama (Junker, 1929, p. 219), and at El Omari (Debono, 1948, p. 568). It has not been determined, however, whether the bones excavated from these major three northern sites were from domesticated or wild herds. Nor can the clay models of cattle found at several Pre-Dynastic sites in lower Egypt (Fig. 3.1) be taken as evidence of domestication, although they show familiarity with cattle. Even at Maadi, a site occupied by settlers who bridged the Pre-Dynastic and Dynastic Periods in the north, the evidence is unclear.

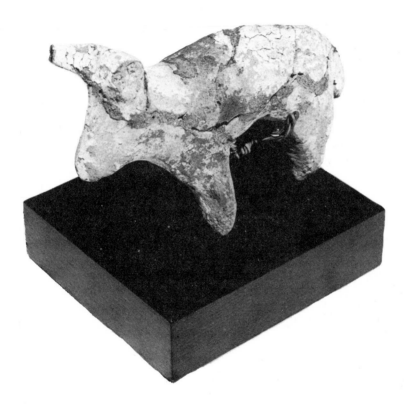

Fig. 3.1. Clay model of a bull; Pre-Dynastic Period, date uncertain. Photographed with permission of the Ministry of Agriculture and the officials of the Agricultural Museum, Dokki, ARE (1969).

Menghin and Amer (1932, p. 52) stated their belief that domesticated cattle were present at Maadi, and they listed the bones of an "ox" among the animal remains. Support for domestication rests more on the connotation of the English word "ox". Although this word may be used to designate any male bovine and, generally, the domestic *Bos taurus*, it is usually applied to castrated bulls, a qualification that may not be warranted by the examination of unearthed bones, but that is well documented in Ancient Egyptian texts.[1]

Similarly, it may be stated that bovines were hunted by early settlers in Upper Egypt. Although scarcer than in the north, bovine bones have been excavated at El-Badari from Early Pre-Dynastic levels throughout Dynastic sequences (Brunton and Caton-Thompson, 1928, pp. 38 and 41), at Abydos (Peet, 1914, p. 6), Armant (Mond *et al.*, 1937, pp. 254–258), and elsewhere. At the Pre-Dynastic cemetery of Gerza, human burials were accompanied by offerings of ribs of meat and shoulder blades of a bovine temporarily identified as an "ox", and by pottery vessels filled with "meat" (Petrie *et al.*, 1912, p. 7). Ivory carvings of cows found in Mahasna cemetery (Pre-Dynastic) offer additional evidence from central Egypt (Ayrton and Loat, 1908, plate. 19, Fig. 2).

Domesticated cattle probably first appeared in the north. The evidence rests, not on excavated material, but on religious and ecological considerations. At an unknown period prior to unification, the dominant role of bovines in the secular religious life of the north is manifest in the emblems of the nomes[2] that composed it; bulls, cows or calves appear in four of these (Table 1), but in none of the southern ones. Even at Dendera, capital of the sixth nome of Upper Egypt and a major centre of cow worship during the Dynastic Period, the emblem was a crocodile, not a cow. On the other hand, Kees (1961, pp. 29–30) attributes the difference in distribution to ecologic factors, rather than to competition between two rival societies, one of which herded cattle, the other not. As long as the two halves of the land were separate,

Table 1

*Emblems of the sixth, tenth, eleventh and twelfth nomes of
Lower Egypt. Redrawn from Engelbach (1961, pp. 75–78)*

Nome	6		Xois
Nome	10		Athribis
Nome	11		Cabasa
Nome	12		Sebennytos

possibly inimical, the wide green expanse of the Delta favoured the development of a cattle industry, whereas the narrowly restricted arable land, bounded by desert and arid cliffs in Upper Egypt, was more adapted to the raising of goats and sheep.

It was only after the unification of Egypt, *c.* 3200 B.C., that cow and bull worship spread throughout the Nile Valley, and that a cattle industry developed in central and southern Egypt.

Egyptian Cattle Industry

mnmnt (a)

Egyptian Vocabulary[3] Relating to Cattle

ꜥwt (b)

The Ancient Egyptians divided herds of domesticated (and wild) animals into two major categories. The term depicted by (a) translated as "large cattle", implied herds of bulls and cows, whereas the term depicted by (b) "small cattle", implied such animals as goats, sheep, and pigs.

Specific words, designating well-defined types of cattle appear in Table 2 with the hieroglyphic names, but it must be noted that the identification of early species of cattle is difficult. Mond and his co-authors (1937, p. 256) illustrate this difficulty in a discussion of a Pre-Dynastic palette from Abydos, which shows a "bovine" attacking a man; this has variously been identified as *Bos primigenius*, "wild ox", Cape buffalo, *Bos indicus*, and "zebu".

On iconographic evidence, the bovines of Ancient Egypt may be classified thus (see Montet, 1910; Andersson, 1912; Ruffer, 1919; Smith, 1969):

1. A long-horned variety called *ngꜣw*, shown as being tall, lean, standing high on muscular haunches, with wide everted horns (Fig. 3.2). This was probably the native wild bull of the Delta marshes. This is supported by the facts that Hathor (Fig. 3.3) and Apis were both such animals, and that only specimens of this variety were mummified, indicating their sacred character. These bulls were not easily tamed. They were captured, controlled, or led, only by lassoeing or under restraint; they are frequently shown cavorting, or jumping with raised tails; never in stalls. Their horns were mutilated or artificially deformed. They were mainly draught animals, only occasionally

Table 2

Additional vocabulary relative to cattle (after Faulkner, 1962)

Cattle:	mnmnt	F.,109	Ox:	tpiw (?)	F.,298
	nfrt	F.,132		iwꜣ	F., 12
	ḫtmw(?)	F.,199	Small cattle:	ꜥwt	F., 39
Cow:	iḫt	F., 28	Short-horn cattle:	wnḏw	F., 63
	idt	F., 35	Sacred cattle:	tntt	F.,306
	ḥmt	F.,191	Milch cow:	iryt	F., 28
Calf:	bḥz	F., 84		mḥit	F.,113
				mnꜥt	F.,108

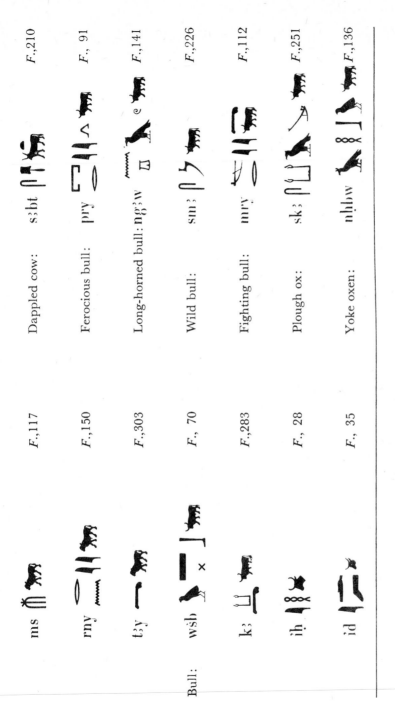

Bull:

ms		*F.*,117
rny		*F.*,150
t3y		*F.*,303
wšb		*F.*, 70
k3		*F.*,283
iḥ		*F.*, 28
id		*F.*, 35

Dappled cow:	s3bt	*F.*,210
Ferocious bull:	ppy	*F.*, 91
Long-horned bull:	ng3w	*F.*,141
Wild bull:	sm3	*F.*,226
Fighting bull:	mry	*F.*,112
Plough ox:	sk3	*F.*,251
Yoke oxen:	nḥbw	*F.*,136

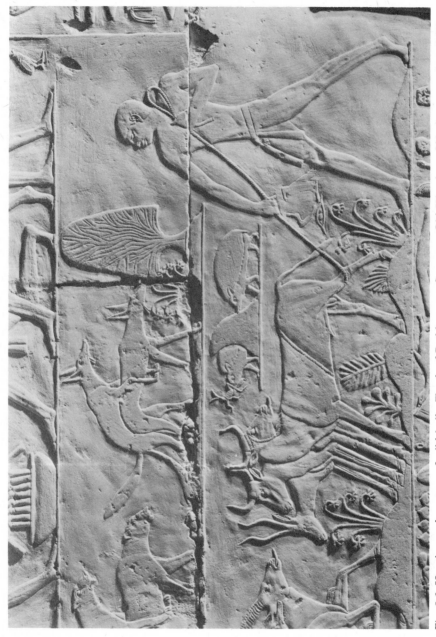

Fig. 3.2. Hunting and capture of wild bulls. Tomb of Ptahhetep at Saqqara; Old Kingdom, fifth dynasty, reign of King Djed-ka-Re, *c.* 2450 B.C. Photograph used with permission of the Ministry of Culture and the officials of the Centre of Documentation, Cairo, ARE (1969).

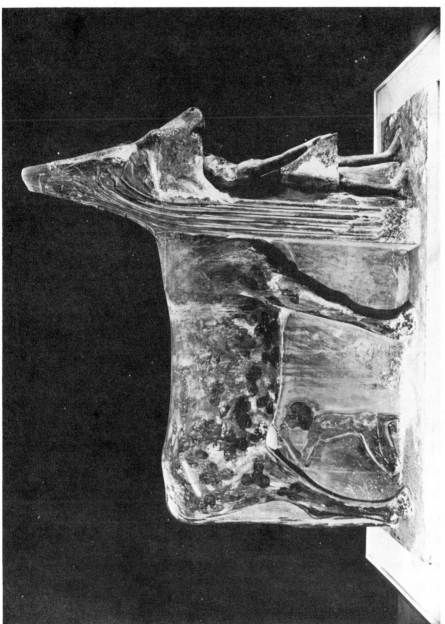

Fig. 3.3. King Amenhotep II drinking from the udder of the goddess Hathor; New Kingdom, eighteenth dynasty, *c.* 1440 B.C. In that kind of statue of which there are other examples, the dead Pharaoh under Hathor's neck is painted black, the colour of death. According to *The Pyramid Texts*, he meets the goddess on his way west to the nether world. The goddess offers him her milk, which is accepted. Now, living again after having drunk of the divine beverage, he is painted at the udder, red, the colour of life. Photograph used with permission of the Ministry of Culture and the officials of the Egyptian Museum, Cairo, ARE (1969).

sacrificed. They were bred in Egypt, and are often shown mating; the cows calving, or being milked. Bones unearthed so far belong to this variety.

2. By way of contrast, $iw\beta$ bulls were butchery animals, exceedingly fat, low on their haunches, with pendulous bellies and wide everted horns that were often artificially twisted asymmetrically or removed during their youth. They are usually depicted standing quietly in their stalls, being fed, fattened, and taken good care of, or quietly following the lead (Fig. 3.4). Cf. the "sleek kine of shambling gait" (*The Odyssey*, Vol. IV, p. 320). Their cows, in contrast to $ng\beta w$ cows, are but rarely represented; and breeding of these animals, which were probably imported from the south, seems to have been uncommon.

3. After the Middle Kingdom, long-horned cattle disappeared and gave way to a short-horned race under the New Kingdom. Literary evidence proves that Syrian short-horned cattle were imported early in Egypt, but the theory that they were introduced after an epidemic had destroyed the long-horned race lacks support.

4. In addition, a hornless race seems to have been abundant under the Old Kingdom (Fig. 3.5). One domain alone is said to have contained 35 long-horned and 220 hornless cattle, but Ruffer (1919) was of the opinion that, until anatomical proof is forthcoming, the existence in Egypt of a race comparable to the modern hornless species remains unproven, as the animals represented as being hornless may simply have been mutilated.

These oxen and cows were of different colours. Kings and queens are often seen, as in Deir el-Bahari, offering four bulls to the god, one red, one white, one black and one spotted (Naville, 1906, Vol. V, p. 7, plate CXXXIV).

The Hunt

Before the development of domestication, hunts were not merely sporting feats but means of obtaining food. It is only later, during the Dynastic Period, that man pitted himself against a bull primarily as a feat of valour and strength, and as a means of rising in status. There was additionally a distinctly religious overtone to these sporting events. The Egyptians, to explain the order that pervades the Universe, imagined it to be continuously imposed by a superior will. According to a

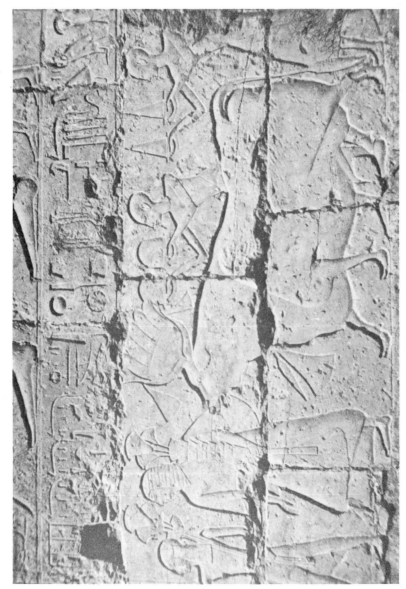

Fig. 3.4. Religious procession. Temple of Luxor; forecourt of King Rameses II, southwest inner wall. New Kingdom, nineteenth dynasty, *c.* 1250 B.C. Photographed 1969.

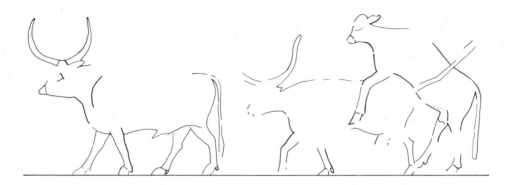

Fig. 3.5. Horned cow serviced by a hornless bull. Tomb of Aba at Deir El Gebrawi; Old Kingdom, sixth dynasty, date uncertain. Redrawn from Davies (1902, plate 7).

further belief, that whatever man did in the visible world or microcosm had an echo in the invisible macrocosm, the king, who was the god's representative on earth, or his nobles, could re-enact the primaeval taming of wildlife in their sporting pursuits, and thus keep the civilized world from falling back into chaos. Similarly, the hunter who killed wild birds was at the same time destroying the evil spirits that hovered around him. Yet, even after the development of agriculture in Egypt (*c.* 5000 B.C.) and the availability of domesticated animals, the challenge remained, and the qualities of strength, virility and fierce aggressiveness attached to the wild bull[4] were often described as attributes of the Egyptian kings

> "I cause them [the enemy] to see thy majesty as a young bull, firm of heart, ready-horned, irresistible" . . .[5] (*A.R.*, II, 659)

Indeed, one of the official titles of the king (*ka-nakht*) meant the "powerful bull",[6] and kings were fond of exhibiting their strength and aggressiveness by participating in bull hunts, or by describing their prowess, for example

> ". . . year two under the majesty of King Amenhotep III given life . . . one came to his majesty [and said] 'there are wild cattle upon the highlands' . . . his majesty appeared upon a horse, his whole army being behind him . . . behold, his majesty commanded to cause that these wild cattle be

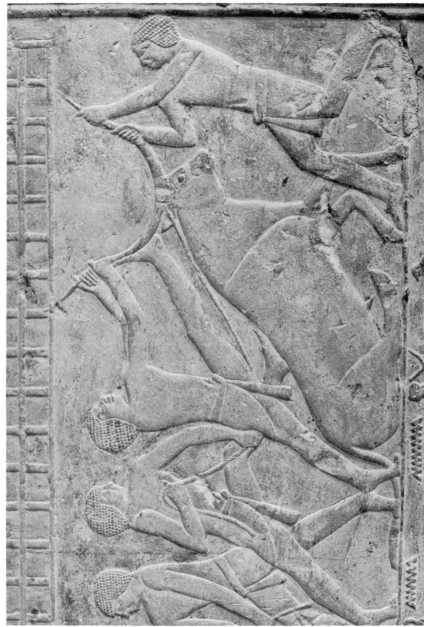

Fig. 3.6. Hunting and capture of wild bulls. Tomb of Mereruka at Saqqara; Old Kingdom, sixth dynasty, reign of King Teti, *c.* 2390 B.C. Photographed 1969.

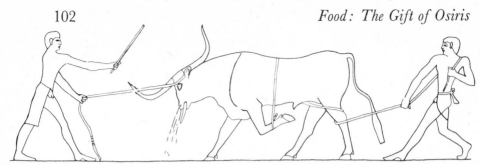

Fig. 3.7. Use of the lasso. Tomb of Senbi at Meir; Middle Kingdom, twelfth dynasty, date uncertain. Redrawn from Blackman (1914, plate 11).

surrounded by a wall with an enclosure . . . his majesty commanded to count all these wild cattle; statement thereof 170 wild cattle . . ." (*A.R.,* II, 864)

Tomb art from the Old, Middle and New Kingdoms from sites scattered throughout Egypt, illustrates a wide variety of techniques used to subdue wild cattle. The tomb of Mereruka, at Saqqara, dated to the sixth dynasty (reign of King Teti, *c.* 2423 B.C.), shows the resisting beasts being overcome with ropes entangling their backs, legs, and horns (Fig. 3.6).

At the Middle Kingdom sites of Meir and Beni Hassan, the lasso (Fig. 3.7) and the bolo[7] (Fig. 3.8) are also depicted.

Of these, the lasso struck very sensitive strings in Egyptian minds and hearts. In the Osireion, an illustration of Pharaoh, where the wild bull symbolize chaos or rebellion, labelled "Taking the wild southern bull with the lasso" resonated with cosmic and political overtones. In a wiser tone, the lasso was an enticing snare to avoid

"Do not fraternize with the passionate man
 Nor go too near him for conversation
 Do not make him cast his speech to lasso you
 Nor be too free with your answer." (Amenemope, 11/13 f., 17f)

An amorous poem compared the ties of love to its noose

"The beloved is expert in the lasso
 She enchains me with her eyes
 She throws it at me with her hair
 She tames me with her attire
 Her red hot seal brands me."

The tomb of Ptahhetep at Saqqara (fifth dynasty), illustrates the use of the lasso also in the northern provinces (Fig. 3.2), but it contains

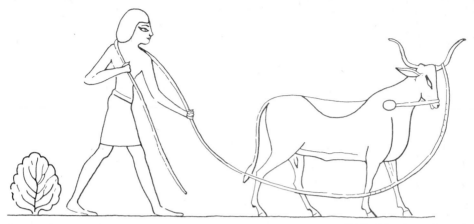

Fig. 3.8. The bolo. Tomb of Baqt III (number 15) at Beni Hassan; Middle Kingdom, eleventh dynasty, date uncertain. Redrawn from Wilkinson (1878, Vol. 2, p. 87, Fig. 353).

a scene that may indicate the utilization of a species of large cat as an aid (Fig. 3.9); unless the hunter had happened by chance on a feline attacking its prey.[8] Saluki dogs are, however, frequently companions to the hunter, either shown by his side, or "worrying", attacking and bringing down desert game, addax, gazelle, hartebeest or oryx. In other tombs, hunters utilize both restraining ropes and arrows. Hunting a wide variety of desert game with bows and arrows is also a common illustration in Middle and New Kingdom tombs.

The dangers of such hunts are aptly registered in Baqt's tomb (Beni Hassan, eleventh dynasty), where a bull gores and tosses over one of the hunters (Fig. 3.10).

Cattle Husbandry

ỉmy-r mnmnt (c)

The bovine life cycle, from mating to birth, is displayed in tomb art from all periods and provinces. Reliefs and paintings from Saqqara, Beni Hassan and elsewhere, show bulls servicing cows. In Aba's tomb at Deir el-Gabrawi (fifth or sixth dynasty) a hornless bull is mating with a lyre-horned cow (Fig. 3.5).[9] According to Herre (1969), crossing as a method of breeding was not practiced before modern times. Were the Ancient Egyptians the remote ancestors of modern cross-breeders, or was this a casual representation of random mating?

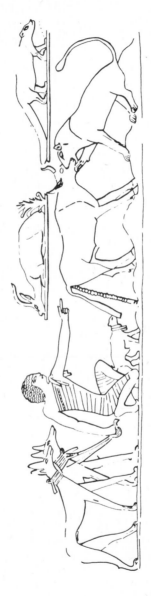

Fig. 3.9. Hunting and capture of wild bulls. Note the loosening of the bull's bowels. Tomb of Ptahhetep at Saqqara; Old Kingdom, fifth dynasty, reign of King Djed-Ka-Re, *c.* 2450 B.C. Redrawn from Davies (1900, plate 22).

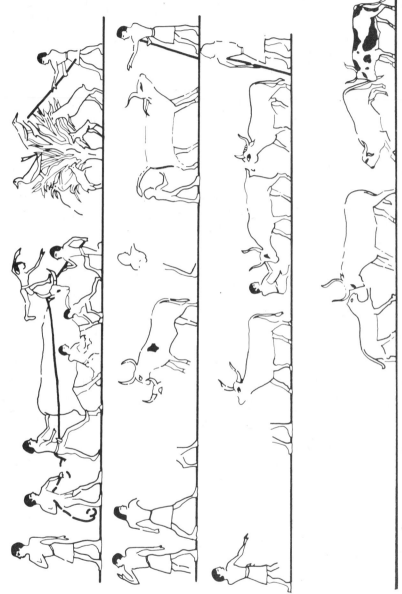

Fig. 3.10. A bull tossing up a herdsman. Tomb of Baqt I (number 29) at Beni Hassan; Middle Kingdom, eleventh dynasty, date uncertain. Redrawn from Newberry and Fraser (1893a, Vol. 1, plate 31).

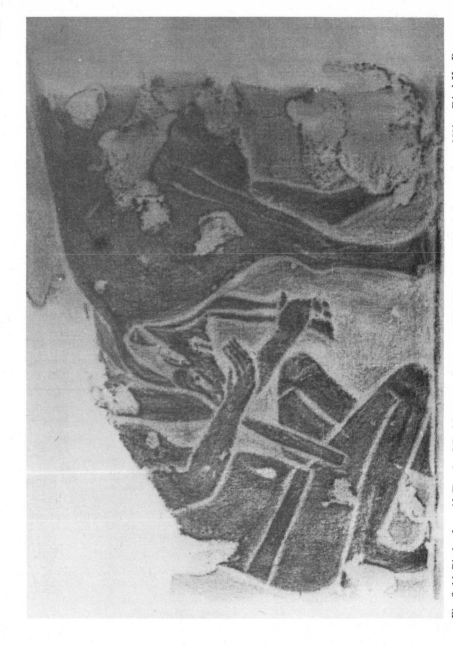

Fig. 3.11. Birth of a calf. Tomb of Ptahhetep at Saqqara; Old Kingdom, fifth dynasty, reign of King Djed-Ka-Re, *c.* 2450 B.C. Rubbing by Ward Patterson, used with permission (1969).

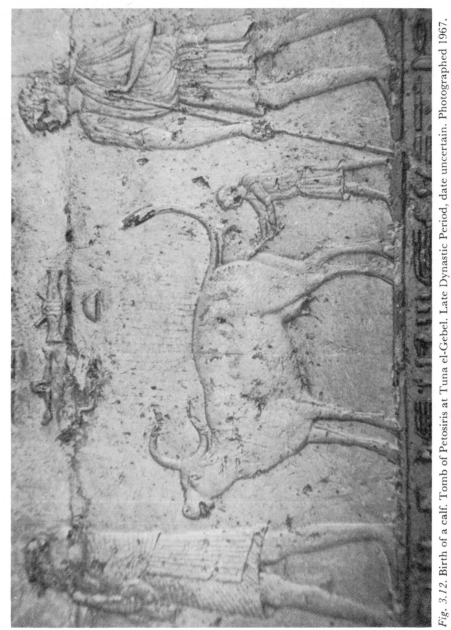

Fig. 3.12. Birth of a calf. Tomb of Petosiris at Tuna el-Gebel. Late Dynastic Period, date uncertain. Photographed 1967.

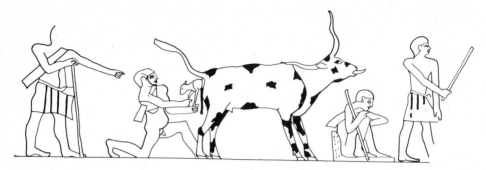

Fig. 3.13. Birth of a calf. Tomb of Senbi at Meir; Middle Kingdom, twelfth dynasty, date uncertain, Redrawn from Blackman (1914, plate 10).

Calving is also portrayed in scattered periods and sites, often with a striking rendition of the physical stress of labour, depicting the wide eyes and out-stretched tongue of the bellowing cow (Figs 3.11 3.12, 3.13). Only an ordinary farmer attended to it, never a medical practitioner (*swnw*). The care, feeding, milking and transport of cattle, though not of majestic importance, figure also among the commonest scenes in Egyptian tombs. Herds were probably controlled by the government and parceled to individual landholders who assumed responsibility for their protection and maintenance. One governmental office, "Overseer of Cattle" (c) (p. 103) was amongst the coveted and influential, for its holder was in a position to levy taxes on the herds (Kees, 1961, p. 89). Such taxes were attached to both living cattle and hides, and periodic "cattle counts" (Fig. 3.14) possibly served to verify the growth (or decrease) of wealth (Winlock, 1955).[10]

In contrast to swineherds (Chapter 4, p. 176), it does not appear that cowherds belonged to a special social class or ethnic group. In most illustrations, they are indistinguishable from other peasants (Fig. 3.15). So-called "Beja" cowherds illustrated at Meir with their gaunt, emaciated forms (Fig. 3.16), and the dwarfs at Giza (Fig. 3.17) do not belong to any set type in the profession.

Cattle in the north, especially the $ng\exists w$ cattle, were undoubtedly allowed to graze in the fields; yet we know of no indisputable illustration of this. Instead, there is substantial evidence from all periods that some cattle, probably the non-working varieties raised for food or sacrifice, were hand fed (Fig. 3.18*a,b*). At Tell el-Amarna (eighteenth dynasty) they are shown raised in stalls (Fig. 3.18*c*).[11] It is not clear whether these were sick or preferentially treated animals. To state that cattle were primarily hand fed is probably an unwarranted generalization.

Herds were identified by some sort of marking. Leclant (1956) cites many examples of "marked" cattle, in some cases with the name of the owner, institution, and a number. He quotes a statement by Kees (1956, p. 485) that an inscription in the tomb of Petosiris entrusts the "priest of Sekhmet" with stamping (*ḥtm*) the animals, and a caption in the famine stele that the beasts "marked with the seal" must be offered to the god Khnum.

Marking by branding is suggested in a painting from the tomb of Nebamun (number 90) at Thebes, dated to the reign of King Thutmose IV, that shows the heating of what appears to be a cattle brand, and its application to the upper right shoulder of two separate bulls (Figs 3.19 and 3.20).[12] This painting is unique in subject matter and, as branding by fire has not to our knowledge been specifically mentioned in texts from the Dynastic Period, one must reserve judgment on the meaning of this scene.

On the other hand, Moustafa (1964) found, buried with the animal bones in an animal cemetery dated 655–630 B.C. (twenty-sixth dynasty), a remarkably large number of horns of all sizes, of which quite a few had markings and etchings on their sides. He made the interesting suggestion that these may have served as marks to distinguish the individuals or the herds, although he could not exclude the possibility that they were associated with magic.

Cows being milked and nursing calves are frequently depicted throughout the Dynastic Period. Milking was not carried out from behind the hind legs as it was in antique Sumer (Tannahill, 1973, p. 41), and artists showed special regard to the cows' feelings. The milch cows at Saqqara and elsewhere were not always docile. They sometimes had to be secured with ropes during the milking (Fig. 3.21) and, once subdued, they are at times seen looking back (Fig. 3.22) or shedding tears (Fig. 3.23) at the removal of their milk, while their thirsty calf is being firmly held.

Moving herds across canals called for tricks. Capitalizing on maternal love, the herdsman would precede the cow with the nursing calf,[13] well knowing that the cow would follow and, in turn, be followed by the remainder of the herd (Figs 3.24 and 3.25), unheeding the ever present threat of crocodiles lurking beneath the murky surface.

As usual, bulls would fight each other; separating them was another routine chore. Wilkinson (1878, Vol. 2, pp. 75–76) published two

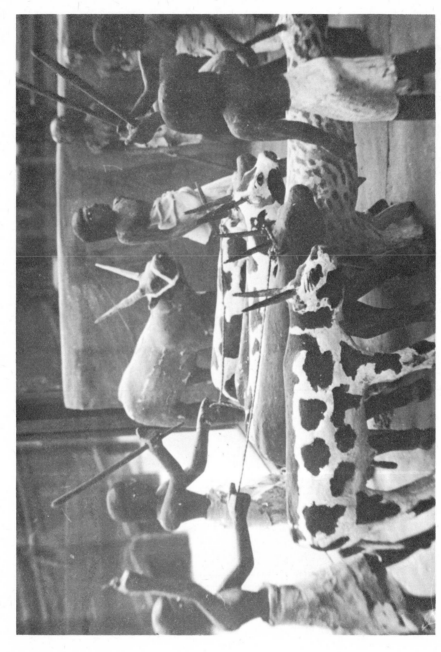

Fig. 3.14. Cattle review. Tomb of Meketre (number 280) at Thebes (Deir El Bahari); Middle Kingdom, eleventh dynasty, date uncertain. Photographed with permission of the Ministry of Culture and the officials of the Egyptian Museum, Cairo, ARE (1967).

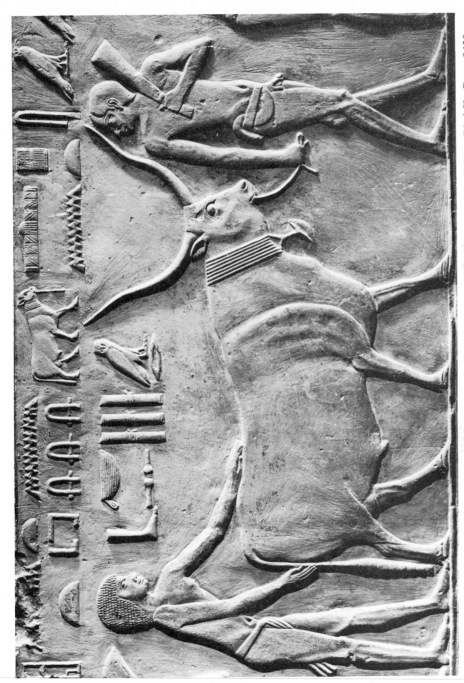

Fig. 3.15. Cattle herdsmen. Tomb of Ptahhetep at Saqqara; Old Kingdom, fifth dynasty, reign of King Djed-Ka-Re, *c.* 2450 B.C. Photograph used with permission of the Ministry of Culture and the officials of the Centre of Documentation, Cairo, ARE (1969).

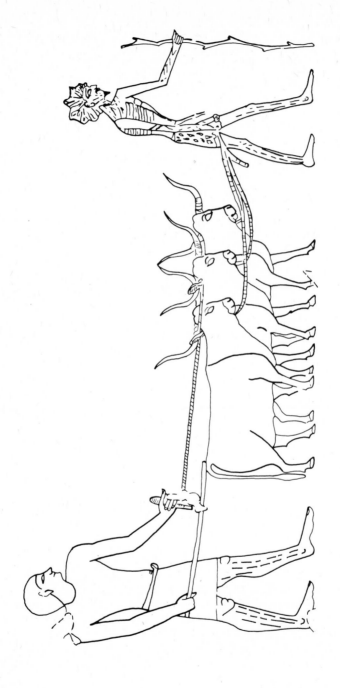

Fig. 3.16. An emaciated herdsman ("Beja" type). Tomb of Ukh-hotp (number 2) at Meir; Middle Kingdom, twelfth dynasty, date uncertain. Redrawn from Blackman (1915a, plate 6).

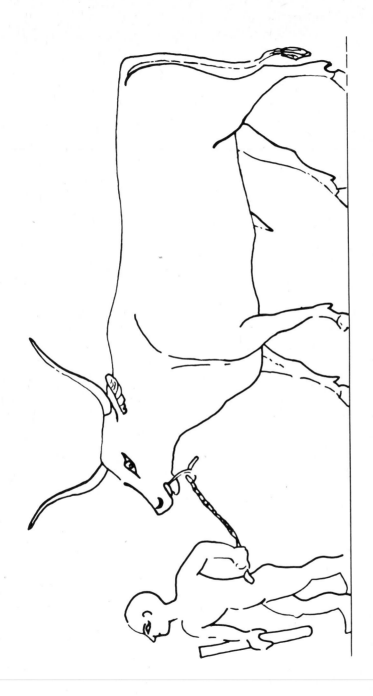

Fig. 3.17. Dwarf herdsman. From a tomb at Giza (?); Old Kingdom, date uncertain. Redrawn from Wilkinson (1878, Vol. 2, p. 444, plate 481).

illustrations of fighting bulls from Thebes; one from an unknown tomb, and the other (Fig. 3.26) from the tomb of Amenemhat (number 82), (reign of King Thutmose III, eighteenth dynasty, *c.* 1480 B.C.). Our examination of the latter tomb in the summer of 1969 revealed several discrepancies between Wilkinson's sketch and the actual painting. We were unable to verify the existence of the painting depicted in the first sketch (Wilkinson, Sketch number 344).

The care of the cattle was thus in the hands of herdsmen and farmers; but the section of the Kahun gynaecological papyrus (Griffith, 1898) which deals exclusively with disease of cattle makes it evident that some physicians, possibly of a distinct class, dealt with animals on the same lines as humans.

In addition, many priests of the goddess Sekhmet, some of them physicians (*swnw*), some not, specialized in cattle care. Thus Hery-shefnekht was both *swnw* and a priest of Sekhmet who "knew" cattle, while Aha-Nakht, another priest of Sekhmet, but who was not a *swnw*, also "knew oxen" (Ghalioungui and Dawakhly, 1963, p. 13, Fig. 26). Besides, some *w'bw* or "pure priests" who, very often, but not always, were also *swnw*, are shown in slaughtering scenes, supervising the whole procedure (Fig. 3.27), or smelling blood and pronouncing on its purity (Fig. 3.28). From the examination of such scenes, Chassinat (1905) concluded that the Egyptians had a special personnel to select beasts for sacred and profane (?) butchery, to direct the killing in accord with the sacred rites, and to examine the flesh for any marks of disease or impurity. We may add to these functions, the veterinary care of living beasts.

Working Cattle

The important role of cattle in the development and expansion of Egyptian agriculture is apparent, not only from tomb and temple art, but also from its religious association with both Osiris and Isis, the gods who reportedly gave agriculture to mankind (Chapter 1). Tomb art distinctly shows that some types of cattle were used for work (ploughing, threshing, pulling loads, and the like), whereas others were raised for religious purposes (see pp. 128–139). A subtle artistic differentiation between the religious and working cattle may be noticed in the long religious processions. Cattle that were carefully tended, fed, and not

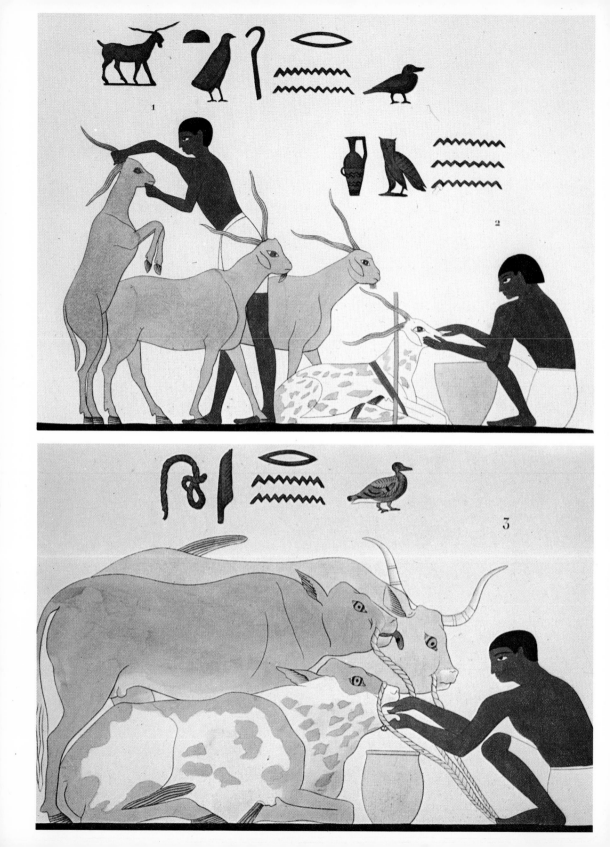

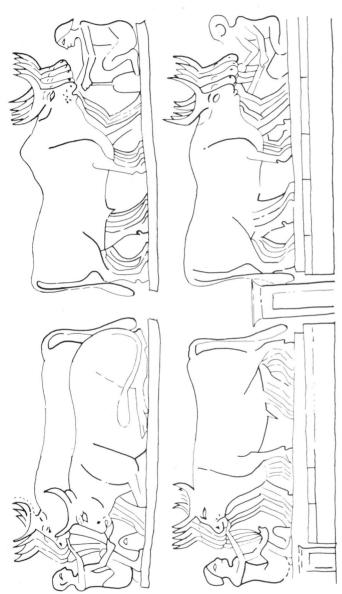

Fig. 3.18a. (Facing page, upper). Care and feeding of goats "Small Cattle"; Beni Hassan. Middle Kingdom. From a painting by Caillaud (1831), Darby Collection.

Fig. 3.18b. (Facing page, lower). Care and feeding of cattle. From an unknown tomb at Thebes; New Kingdom, date uncertain. From a painting by Caillaud (1831) Darby Collection.

Fig. 3.18c. (This page). Bovines hand-fed in stalls. Tomb of Merya at Tell el Amarna, New Kingdom, eighteenth dynasty, reign of King Amenhotep IV (Akhenaten), *c.* 1360 B.C. Redrawn from Davies (1903, plate 29).

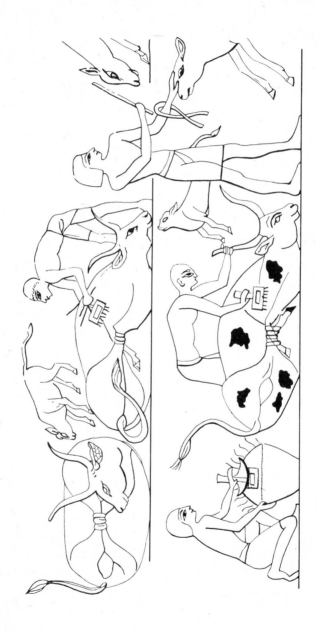

Fig. 3.19. Branding cattle. Tomb of Nebamun (number 90) at Thebes (Upper Enclosure); New Kingdom, eighteenth dynasty, reign of King Thutmose IV, *c.* 1420 B.C., Redrawn from Wilkinson (1878, Vol. 2, p. 84, Fig. 349).

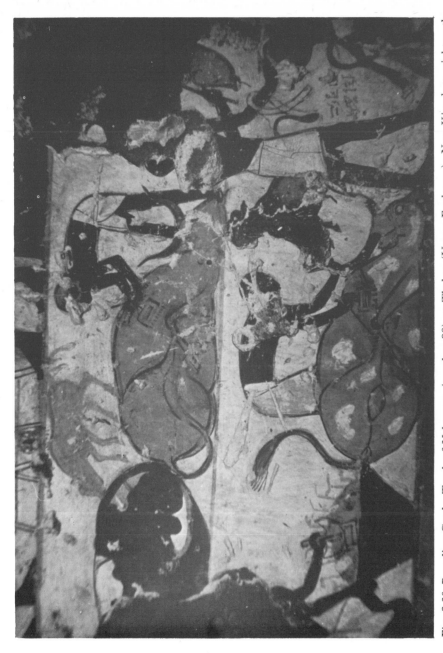

Fig. 3.20. Branding Cattle. Tomb of Nebamun (number 90) at Thebes (Upper Enclosure); New Kingdom, eighteenth dynasty, reign of King Thutmose IV, *c.* 1420 B.C. Photographed 1969.

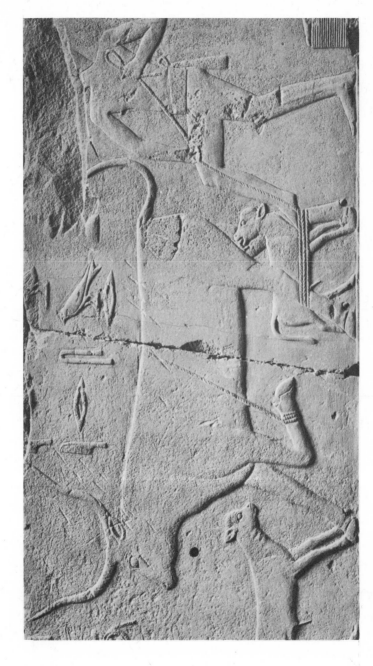

Fig. 3.21. Techniques of milking. Securing legs of cow. Tomb of Ka-Gem-Ni at Saqqara; Old Kingdom, sixth dynasty, reign of King Teti, c. 2390 B.C. Photographed 1969.

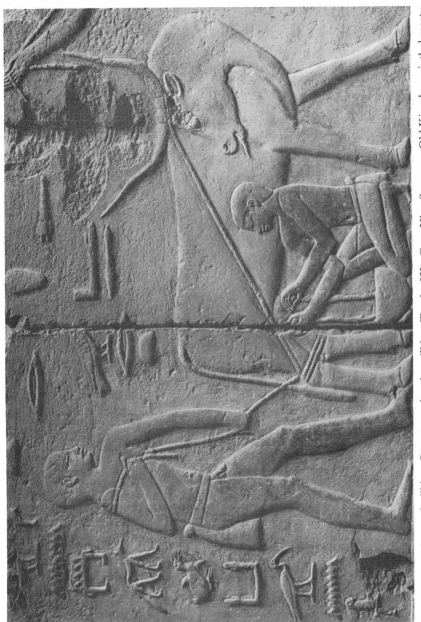

Fig. 3.22. Techniques of milking. Cow protesting the milking. Tomb of Ka-Gem-Ni at Saqqara; Old Kingdom, sixth dynasty, reign of King Teti, *c.* 2390 B.C. Photographed 1969.

allowed to graze developed long spurs along their hoofs, whereas working animals are not so depicted (Fig. 3.4).

The accurate anatomical drawings of Egyptian artists clearly show also that for work, ploughing or threshing, castrated oxen[14] were utilized, not bulls; and harnesses, as we know them today, were unknown. A brace or rope attached to their horns or necks connected a team of animals that pulled the plough by a line attached to it. Oxen also pulled heavy loads such as sarcophagi (especially in funerary scenes at Thebes), sleds filled with quarried stones, or carts for human transport. In all these scenes the artists left their individual touches. Such pictures did not lack humour. Encouragement with a stout club sometimes reactivated a tired ox that had laid down while ploughing (Fig. 3.29); oxen, driven in circles around the threshing floor, stoop to nibble some grain (Fig. 3.30); or a cow is drawn shedding tears as her mate is being slaughtered.

Religious Patterns and Their Impact on the Consumption of Beef

It has been stated that the Egyptians avoided the flesh of cows. Porphyry in the third century A.D. wrote

"... with the Egyptians, therefore, and Phoenicians, any one would sooner taste human flesh than the flesh of a cow ..." (2, 11)

Many contradictory facts, however, make it necessary to weigh critically the available evidence. Such a study must be related to the different periods of Egyptian history, and must be made from three distinct but intertwined viewpoints:

1. cow and bull worship;
2. cattle sacrifice;
3. consumption/avoidance of beef in the diet.

Sacred Cattle: Cows

"... you worship the cow, but I sacrifice it to the gods ..." (Anaxandrides of Cameirus, according to Athenaeus 7, 299, F)

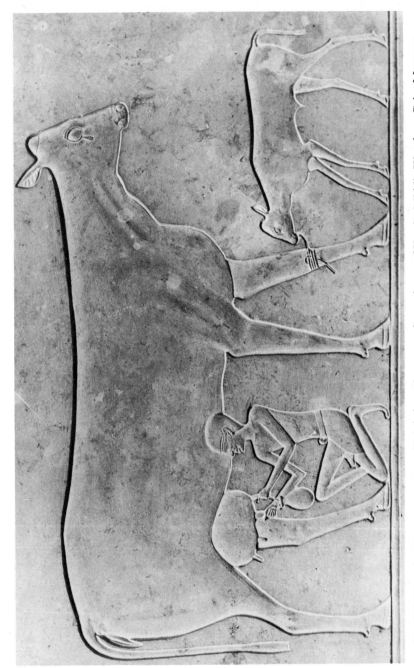

Fig. 3.23. Cow shedding tears as her milk is being taken away. Sarcophagus of Kawit; Middle Kingdom, Cairo Museum.

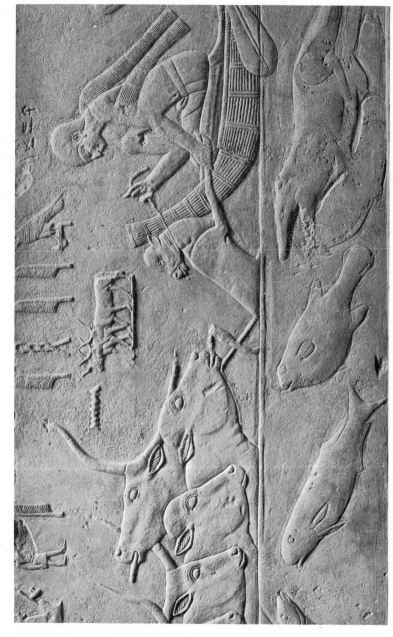

Fig. 3.24. Transport of cattle across a canal. Tomb of Ka-Gem-Ni at Saqqara; Old Kingdom, sixth dynasty, reign of King Teti, c. 2390 B.C. Photographed 1969.

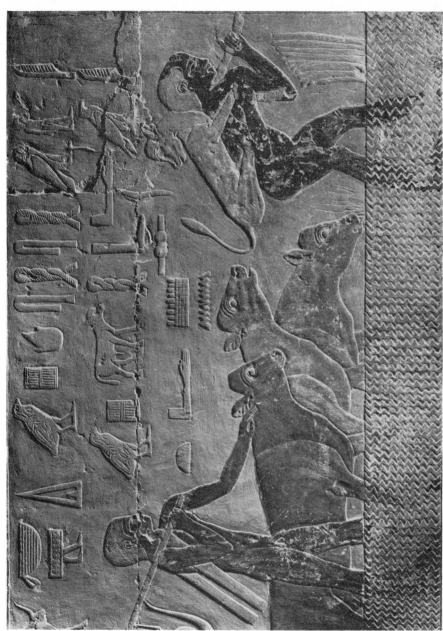

Fig. 3.25. Transportation of cattle across a shallow canal (or rescue during flood season). Tomb of Ti at Saqqara ; Old Kingdom, fifth dynasty, reigns of King Nefer-ir-ka-Re and Ne-Woser-Re, *c.* 2500 B.C. Photograph used with permission of the Ministry of Culture and the officials of the Centre of Documentation, Cairo, ARE (1969).

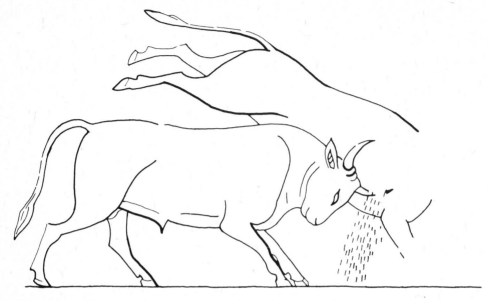

Fig. 3.26. Tomb of Amenemhat (number 82) at Thebes (Upper Enclosure); New Kingdom, eighteenth dynasty, reign of King Thutmose III, *c.* 1475 B.C. Redrawn from Wilkinson (1878, Vol. 2, p. 75, Fig. 343).

The cow was considered sacred[15] throughout much of the Dynastic Period, and was associated primarily with the goddess Hathor (Fig. 1.5); at other times, with both Isis (Fig. 1.6*b*) and Nut (Figs 1.9 and 1.10).

In Egyptian cosmology Hathor was the mother (or daughter) of the sun, Ra, and was viewed then as a distinct entity; but, in other instances, she was identified or confused with Isis, Nut or other goddesses. Both she and Nut were sometimes visualized as "celestial cows" standing with their feet at the four corners of the earth and with golden stars upon their bellies.[16]

In her commonest bovine form, Hathor was a mother goddess, the mother of mankind and the personification of mirth and love, constantly giving of herself and nourishing the living with an endless supply of her divine milk (Figs 1.5, 3.3). However, possibly as a result of the religious syncretism of which the Egyptians were fond, she was also the avenging "eye" of her father Ra who sent her to punish mankind. The tale as told in the Theban tombs of Seti I and Rameses III is summarized here:

Ra, the sun, became old; his bones changed to silver, his flesh to gold, and his hair was coloured the blue of lapislazuli. Mankind, aware of his weakness, plotted against him, but Ra learned of the plan and gathered Hathor (his eye), along with the four primordial gods and goddesses; Shu (wind), Tefnut (water), Geb (earth) and Nut (sky). Nun, god of the primordial sea and the deity which existed before all else, advised Ra to direct his "eye" at mankind. Thus Hathor began the slaughter and accomplished it with such fury and thoroughness that Ra was taken with compassion and feared that mankind would be entirely destroyed. He, therefore, concocted a mixture of beer that he coloured blood-red, and spread it over the flooded fields, on which it shone like a giant mirror.[17] Hathor, vain like most women, paused to admire herself in it and was attracted to the mixture. She drank it, was intoxicated, and forgot her avenging task. Man thus survived to repopulate the earth.[18] (See Erman, 1966, pp. 47–49; Maystre, 1941, pp. 53–115.)

Sacred Cattle: Bulls

". . . the sacred bulls—I refer to the Apis and the Mnevis—are honoured like the gods, as Osiris commanded, both because of their use in farming and also because the fame of those who discovered the fruits of the earth is handed down by the labours of these animals to succeeding generations for all time . . ." (*Diod.*, 1, 88, 4)

The worship of bulls in Ancient Egypt has been well described by Greek and Roman visitors.[19] In some instances the bulls were indeed gods, for example, Apis, Mnevis and Buchis. In other instances, in the opinion of Strabo (17, 1,22), they were only held in religious veneration

". . . now these [Apis, Mnevis, Buchis] are regarded as gods, but those in the other places, for in many places, indeed, both in the Delta and outside of it, either a bull or cow is kept, those others, I say, are not regarded as gods though they are held sacred . . ."

Although adored throughout Egypt, it is in the Delta that the cow and bull were a major focus of worship. The Israelites, who spent long years there, were at least in part contaminated by this practice

". . . they broke off the golden earrings which were in their ears, and brought them unto Aaron. And he received them at their hand, and

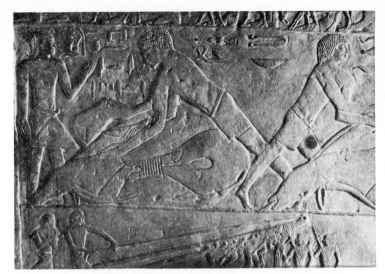

Fig. 3.27. A "pure priest" overseeing butchery. Tomb of Sabu. Old Kingdom. Cairo Museum.

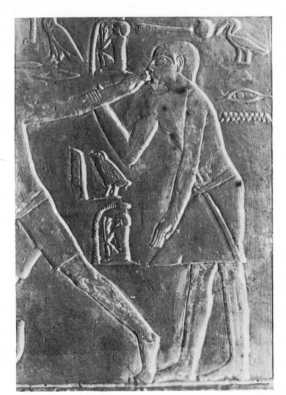

Fig. 3.28. The "pure priest" and physician (*swnw*) Ire-nakhty smelling blood presented on the fingers of the butcher and saying: "It is pure". Tomb of Ptahhetep. Old Kingdom Saqqara.

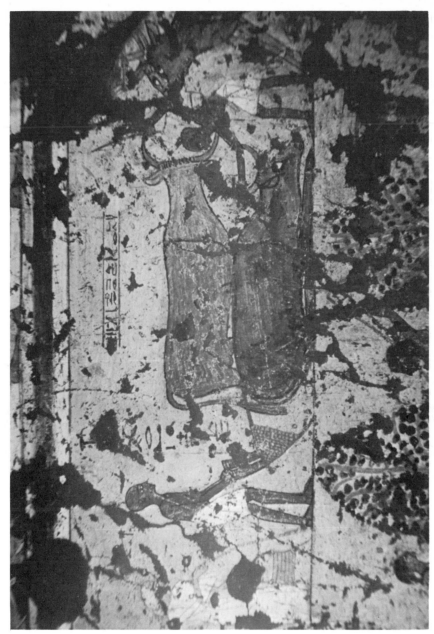

Fig. 3.29. Reluctant ox coaxed to resume ploughing. Tomb of Penehsi (number 16) at Thebes (Drah Abul Naga); south-ern tombs; New Kingdom, nineteenth dynasty, reign of King Rameses II, *c.* 1250 B.C. Photographed 1969.

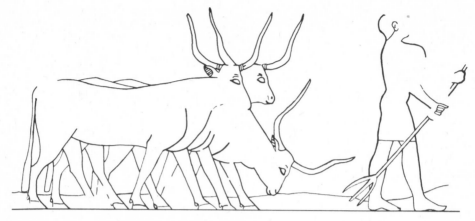

Fig. 3.30. Feeding from the threshing floor. Tomb of Senbi at Meir; Middle Kingdom, twelfth dynasty, date uncertain. Redrawn from Blackman (1914, plate. 4).

fashioned it with a graving tool, after he made it a molten calf; and they said, 'These be thy gods, O Israel, which brought thee up out of the land of Egypt' . . ." (Exodus, 32, 3, 4)

Later, images of bulls were erected in the sanctuaries of Israel by Jeroboam, and this was regarded as a great sin (Kings, I, 12, 28–33; II, 10, 29; Hosea, 8, 5–6, etc.). According to Simoons (1961, p. 163), the use of bull figures to support the brazen sea in Solomon's temple (Kings, I, 7, 25) suggests a survival of the ancient belief in the sacredness of bulls.

To understand the interplay between religion and beef avoidance a short account of these three major sacred bulls might be helpful.

Apis

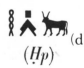 (d)

($\underset{.}{H}p$)

The bull known by the Egyptians as depicted by (d) (Faulkner, p. 168), and by the Greeks as Apis, was worshipped at Memphis. No succession of Apis bulls beginning with the earliest dynasties has been discovered and all the mummies buried in the Saqqara Serapeum date only to the New Kingdom. Nevertheless, its cult was said to have been introduced by Mena, the first pharaoh. Manetho[20] attributed it to Kaiechos[21] of the second dynasty

". . . in his reign the bulls, Apis at Memphis, and Mnevis at Heliopolis, and the Mendesian goat were worshipped as gods." (Fragment 8, 1940, p. 35)

His statement as to this early worship is confirmed by an inscription on the Palermo stone[22]

". . . [first dynasty] year $x + 12$[23] King (?) born of Meret–Neit:[24] first occurrence of 'running of Apis'." (*A.R.*, I, 114)

In addition, an ivory from the Hierakonpolis deposit in the Petrie Collection in the University of London has recently proved, after cleaning, to show a bull with a disc between its horn, probably Apis or Mnevis (Otto, 1964).

One may conclude therefore, that the Apis cult was indigenous in origin and reject the suspicion that it was a creation of the New Kingdom, or that Manetho was coerced to give it an antique origin in order to bring it in line with Greek legends concerning several different personages called Apis in their mythology.

Of these legends, the myth of Io suggests a possible link between the two cultures. This Io, beloved by Zeus was changed by him into a cow to spare her the ire of his wife Hera, and carried to Egypt where she was restored to human form. There, she married Telegonus, King of Egypt, and gave birth to Epaphus, her son by Zeus. Epaphus, believed by some to have been the sacred bull Apis, then received the throne of Egypt (see Graves, 1955, Vol. 1, 56B; Apollodorus 2, 1, 3).

Diodorus (1, 21, 9–11) was interested in the origins of Apis worship and believed it to have stemmed from an association between agriculture, bulls and oxen, a belief shared by Columella of Gades (6, P, 7) who expressed a similar thought

". . . the ox too is said to have been the attendant of Demeter and Triptolemus[25] . . . and it is still man's most hardworking associate in agriculture . . ."

Similar associations were discovered by foreign travellers to Egypt who, in discussing religion with priests, were informed that the god Osiris had taught agricultural methods to mankind. On the origin of the link between the agricultural bull and Osiris, Diodorus recorded two versions

". . . some explain the origin of the honour accorded this bull in this way, saying that at the death of Osiris his soul passed into this animal and therefore up to this day has always passed into its successor . . ." (1, 85, 4–5)

and

"... but some say that when Osiris died at the hands of Typhon [Seth], Isis collected the members of his body and put them in an ox made of wood covered over with fine linen ..." (1, 85, 5)

Plutarch (*I. and O.*, 362, 29, D) concurred

"... most of the priests say that Osiris and Apis are conjoined into one, thus explaining to us and informing us that we must regard Apis as the bodily image of the soul of Osiris ..."

This agricultural association was perpetuated by Aelian (11, 10) who confused, however, the relationship, and identified Apis with Horus, son of Isis and Osiris

"... the Egyptians liken Apis to Horus whom they believe to be the prime cause of the fertility of their crops and of every good season ..."

As Greek and Roman traditions relative to Apis were mixed with Egyptian beliefs, the origins and function of the Memphite bull became confused. By the first century A.D. several mythological variants were subjects of dispute and Plutarch, aware of these divergences, attempted to separate religious dogma from fiction

"... it is not worth while to pay attention to the Phrygian[26] writings, in which it is said that Serapis[27] was the son of Heracles,[28] and Isis was his daughter, nor must we fail to condemn Phylarchus,[29] who writes that Dionysus[30] was the first to bring from India into Egypt two bulls, and that the name of one was Apis and the other Osiris ..." (*I. and O.*, 362, 29, B–C)

Aelian, who related the standard Greek belief concerning the parentage of the Egyptian Apis "... the Greeks call him Epaphus" and trace his descent from "... his mother, the Argive Io, daughter of Inachus ..." (see above), recorded Egyptian objections to this parentage

"... the Egyptians, however, reject the story as false, and appeal to time as their witness, for they maintain that Epaphus was born late down the ages, whereas the first Apis visited mankind many, many thousands of years earlier ..." (11, 10)

This tradition focused upon an interesting "immaculate [?] conception"; it is related that Zeus slept with the beautiful Io and "touched her for some purpose" probably a physiological understatement reflected in the name of their offspring, for Epaphus (Apis) translates as "he-of-the-touch" (Graves, 1955, Vol. 1, 56B).

Since Apis was thus considered the incarnate soul of a god, one might anticipate that the Apis bull would be distinct from all others. Egyptian tradition, as recorded by Greek visitors, indeed sets it apart, both in its conception and in its shape

"... now this Apis, or Epaphus, is the calf of a cow which is never afterwards able to bear young. The Egyptians say that fire comes down from heaven upon the cow, which thereupon conceives Apis . . ." (*Her.*, III, 38)

Aelian (11, 10) and other writers perpetuated this Egyptian belief, and Plutarch (*I. and O.*, 368, 43, C) differed but slightly

"... Apis, they say, is the animate image of Osiris, and he comes into being when a fructifying light thrusts forth from the moon and falls upon a cow in her breeding season . . ."

The calf of miraculous birth, Apis, had well-defined marks of identification as additional evidence of its divine origin

"... the calf which is so called has the following marks: he is black, with a square spot of white upon the forehead, and on his back the figure of an eagle,[32] the hairs in his tail are double,[33] and there is a beetle[34] under his tongue . . ." (*Her.*, III, 28)

Other writers agreed, or added new information

"... his forehead and certain other small parts of his body are marked with white, but the other parts are black; and it is by these marks that they choose the bull suitable for the succession when the one that holds the honour has died . . ." (Strabo, 17, 1, 31)

Pliny (8, 71, 184) added

"... its distinguishing mark is a bright white spot in the shape of a crescent on the right flank, and it has a knob under the tongue which they call a beetle [*cantharum*] . . ."

Aelian (11, 10) wrote of twenty-nine marks of identification[35] but did not describe them. Plutarch (*I. and O.*, 368, 43, C) stated

"... there are many things in the Apis that resemble features of the moon, his bright parts being darkened by the shadowy . . ."

Small wonder that Egyptologists, archaeologists, and mythographers are divided over the colour and markings of the Apis bull!

Since the marks of identification were multiple and unusual, the search for each new "true" Apis calf would be expected to have taken a long time, and any period without a living Apis would contradict the belief in the continuity of the god. Hence, the search for a replacement calf may have begun long before the death of the adult bull. Aelian (11, 10) noted that

> ". . . the man in whose herd this divine animal was born is counted fortunate and is so, and the Egyptians regard him with admiration . . ."

The events that followed the discovery and recognition of the new Apis calf were described by Diodorus (1, 85, 1–3)

> ". . . when it has been found the people cease their mourning and the priests who have the care of it first take the young bull to Nilopolis[36] where it is kept forty days, and then, putting it on a state barge fitted out with a gilded cabin, conduct it as a god to the sanctuary of Hephaestus [Ptah] at Memphis . . ."

Diodorus further reported on the strange homage paid by Egyptian women to the bull during its stay at Nilopolis (Fig. 14.11)

> ". . . during these forty days only women may look at it; these stand facing it and pulling up their garments to show their genitals,[37] but henceforth they are forever prevented from coming into the presence of this god . . ." (1, 85, 3)

Aelian (11, 10) described in greater detail the transport of Apis to Memphis

> ". . . at the rising of the new moon the sacred scribes and priests go out to meet it—year by year [they make] ready a sacred vessel for this god and transport him on board to Memphis, where he finds abodes after his heart and delightful spots to linger in, and places where he may amuse himself, where he may run and roll in the dust and exercise himself, and the homes of beautiful cows . . ."[38]

He then describes the garlands and ornaments placed on the cows offered to Apis.

Once enshrined at Memphis, Apis was the object of reverence and devotion. Visitors came from all parts of Egypt and abroad to view the god

> ". . . in front of the sanctuary is situated a court, in which there is another sanctuary belonging to the bull's mother. Into this court they set Apis loose at a certain hour, particularly that he may be shown to foreigners; for

although people can see him through the window in the sanctuary, they wish to see him outside also, but when he has finished a short bout of skipping in the court they take him back again to his familiar stall . . ." (Strabo, 17, 1, 31)

Foreigners delighted in observing the cavorting Apis, but the main purpose of their visit stemmed from the proclaimed oracular powers with which Apis was endowed

". . . Apis, it seems, is in effect a good prophet; he, to be sure, never sets girls or elderly women on tripods,[39] never fills them with some sanctified draught, but a man prays to this god, and children without, who are playing and dancing to the music of pipes, become inspired and proclaim in time with the music the actual response of the god . . ." (Aelian, 11, 10)

Pliny (8, 71, 185) reported, however, a somewhat different technique of oracular delivery

". . . and companies of boys escort it singing a song in its honour; it seems to understand, and to desire to be worshipped. These companies are suddenly seized with frenzy and chant prophecies of future events . . ."

Apis delivered his "prophecies" also in other fashions

". . . it has a pair of shrines, which they call its bedchambers, that supply the nations with auguries: when it enters one this is a joyful sign, but in the other one it portends terrible events . . ."

Personal consultation with Apis was also sought

". . . it gives answers to private individuals by taking food out of the hand of those who consult . . ."

We are not informed what foods Apis preferred; perhaps the priests withheld this secret, fearing the knowledge might unduly prejudice the "selective blessing" of the bull. But its oracular fame was fortified and spread afar when he turned away from food held by Germanicus Caesar,[40] who, indeed, met an untimely death shortly later (Pliny, 8, 71, 185).

Apis was not allowed to become fat or senile. Plutarch (*I. and O.*, 353, 5, A) and Aelian (11, 10) both record a belief relative to Apis and Nile water. The bull was watered from a special well of its own as the priests did not want him to become obese by drinking fattening Nile water.[41] The "senility" of Apis was, likewise, cause for concern, and before the rigours of old age overtook the bull he was ritually slain[42]

". . . it is not lawful for it to exceed a certain number of years of life,[43] and they kill it by drowning it in the fountain of the priests . . ." (Pliny, 8, 71, 184)

When Apis died, either by natural or induced causes, widespread grief and mourning filled the land

". . . they mourn for it as deeply as do those who have lost a beloved child and bury it in a manner not in keeping with their ability, but going far beyond the value of their estates . . ." (*Diod.*, 1, 84, 7–8)

Lucian (*On Sacrifices*, 15) reported an interesting display of personal mourning for the Apis

". . . and if Apis, the greatest of their gods, dies, who is there who thinks so much of his hair that he does not shave it off and boldly shows his mourning on his head."

In this description, however, Lucian unwittingly contradicted an earlier report of Herodotus[44]

". . . with all other men, in mourning for the dead those most nearly concerned have their heads shaven; Egyptians are shaven at other times, but after death they let their hair and beard grow . . ." (II, 36)

The Apis bull was embalmed upon a slab or table of polished alabaster (see Dimick, 1958) and the funerary procession proceeded from Memphis westward to the necropolis of Saqqara where Apis was interred in a huge granite sarcophagus inside the vast subterranean galleries of the Serapeum[45]

". . . when they convey his body on an improvised bier . . . they fasten skins of fawns about themselves, and carry Bacchic wands and indulge in shoutings and movements exactly as do those who are under the spell of the Dionysiac ecstasies . . ." (*I. and O.*, 364, 35, E–F)

Apis, thereafter merged with Osiris, whereupon he was called Osiris–Apis (e), pronounced by the Greeks *Osirapis*.

(e)

Wsr Ḥpw

When Ptolemy I, first of the Greek rulers on Egypt after Alexander, introduced into Egypt the Asiatic god Serapis,[46] in an attempt to proclaim a Graeco-Egyptian deity that would unite both peoples in the same worship, this god soon became confused with Osirapis, and the name Serapis was applied to both. But the early pure form of Serapis worship centered at Alexandria, where his temple was one of the local wonders, while Memphis was the Mecca of the Serapis–Osirapis cult, and its necropolis at Saqqara, later called the "Serapeum", was the site of internment of the Apis bulls. This holy place was also somewhat connected with Imhotep, the god of medicine, and became, even into the Christian period, a centre of pilgrimage and temple healing.

After the Roman conquest, the cult of Serapis spread throughout much of the eastern Mediterranean where the once distinct entities of Osiris, Apis, Serapis and Horus, were merged into several syncretic beliefs. But in Rome, Isis, rather than Apis, emerged as the principal deity, and her priests spread her fame and worship to the limits of the Roman Empire.[47]

Mnevis

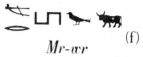

Mr-wr (f)

The Mnevis[48] bull, worshipped at Heliopolis, received less attention in Greek and Roman writings than its counterpart, Apis, enshrined at Memphis across the Nile. According to Ames (1965, p. 128), Mnevis was the Greek phonetic equivalent of the hieroglyph (f)[49] and this god was associated with the god Ra-Atum.[50] Plutarch (*I. and O.*, 364, 33, C) relates, however, that the Mnevis bull was sacred to Osiris, not to Ra-Atum, and some Egyptians thought him the sire of Apis. Aelian (11, 11) described Mnevis as bearing unique features

". . . and he, say the Egyptians, is sacred to the sun, whereas Apis, they say, is dedicated to the moon, and accordingly, to the Egyptians, he also bears a special mark to show that he is no counterfeit, no bastard, but beloved of the aforesaid god . . ."

Little information has survived relative to Mnevis except for a tale linked to the Egyptian King Bochchoris[51]

". . . this is how, from a desire to cause pain to the people of Egypt, he treated Mnevis. He sent a wild bull against him. And then the stranger rushed forward in anger intending to fall upon the bull beloved of the god, but tripped, and falling against the stem of a Persea tree, broke his horn, whereupon Mnevis wounded him in the flank. Bochchoris was put to shame, and the Egyptians loathed him . . ." (Aelian, 11, 11)

Buchis

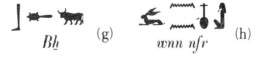

Bḫ (g)   *wnn nfr* (h)

A third bull, believed to be a manifestation of the god Mont, was worshipped at Hermonthis, the modern Armant. Like Apis and Mnevis, this bull, called by the hieroglyph (g) caused confusion to a number of writers. Aelian (12, 11) reports his name as Onuphis, perhaps the Greek phonetic equivalent of the Egyptian hieroglyph (h) (Gardiner, 1950, p. 561), "he-who-is-continually-happy", one of the attributes of the god Osiris. Modern writers have variously transliterated the bull's name as *Basis, Pakis* (Wilkinson, 1878, Vol. 3, p. 307), and *Bukhe* (Ames, 1965, p. 128). The burial site of the Buchis bulls (the Bucheum) has been excavated near the village of Armant (Ancient Hermonthis) in Upper Egypt. It contained the graves of the bulls that were worshipped between the reigns of King Nektanebo II and of the Roman Emperor, Diocletian (see Mond *et al.*, 1934).

The distinctive nature of Buchis was described by Macrobius of Parma, a writer of the fifth century A.D.

". . . in the city of Hermonthis they adore the bull Bacchis, which is consecrated to the sun, in the magnificent temple of Apollo [Mont]—for every hour it is reported to change its colour and to have long hairs growing backward contrary to the nature of all other animals[52] whence it is thought to be an image of the sun shining on the opposite side of the world . . ." (Wilkinson, 1878, Vol. 3, pp. 307–308)

Cattle Sacrifice

". . . all Egyptians sacrifice unblemished bulls and bull-calves; they may not sacrifice cows; these are sacred to Isis . . ." (*Her.*, 2, 41)

No surviving Ancient Egyptian texts reveal the origin and development of cattle sacrifice or specifically discuss the techniques and methodology involved. Numerous descriptions of the varieties of sacrificial cattle, of donations, and of the numbers offered to various temples and gods are available from most of the Dynastic and Post-Dynastic Periods, but they shed no light on specific procedural matters. Egyptian tomb and temple art throughout the Dynastic and Graeco-Roman Periods, likewise, offers profusely illustrated scenes of sacrifice, and butchery, but the accompanying texts are nearly always short, cursory, and deficient in explanatory detail.

The most complete descriptions of cattle sacrifice as practiced during the late phases of the New Kingdom were left by Greek travellers. These observations, made during visits far separate in time are sometimes contradictory. Nevertheless, comparison with tomb and temple artifacts permits some assessment of relative reliability. One observes, for example, close parallels between the Ancient Egyptian tomb illustrations and the later Greek literary descriptions, with basic similarities that extend across a vast span of time. Yet, in regard to the details of selection or certification of the kine, it is less clear whether the later Greek reports form a valid basis for interpretation of more ancient methods.

According to Herodotus (II, 38), selection of sacrificial cattle was carefully conducted

". . . one of the priests appointed for the purpose searches to see if there is a single black hair on the whole body, since in that case the beast is unclean. He takes the tongue out of the [animal's] mouth to see if it be clean in respect of the prescribed marks—he inspects the hairs of the tail to observe if they grow naturally—after passing the prescribed examination of the priest they certified the victim pure for sacrifice . . ."

Such an inspection would have certainly prevented the unintentional sacrifice of an Apis bull (see p. 131) which was supposed to bear identification marks under the tongue[53] and on the hairs of the tail.

Sacrifice of reddish-brown cattle posed a different problem

". . . the Egyptians, because of their belief that Typhon [Seth] was of a red complexion, also dedicate to sacrifice such of their meat cattle as are of a red colour,[54] but they conduct the examination of these so scrupulously that, if an animal has but one hair black or white, they think it wrong to sacrifice it . . ." (Plutarch, 363, 31, B)

As remarked by Ruffer (1919, p. 10) the description parallels the Jewish sacrifice of cattle

"Speak unto the children of Israel, that they bring thee a red heifer without spot, wherein is no blemish, and upon which never came a yoke . . ." (Numbers, 19, 2)

Chaeremon of Alexandria (first century A.D.) added further restrictions

". . . thus, for instance, of oxen they reject the female and also such of the males as were twins, or were speckled or of a different colour" (according to Porphyry, 4, 7)

Nevertheless, red cattle, spotted calves, and multi-coloured bovines are abundantly illustrated on sarcophagi, on the tombs and on temple walls, thus seemingly casting doubt on these reports.

After passing the "prescribed examination" the sacrificial animal was declared ritually pure

"... the priest marks him by twisting a piece of papyrus round his horns and attaching thereto some sealing-clay, which he then stamps with his own signet-ring[55]—it is forbidden, under penalty of death, to sacrifice an animal that has not been marked in this way." (*Her.*, II, 38)

According to the Greeks, the mark stamped by these priests, whom they called "sphragists", represented a kneeling man, his hands tied behind him, with a sword pointed at his throat. Now this is exactly the hieroglyphic determinative of words like "impious" and "evil", which would indicate that the victim was thereby identified with Seth and his companions (Chassinat, 1905).

Also according to Herodotus (II, 39, 40), the priests, prior to the initiation of the sacrificial rite, fasted and took the victim to the altar and,

"... setting the wood alight [they] pour a libation of wine upon the altar in front of the victim, and at the same time invoke the god. Then they slay the animal and cutting off his head, proceed to flay the body ..."

(i)

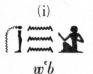

w'b

Subsequent steps are well illustrated in many tombs where a "pure priest" depicted by (i) who often was a physician (*swnw*) as well, examines the kill and tests the blood to declare its fitness[56] (see also p. 109 and Figs 3.19, 3.20, 3.27, 3.28).

Although the sacrificial animal was certified pure, the head, said Herodotus (II, 39) was seen in a different light

"... next they take the head, and heaping imprecations upon it, if there is a market-place and a body of Greek traders in the city, they carry it there and sell it instantly; if, however, there are no Greeks among them, they throw the head into the river ..."

This Egyptian custom is almost identical to the Biblical way of ridding the community of impure meat

"... thou shalt give it unto the stranger that is in thy gates, that he may eat it; or thou mayest sell it unto an alien; for thou art an holy people unto the Lord thy God." (Deuteronomy, 14, 12)

Herodotus (II, 39) further elaborated on Egyptians' customs relative to the head of sacrificial animals

"... these practices, the imprecations upon the heads, and the libations of wine, prevail all over Egypt, and extend to victims of all sorts; and hence the Egyptians will never eat the head of any animal ..."

These statements, however, do not agree with Mustapha's finding of heads, sawed along their middle, presumably to extract their brains

(1964), or with the tomb illustrations from all periods that show calves' heads among the food offerings presented to both the gods and the deceased (Figs 3.31 and 3.32). Rawlinson (1885, Vol. 2, pp. 59, 60) explained this inconsistency by supposing that the head was avoided only during special religious festivals, not throughout the year. According to Erman (1934) the head was then treated as a "scapegoat". On the other hand, the head may have stood metaphorically for the whole animal. This was a common form of language in animal lists, where the number of "heads" stood for the number of animals (*A.R.*, IV, 223–225, 280, 338, and 365–369).

After removal of the head

". . . when they have flayed their steer they pray, and when their prayer is ended they take the paunch of the animal out entire, leaving the intestines and fat inside the body; they then cut off the legs, the ends of the loins, the shoulders, and the neck; and having so done, they fill the body of the steer with clean bread, honey, raisins, figs, frankincense, myrrh, and other aromatics. Thus filled they burn the body, pouring over it great quantities of oil . . ."[57] (*Her.*, II, 40)

While the altar fire consumed the sacrificial offerings the priests scourged themselves. At the conclusion of the ceremony the remaining portions of meat were served to the priests and temple attendants (*Her*, II, 40).

Evaluation

Priests, because of their role as sacrificers, were most likely the major consumers of beef

". . . they consume none of their own property, and are at no expense for anything; but everyday bread is baked for them of the sacred corn[58] and a plentiful supply of beef and of goose's flesh is assigned to each . . ." (*Her.*, II, 37)

We agree with Montet's opinion (1958, p. 89) that consumption of beef was in general limited, and restricted to the upper sections of Egyptian society, the large landholders, priests and royalty. This was more a function of economics than of religious restriction. The eating of beef by others could take place only during feasts, when the entire slaughtered animal could be consumed collectively within a few days, before it spoiled. Otherwise, the meat more commonly eaten by peasants was that of smaller species—lamb, goat, pork, fowl or fish, which could be

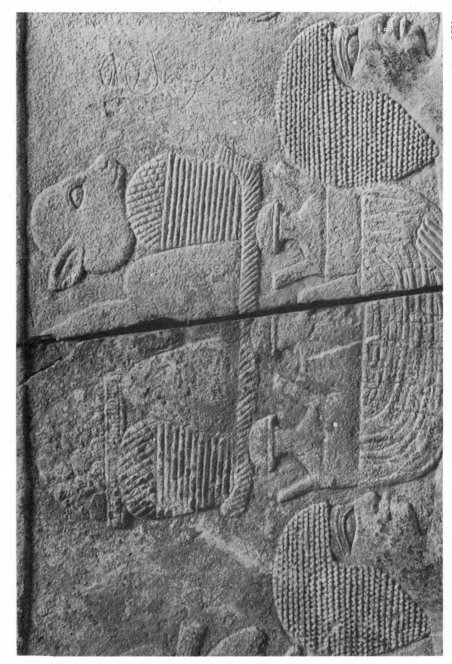

Fig. 3.31. Severed head as desired food offering. Tomb of Ka-Gem-yi at Saqqara; Old Kingdom, sixth dynasty, reign of King Teti, *c.* 2390 B.C. Photographed 1969.

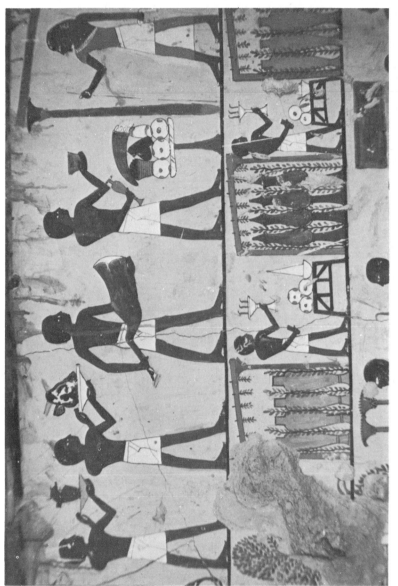

Fig. 3.32. Severed head and hind limb offerings. Tomb of Minnakht (number 87) at Thebes (Upper Enclosure); New Kingdom, eighteenth dynasty, reign of King Thutmose III *c.* 1475 B.C. Photographed 1969.

eaten in a single day. Nevertheless, although to be denied a food because it is "too expensive" is not related to cultural or religious history, if the same conditions persist for centuries, a class attitude may develop towards it and turn into an avoidance pattern.

Herodotus (II, 41), (p. 136) offered the first classical evidence of beef avoidance in Egypt. He defined the avoidance as one associated with the flesh of cows and stated that this pattern extended geographically beyond the limits of Egypt into Libya

> ". . . thus from Egypt as far a Lake Tritonis,[59] Libya is inhabited by wandering tribes whose drink is milk and their food the flesh of animals. Cow's flesh, however, none of these tribes ever tastes, but abstain from it for the same reason as the Egyptians—even at Cyrene, the woman think it wrong to eat the flesh of the cow—the Barcaean[61] woman abstain, not from cow's flesh only, but also from the flesh of swine . . ." (IV, 186)

Was then beef rejected in Ancient Egypt? The critical point in favour of rejection centres on the above statement by Herodotus and by the later assertion of Porphyry (see p. 120). Earlier writers, without the benefit of the improved translations now available, accepted this point of view and have gone to great lengths to base it on historical or religious reasons. Two orders of motives are usually offered. One relates avoidance to ecological motives

> ". . . by a prudent foresight, in a country possessing neither extensive pasture lands, nor great abundance of cattle, the cow was held sacred and consequently was forbidden to be eaten." (Wilkinson, 1854, Vol. 1, p. 166)

This was merely a repetition of an argument known from antiquity. Philochorus of Athens in the third century B.C., wrote

> ". . . at one time, also when there was a dearth of cows, a law was passed, on account of the scarcity, that they should abstain from these animals since they wished to amass them and fill up their numbers by not slaughtering them . . ." (according to Athenaeus, 9, 375, C)

It seems, however, doubtful that available acreage could have had any influence on the selection of sacred animals. Deification did not arise because of threatened extinction. This was more probably a function of physical characteristics, since the criteria of totemistic identification, even in agricultural economies, had already been established when man was still struggling in a pre-agricultural hunting-gathering economy, long before domestication.

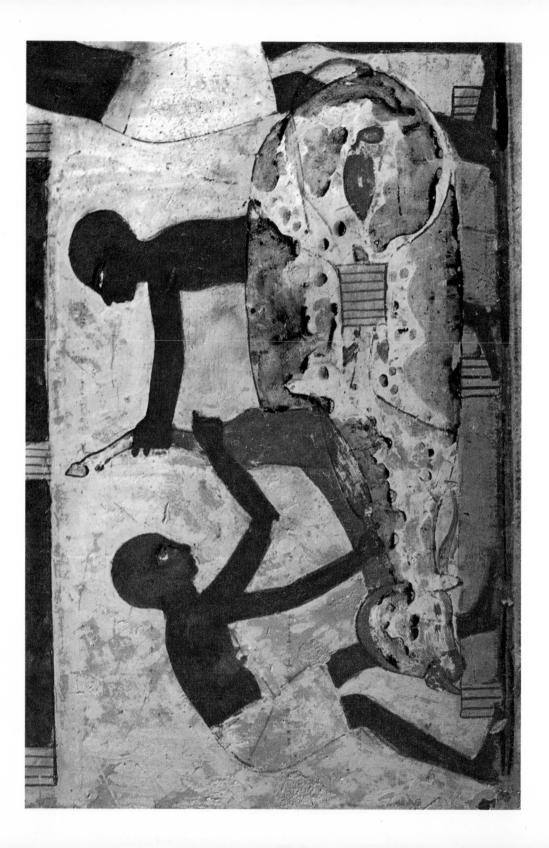

The second motive invoked to explain rejection is the religious association and identification with Hathor (Rawlinson, 1885, Vol. 2, p. 23). But this hypothesis raises more difficulties than it solves, for the same logic, if applied to the sacred bulls, Apis, Mnevis and Buchis, would have forbidden the slaying or eating of bulls and oxen.

Egyptian records, however, offer no support for either of these theses. Rawlinson, considering the evidence, stated, in contradiction to his previous assertions

". . . not only do cows and heifers appear among the sacrificial animals presented to the temple by the Egyptian monarchs, but it is distinctly stated in numerous passages that cows were actually offered in sacrifice . . .!"

Reports attributed to King Rameses III (nineteenth dynasty, *c.* 1198 B.C.) confirm this

". . . and there was offered to thee a festival offering consisting of numerous ablations of bread, wine, shedeh [*šdh*], vegetables, bulls, bullocks, calves by the hundred thousand, cows by the ten thousand, without number . . ." (*A.R.*, Vol. IV, 335)

It is, therefore, reasonable to conclude that, although some kind of taboo was in effect during the Late Dynastic Period through the Graeco-Roman Period, it is not clear whether it was applied to all varieties of beef, or only selectively to cows, to female calves, to bovine "heads", or to some species of bovines. It is, consequently, erroneous sweepingly to conclude that Egyptians of all periods avoided beef.

Some have interpreted one Biblical passage as indicating beef avoidance.

". . . and Pharaoh called for Moses and for Aaron, and said, go ye, sacrifice to your God in the land. And Moses said, it is not meet so to do; for we shall sacrifice the abomination of the Egyptians before their eyes, and will they not stone us? We will go three days journey into the wilderness and sacrifice to the Lord our God, as He shall command us . . ." (Exodus, 8, 25–27)

Fig. 3.33 (Facing page). Butchering cattle. Tomb of Nakht (number 52) at Thebes (Lower Enclosure); New Kingdom, eighteenth dynasty, reign of King Thutmose IV, *c.* 1420 B.C. Photographed 1969.

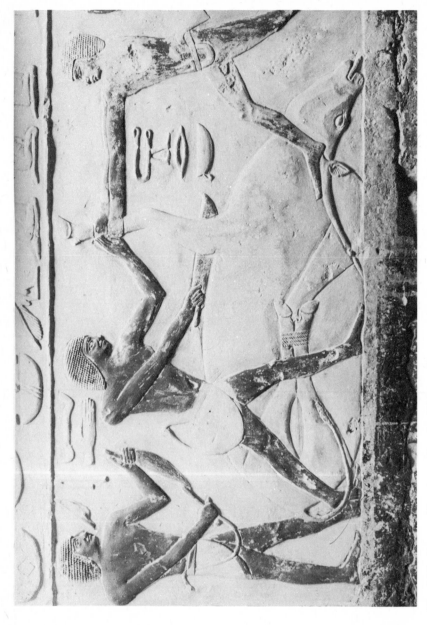

Fig. 3.34a. Scene of butchery. Tomb of Idut at Saqqara; Old Kingdom, fifth dynasty, reign of King Unas, *c.* 2423 B.C. Photographed 1969.

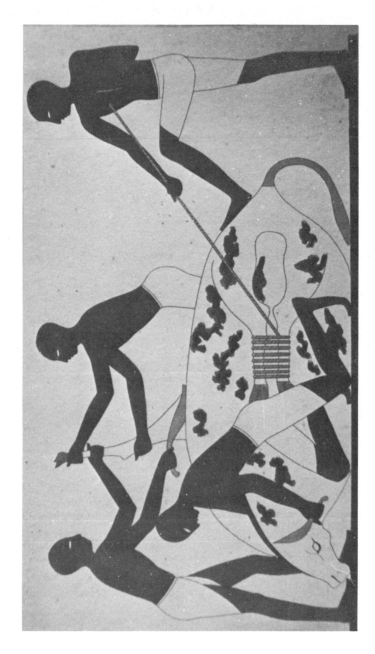

Fig. 3.34b. Scene of butchery. From unknown tomb at Thebes; New Kingdom, date uncertain. From a painting by Frederic Caillaud (1831), Darby Collection.

This animal, the sacrifice of which was considered an abomination in the eyes of the Egyptians, and whose flesh was avoided, might have been a calf, for the Egyptian nobility and peasantry would not have been upset over the sacrifice of a lamb or goat. This is conjectural, however, and has not been substantiated.[61]

Another avoidance, extending to beef, was current in Egypt during the Late Periods

> ". . . no native of Egypt, whether man or woman, will give a Greek a kiss, or use the knife of a Greek, or his [squewer], or his cauldron, or taste the flesh of an ox, known to be pure, if it has been cut with a Greek knife . . ." (*Her.*, 41)

The Egyptian practice was to slay cattle and other large mammals by cutting the throat. The avoidance of meat cut with a Greek knife may have reflected an unorthodox method used by the Greeks to slay their sacrificial victims. It might, on the other hand, have reflected the Egyptians aloofness towards the visiting or ruling Greeks or Romans. They felt themselves superior in nearly every way to the Greeks (pp. 29–30); hence the Egyptian avoidance of meat butchered by Greeks may have simply reflected this attitude.

Butcher Shops, Slaughtering and Butchery

As discussed in the preceding pages, it is difficult to separate aspects of religious ceremonial from everyday butchering. The slaying, skinning and quartering of animals, usually cattle and desert game, is an oft-repeated motif in Egyptian art from all periods and provinces.

Butchers are portrayed in the dress of commoners (Figs 3.33 and 3.34) and were, most probably, servants of the nobility, supervised by priests or priest-physicians. Cattle were slain by cutting the throat with knives; they were bled, then skinned (Figs 3.35, 3.36). Blood was not considered taboo nor avoided by the Ancient Egyptians. The pictures that show their priest-physicians smelling it to pronounce on its purity (Fig. 3.28) and a paragraph in the *Ebers Papyrus* (XXXIV, 198) that compares melaena to cooked blood indicate that they did not scorn at "blood pudding" or "blutwurst". This is in marked contrast with Mosaic and Islamic traditions

> ".. it shall be a perpetual statute for your generations throughout all

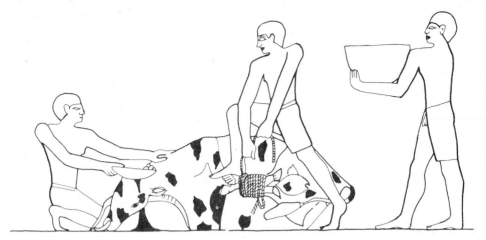

Fig. 3.35. Bowl for collecting blood. Tomb of Senbi at Meir; Middle Kingdom, twelfth dynasty, date uncertain. Redrawn from Blackman (1914, plate 11).

your dwellings, that ye eat neither fat nor blood . . ." (Leviticus, 3, 17; 7, 26; 17, 10–14; 19, 26; Deuteronomy, 12, 16)

". . . these things only has He forbidden you: carrion, blood, the flesh of swine . . ." (Holy Koran, 2, 168; 5, 4; 6, 147; 16, 116)

After the animal was skinned, it was disemboweled and the butchers then dismembered the various parts, which are illustrated with fair accuracy (Figs 3.37, 3.38). Select pieces were presented as offerings (Fig. 3.39) or exhibited as "filets" or joints suspended from ropes in "meat shops".[62] Representations of butchers in association with "meat shops" are known from the Old, Middle and New Kingdoms (see Montet, 1910). A recently excavated tomb at Saqqara belonging to the fifth dynasty noble, Nefr, shows one such early example in which ribs, filets and legs of beef are suspended inside a shelter. Old and Middle Kingdom tombs at Meir depict similar meat shops (Fig. 3.40), and the subject is also shown in Theban Middle and New Kingdom tombs (Figs 3.41 and 3.42).

The brains of these animals were also eaten. Moustafa (1964) found in a bovine cemetery (twenty-sixth dynasty) skulls split along the median basicranial axis, apparently to permit access to their brains. Joints of dried preserved meats have been found in Theban tombs (Fig. 3.43).

During the very late and Post-Dynastic Periods most Greek and

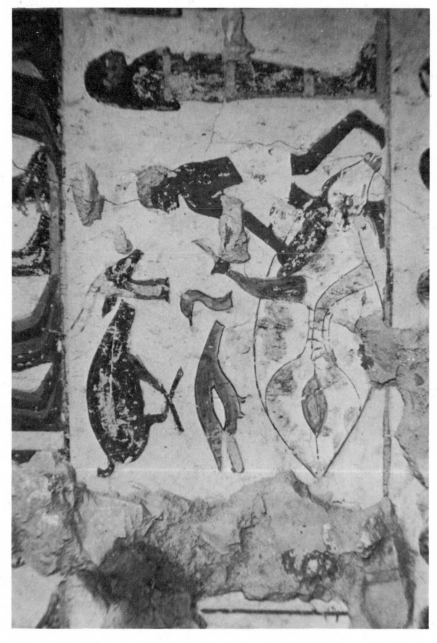

Fig. 3.36. Desert game, fowl, and cattle slain by cutting the throat. Tomb of Suemnut (number 92) at Thebes. (Upper Enclosure); New Kingdom, eighteenth dynasty, reign of King Amenhotep II, *c.* 1440 B.C. Photographed 1969.

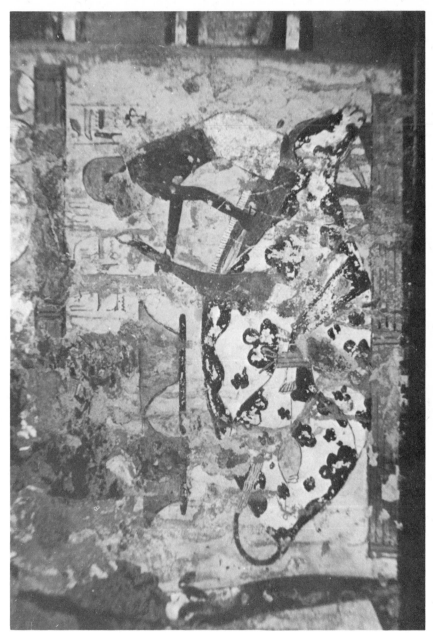

Fig. 3.37. Exposed trachea. Tomb of Amenmose (number 89) at Thebes (Upper Enclosure); New Kingdom; eighteenth dynasty, reign of King Amenhotep III, *c.* 1370 B.C. Photographed 1969.

Roman authors did not report or discuss meat shops except by passing reference

"... the ibis is useful because it singles out every animal and the refuse in the meat-shop and bakeries ..." (Strabo, 17, 2, 4)

Athenaeus (3, 94, C) likewise described a variety of meat shops, one of which specialized in offal and other inexpensive cuts of meat

"... many kinds of meat prepared with water: feet, heads, ears, jawbones, besides guts, tripe, and tongues in accordance with the custom in shops at Alexandria called 'boiled meat' shops."

Hunt and Edgar (1932) translated a meat bill, dated to the third century A.D. (approximate period of Athenaeus), that could have been supplied from such a shop

"... 4th [day]: four minae[63] of meat, two trotters, one tongue, one snout; 6th [day]: half a head with tongue; 22nd [day]: one paunch, two kidneys; 25th [day]: for Tryphon, two minae [of meat], one ear, one trotter, two kidneys ..."

It may be remarked in passing that such offals are still appreciated in Egypt. They are sold for popular prices in the *masmat* shops that serve such delicacies as feet, lungs, spleen, liver, kidneys, pancreas, thymus, brain, tripe, sausage, testicles, and "calf's foot soup", but no vegetables or usual cuts of meat. The prestige of "noble" cuts, however, is expressed in a popular proverb

"An arpent of meat rather than an acre of tripes."

In Pre-Islamic Arabia, a similar hierarchy graded camel flesh into "noble" and common cuts. In one of his songs Abul Farag al-Isfahâny (1936) related how a noble woman distinguished her suitor, the prince-poet Imru' ul-Qeiss, from a plebeian impersonator by his insistence on having nothing but the hump, the liver, and the sirloin strip.

Cooking

Despite considerable evidence relative to all aspects of cattle, beef and butchering, little is known about the cooking of beef in Ancient Egypt. One might expect roasted beef to have been the most common method of preparation, considering the numerous scenes of Egyptian cooks roasting fowl (Fig. 6.24). But presentations of roasting beef are rare;

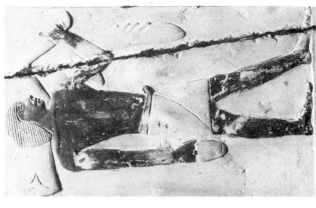

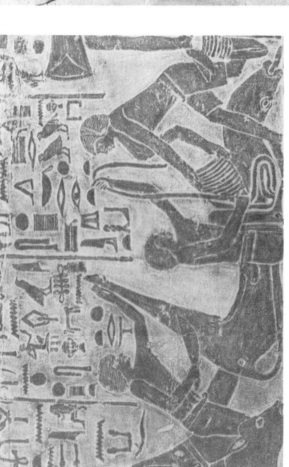

Fig. 3.38. (Left.) Removal of rib cage and intestines. Tomb of Ankh-ma-Hor at Saqqara; Old Kingdom, sixth dynasty, reign of King Teti, c. 2390 B.C. Rubbing by Ward Patterson; used with permission (1969).

Fig. 3.39. (Right.) Offering of a haunch and select organs. Tomb of Idut at Saqqara; Old Kingdom, fifth dynasty, reign of King Unas, c. 2423 B.C. Photographed 1969.

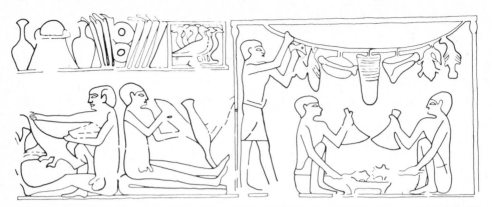

Fig. 3.40. The preparation, cooking and drying of beef and various fowl. Tomb of Pepi-Onkh at Meir; Old Kingdom, sixth dynasty, reign of King Pepi II, *c.* 2300 B.C. Redrawn from Blackman (1924, plate 8).

one example known to us is from the tomb of Ukh-hotp, son of Ukh-hotp at Meir (Fig. 3.44). The cooking method most commonly depicted was boiling (Figs 3.45 and 3.46). Egyptian terminology, however, indicates that roast "meat" was more common than its portrayal would suggest.[64]

It is most difficult to determine the reasons that would account for the practices of roasting fowl, as opposed to boiling beef and "meats". According to the Terabiyin bedouins, whose origins stem from northern Sinai, and who were interviewed by us in the summer of 1969, their women boil all meats (lamb, goat, desert game or beef when available), but roast fowl. This interesting custom, parallel with past practices, does not indicate a carry-over of Ancient Egyptian usage, and the reasons given for the custom by the Terabiyin are presented here out of interest. These Bedouins believe that boiling kills evil, possibly by removing it in the broth—hence, the supposed wholesomeness of boiled meat. Roasting is believed to preserve evil, possibly by hardening the crust over it. On the other hand, boiling may be preferred because it is less messy, and easier to carry out, especially when dealing with small morsels. These explanations, however, do not explain why Terabiyin roast fowl.

In concluding these remarks on cooking, one might mention that a new interpretation is now given by some archaeologists to a scene usually cited as "An Egyptian Kitchen from the Tomb of Rameses III" (Wilkinson, 1878, Vol. 2, p. 32), (Figs 3.47 and 3.48).

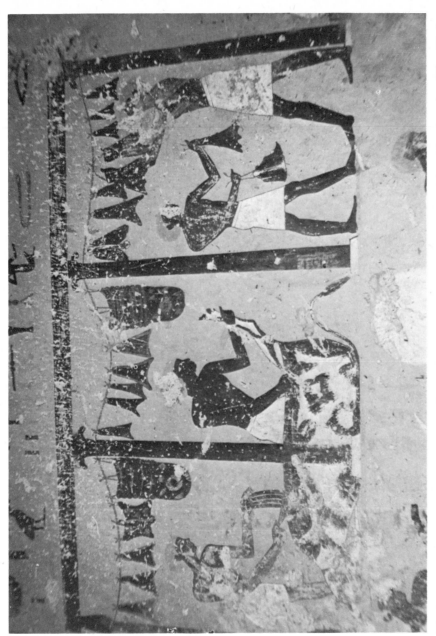

Fig. 3.41. The preparation and drying of cuts of beef including ribs and liver (?). Tomb of Antefoker (number 60) at Thebes (Upper enclosure); Middle Kingdom, twelfth dynasty, date uncertain. Photographed 1969.

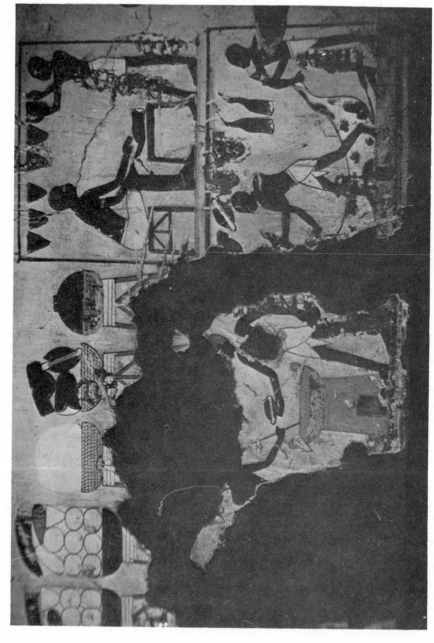

Fig. 3.42. The preparation, cooking, and drying of beef. Tomb of Menkheper (number 79) at Thebes (Upper Enclosure) New Kingdom, eighteenth dynasty; reign of King Thutmose III, *c.* 1475 B.C. Photographed 1969.

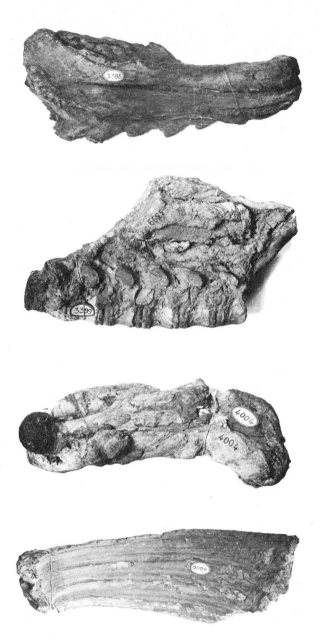

Fig. 3.43. Four preserved joints of beef. Dokki Agricultural Museum numbers 3398, 3399, 4000 and 4004; attributed to the tomb of Maher-Ra at Thebes; date uncertain. Photographed with permission of the Ministry of Agriculture and the officials of the Agricultural Museum, Dokki, ARE (1969).

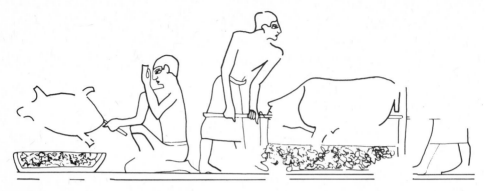

Fig. 3.44. Roasting. Tomb of Ukh-hotp son of Ukh-hotp at Meir; Middle Kingdom, date uncertain. Redrawn from Vandier (1964, Vol. 4, Fig. 121), after Blackman (1915b, pl. 23).

The original painting has suffered considerable damage since the time of Wilkinson, but it is still recognizable, and is being now regarded as a picture of a "candle-makers' shop".

Cattle and Medicine

Numerous medical prescriptions utilized diverse parts of the ox—liver, blood, horn, brain, spleen, grease and raw flesh. One of the most frequently encountered substances in the Egyptian medical papyri[65] is "ox-grease" (j).

In certain prescriptions it was to be ingested

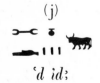

"... *To expel cough:* honey, ox-grease, yeast-water, roasted ammi, gum of acacia are ground together, boiled, and eaten at finger-warmth ..." (*Eb.*, LIV, 323)

More frequently, however, it was applied externally

"... *Remedy against burns:* manna, barley, rush-nut from the field, northern salt, *dbjt*,[66] papyrus, burnt leather, grease-of-ox, oil, wax, applied thereto after it is cooled; it is applied every day ..." (*Eb.*, LXVIII, 484)

Organs and blood of oxen were also important, and sometimes more than one was incorporated into the same formula

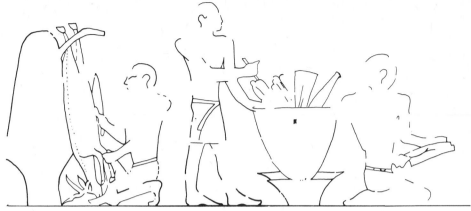

Fig. 3.45. Boiling. Tomb of Aba at Deir el Gebrawi; Old Kingdom, sixth dynasty, date uncertain. Redrawn from Davies (1902, plate 9).

"... *To soften the knee: ssk₃*,[66] lees of date-wine, fruit of *thw₃*,[66] northern salt, grease-of-ox, marrow-of-ox, meat-of-ox, spleen-of-ox, dregs of sweet beer, honey,*'f₃*,[66] myrtle (?); are closed together and [it] is bandaged therewith ..." (*Eb.*, LXXVII, 608)

One of these applications is of special interest

"... *For night blindness in the eyes:* liver-of-ox, roasted and crushed, is given against it. Really excellent! ..." (*Eb.*, LVII, 351)

In another papyrus, juice of pressed liver was similarly applied (*L.*, 35).

Unknown to the ancients, animal liver contains high quantities of vitamin A, which is effective against some forms of "night-blindness"; hence, application of "ox-liver" as stated in the *Ebers Papyrus* could have alleviated the disorder through local absorption of the vitamin, and given cause for the enthusiastic phrase inserted at the end of that specific prescription.

Raw meat, most commonly from oxen, was applied directly to wounds in order to keep them moist and supple. Such an application was an ideal haemostatic. It was especially popular in cases of animal bites.

"... *What is done for bites by a crocodile:* if thou examinest a crocodile bite, and thou findest that its flesh has been thrown aside and its two sides are separated, then thou shalt bandage it with fresh meat the first day ..." (*Eb.*, LXIV, 436)

Cow's milk was considered a powerful ingredient

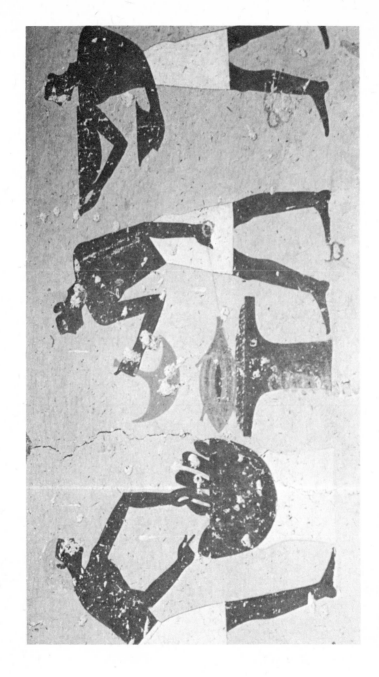

Fig. 3.46. Boiling meat and roasting fowl. Tomb of Antefoker (number 60) at Thebes (Upper Enclosure); Middle Kingdom. twelfth dynasty, date uncertain. Photographed 1969.

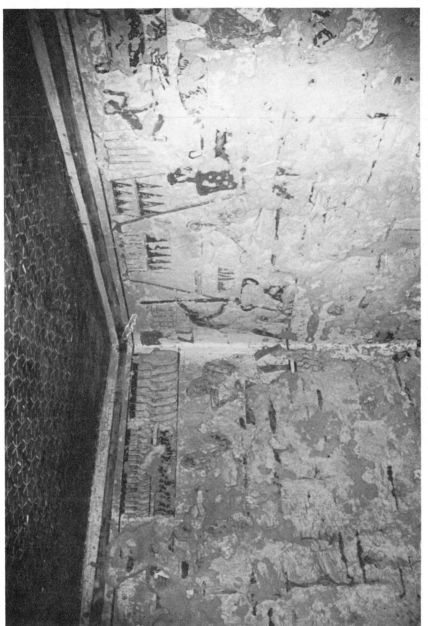

Fig. 3.47. "An Egyptian Kitchen"—Tomb of King Rameses III, at Thebes (Valley of the Kings). New Kingdom, twentieth dynasty, *c.* 1166 B.C., Possible modern interpretation: "An Egyptian candle-maker's shop". Photographed 1969.

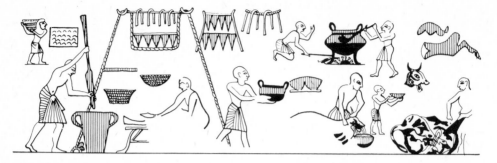

Fig. 3.48. "An Egyptian Kitchen"—Tomb of King Rameses III at Thebes (Valley of the Kings);
New Kingdom, twentieth dynasty, *c.* 1166 B.C. Redrawn from Wilkinson 1878, (Vol. 2, p. 32,
Fig. 300).

> "... *To empty the belly:* cow's milk, sycamore-fruit, honey, are ground fine,
> boiled,[67] and taken for four days ..." (*Eb.*, V–VI, 18)

Other prescriptions associated cow's milk with grease-of-ox in the
treatment of mouth disorders, for example, against a

> "tongue which is ill" (*Eb.*, LXXXV, 698)

and ulcers adjacent to the mouth

> "... *To expel eating ulcer on the gums and make the flesh grow:* cow's milk, fresh
> dates, manna, [it] remains during the night in the dew,[68] rinse the mouth
> for nine days ..." (*Eb.*, LXXXIX, 746)

Unspecified Meats

iw3 (k)   *iwf* (l)

References to the term "meat" are frequent in the literature of Ancient
Egypt and the reports of Greek and Roman visitors. Several terms, for
example, Egyptian hieroglyphs (k) and (l), and Greek *kreos*, were
used in an unspecific context and considered distinct from fowl and
fish. It may be justifiable to conclude that the term "meat" most usually
referred to beef.

Hayes (1964, p. 48), believed that meat was the primary component
of man's diet in Egypt before the agricultural revolution (prior to
5000 B.C.). This conforms to an interesting observation by Diodorus
(1, 43, 4) made during the first century B.C.

". . . they [the earliest Egyptians] also ate the flesh of some of the pasturing animals, using for clothing the skins of the beasts that were eaten . . ."

If one accepts the connotation of the English word "stew" as a preparation of vegetables with varying amounts of meat, and not as a technique of cooking, it might be proper here to include a report relative to the diet of Egyptian children of the first century B.C.

". . . they feed their children in a sort of happy-go-lucky fashion that, in its inexpensiveness, quite surpasses belief; for they serve them with stews made of any stuff that is ready to hand and cheap . . ." (*Diod.*, 1, 80, 5)

Unfortunately, Diodorus does not further discuss the ingredients of such preparations, and it might be argued that these were non-meat dishes; hence "meat-stew" as a component of Ancient Egyptian diet is still problematical.

One might well include sausage among the varieties of non-specific meat. The historical record concerning this food preparation is amazingly blank; no record known to us from the Dynastic Period discusses it. But during the Late Byzantine Period in Egypt, just prior to the Arab conquest in A.D. 641, a thriving "sausage-industry" existed in Middle Egypt, perhaps indicative of a longer history than the record immediately shows

". . . I accept at your hands the charge and responsibility for Aurelius, sausage-maker, of Antinoë, engaging that he shall remain here in Antinoë pursuing his trade of sausage-making without fault . . ." (*S.P.*, II, 364)

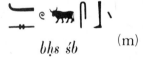

bḥs šb   (m)

Notes: Chapter 3

1. Castration of bulls, in Egyptian (m), has an ancient religious history and is mentioned in the Egyptian *Book of the Dead* ". . . I have come, and I have smitten for thee emasculated beasts . . ." (Budge, 1949, p. 591). It is also mentioned in the *Leyden Papyrus* (350, Rs 2, 5, D19), *Anastase Papyrus* (IV, 15, 5), and in a New Kingdom command to make preparations for Pharaoh's arrival ". . . oxen, five castrated, short-horned cattle of the west . . ." (Caminos, 1954).

2. Egypt was divided into regional districts as early as the Old Kingdom. The Egyptian word for "district" or "province" was (n), *spt* or (o). The word nome, today used in Egyptology, stems from the Greek *Nomos*.

(n)   (o)

iš

3. See also Chapter 1, pp. 30–36.
4. Egyptian princes and army commanders were deprecated by the Ethiopian King Piʿ-Ankhi who invaded Egypt *c.* 716 B.C. in a phrase that appears on his triumphal stele "... thou makest bulls into women ..." (Breasted, 1906, Vol. 4, p. 883); see also Chapter 7, p. 394.
5. Attributed to King Thutmose III (eighteenth dynasty, *c.* 1475 B.C.).
6. Nilotic tribes to honour a guest or a chief still grant him a "bull's name".
7. A rope secured to a weight which, when twirled, entangles the feet of running game.
8. Cats (*Felis chaus*) appear to have been used by Egyptian fowlers during the New Kingdom.
9. Al Demiry (I, 186) wrote in the fourteenth century A.D. "There are in the land of Egypt cows called *Baqar el kheiss* with long necks, crescentic horns and giving abundant milk."
10. It is difficult to ascertain the relative barter or trade value of a bull, calf, cow or ox. One record dated to the New Kingdom states that a bull fetched between 30 and 120 deben (1 deben = approximately 91 grams) of copper, depending upon quality (Kees, 1961, p. 89); see also Chapter 2, pp. 53, 54.
11. Ruffer (1919, p. 9) states that animals to be slaughtered for daily consumption were often stable fed.
12. Compare the obvious discrepancies between the photograph taken in the summer of 1969 and the sketch by Wilkinson (Figs 3.18 and 3.19).
13. Shallow papyrus boats, the variety commonly illustrated in Egyptian tombs, were not used for normal Nile river transport, but were generally restricted to the marshy Delta regions.
14. See Note 1.
15. Investigation into the origins of cow worship is ancient. Plutarch (*I. and O.*, 380, 74, F) during the first century A.D., wrote "... It is clear that the Egyptians have honoured the cow, the sheep, and the ichneumon [mongoose] because of their need for these animals and their usefulness ..."

16. Another image described the floor of heaven as a pierced plate of iron through which were hung the "Lamps of Heaven" (Budge, 1960, p. 131). A parallel modern Turkish tradition regards stars as the shining heads of the countless nails inserted into the sky to hold it up (Reynolds, 1969, personal communication).

17. The golden sun, reflecting its light upon the Egyptian fields flooded with the reddish inundation waters, sometimes appears dazzling red. This is perhaps one origin for this myth.

18. A similar tale is told regarding the goddess Sekhmet. Sekhmet, the wind, came into Egypt from Nubia, blowing with rage. But as she reached Upper Egypt, she was gradually calmed and transformed herself into the kind and merry Hathor. Clark (1959, p. 182) comments that Sekhmet represents a pun on the word depicted by (p) that meant power or control.

(p)

shm

19. Aelian, who discussed at length various aspects of the Egyptian sacred bulls, suspected that some of his readers would doubt his veracity. ". . . for I am stating what the practice is with these bulls, and what then occurred, and what I hear the Egyptians say—[for] a lie to them is an abomination . . ." (11, 11).

20. Chapter 1, p. 43.

21. Kaiechos is the Greek phonetic equivalent of the Egyptian king, Kakau. The chronologic position of this king is uncertain for it is not known whether he belonged to the first or second dynasty. He is tenth on the Abydos King list, and fourth on the Saqqara Tables.

22. Chapter 1, p. 43.

23. Meaning the twelfth year of that particular reign.

24. Breasted suggested restoring the name of Mievis

25. Persephone, daughter of the goddess Demeter was abducted by Hades. The distressed Demeter, in her search for her missing girl, came to Eleusis where Triptolemus (Table 3, p 164), son of King Celeus, came to her aid For his help, he was given the gift of agriculture, and sent on a world-wide journey to bring this knowledge to mankind (summarized from Graves, 1955, 24, A–M).

26. From Phrygia, a country of Asia Minor.

27. See p. 134.

28. There were apparently several heroes of this name, the best known being the son of Alcmene, famed for his vast progeney and for this "twelve labours" But an "Egyptian" Heracles was also the subject of Ancient Greek writings ". . . Heracles, for instance, was by birth an Egyptian who, by virtue of his manly vigour, visited a large part of the inhabited world—the son of Alcmene, who was born more than ten thousand years later was called Alcaeus at birth—Heracles cleared the earth of wild beasts . . ." (*Diod.*, 1, 24, 1–8).

29. Phylarchus of Naucratis (?) flourished during the third century B.C.

Table 3

Interplay between Egyptian, Greek, and Phoenician mythology

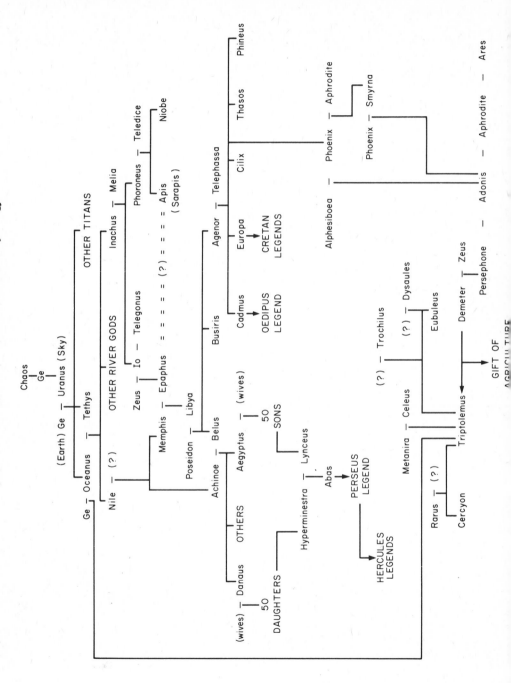

30. Dionysus and Osiris were repeatedly equated by Ancient Greek and Roman authors, for both myths sprang from the same human experience with suffering and hope. Both Osiris and Dionysus suffered tragic deaths from which they arose, like their incarnations the vine and wheat. Thus through their birth-death-rebirth, they offered mankind the consoling beliefs in immortality and in a better life thereafter.

31. Among the Ancient Egyptians celestial fire had long been believed a divine impregnating agent. A coffin text has recently been interpreted to mean that Isis was impregnated by fire or lightning (Faulkner, 1968, p. 40.)

32. Bronze statues of Apis show the protective bird not as an eagle but as a vulture (see also Chapter 6, p. 326).

33. Compare with the report for Buchis, p. 136.

34. The Egyptian "Dung Beetle" was personified by the god, Kheper, who was visualized as a gigantic invisible beetle that rolled the sun across the sky (Fig. 1.10)

35. Such a large number possibly represents later astronomic interpretations, each mark representing a day of the lunar month.

36. Ball (1942, p. 51) situates Nilopolis at modern Ballas.

37. Such women were possibly barren, and believed that exposing themselves to the bull facilitated conception. Similar parallels are known throughout Egypt and the Middle East today. In the Egyptian city of Tanta, barren women make a pilgrimage to the shrine of Sheik Ahmad el Badawi where the walls inside the burial room have been heavily polished, rubbed by women who wish to conceive. Others surreptitiously enter the Cairo Museum or an Egyptian tomb where they may step over a mummy. Some spend the night in a holy place, as they did, until recently in the tombs of the Bektashi, east of Cairo, at the edge of the Moqattam Hills. A common belief among Kuwaity sailors and pearl fishermen holds that a barren woman will conceive if she steps over the first timber laid for the keel of a new ship. If this be allowed, however, it is believed that one of the crew must forfeit his life in exchange for the new life of the child—hence the keels are heavily guarded during construction (Freeth, 1956, p. 106).

    This behaviour of Egyptian women had notable antecedents. Hathor uncovered herself in front of her father Ra; and this may be the origin of the legend, told by Clement of Alexandria, of the Eleusian goddess Baubo unveiling her nakedness in front of the mourning Demeter to distract her sorrow. Could it also account for the eighth century A.D. story of the Japanese dancer, Uzume, who rejoiced by the same sight the eight hundred myriads of gods? (Lefebvre, 1949, p. 181).

38. Pliny (8, 71, 186) reported a slightly different version: "... once a year a cow is displayed to it, she too with her decorations, although they are not the same as his, and it is traditional for her always to be found and put to death on the same day ...".

39. A reference to the Pythoness, high priestess of Apollo at his temple at Delphi, who was reported to rest astride a religious tripod suspended over a rock cleft, from which vapours arose sending her into prophetic trances.

40. Germanicus Caesar was victorious in Europe, which led to his being declared Emperor of the East. His success caused suspicion and envy in Tiberius, and the Roman emperor ordered him to be poisoned (Lemprière, 1963, p. 252). When Germanicus was rebuffed by Apis during his visit to Egypt in A.D. 19 prior to the mysterious poisoning, the reported "prophecy" brought increased fame to Apis.

41. Aelian (11, 10) also makes this observation in regard to Nile water. Some Egyptian peasants today believe in the nurturing effects of Nile water. They regret the clearing effect produced by the Nile dams which eliminate some of the suspended solids; they believe filtered water causes impotence.

42. The "king-must-die" motif where the god (or ruler) is slain before senility is a facet of Egyptian religious thought dating to the earliest times (see Chapter 1, note 4).

43. According to Plutarch, *I. and O.*, 374, 56, A–B) Apis was not allowed to live more than twenty-five years ". . . five makes a square of itself as many as the letters of the Egyptian alphabet, and as many as the years of the life of the Apis . . ."

44. The discrepancy may represent a shift in custom through time, for over 500 years separated Herodotus from Lucian.

45. The name "Serapeum" is a late appellation. It is unclear how the Ancient Egyptians of the New Kingdom termed this burial site.

46. Both Plutarch, (*I. and O.*, 362, 28, A) and Clement of Alexandria (*Exhortation to the Greeks*, 4, 42) state that Serapis was a god native to Sinope, a seaport city of Asia Minor.

47. Ames (1965, p. 149) offers as an interesting possibility that the emphasis placed by the earliest Christians on the role of Mary, mother of Christ, was a reflection of widespread beliefs and acceptance of Isis worship during the Roman Period. Throughout their history, Egyptians viewed new gods simply as manifestations of older ones, and easily fused them with older deities into new synthetic ones, like Amon-Ra, etc. This custom avoided many problems that plagued less tolerant faiths. The only exception occurred under the eighteenth dynasty rise of Aten worship, when Akhenaten declared Aten the only god, with resulting widespread religious unrest and open revolution. Naturally, such syncretic tendencies as manifested themselves in the Serapis-Apis cult, facilitated Christian development and expansion in Egypt. The tolerant Egyptians readily adopted the Christian concept of resurrection and immortality, that was already a solid part of this faith, and explained several observable natural cycles, such as the daily birth, disappearance,

and rebirth of the sun, and the lore of the dung beetle carrying every morning out of its burrow a ball of dung, that was compared to the sun disc (note 34). Even seeds, seemingly dead, could grow again and flourish. In Egypt today there is a tradition, especially among Copts, Greeks, Armenians and other groups, of planting between Christmas and the New Year, quick sprouting seeds such as lentils, wheat, or barley, in shallow pans or clay pots which are then watered and allowed to sprout; and the many such tiny "gardens", prominently displayed in season in homes, offices, and shops, curiously remind one of the "vegetating Osiris" beds.

48. According to Ames (1965, p. 128) two bulls bore this name, one at Heliopolis and the other at Meroe in the Sudan.

49. *F.*, 112.

50. A combination of the sun gods, Ra and Atum, the latter a creative god and a manifestation of the "accomplished" or setting sun.

51. Possibly Bekenranef (twenty-fourth dynasty, *c.* 720 B.C.).

52. Compare with p. 131.

53. Tongue examination is the classic manner by which cysticercosis is now diagnosed. Noting the mark which "identified" the Apis would not only have prevented the sacred bull from being slaughtered but, possibly also, an infected animal from being consumed.

54. Diodorus believed that the red oxen were sacrificed by the Egyptians as a revenge from Seth: ". . . this was the colour of Typhon [Seth] who plotted against Osiris and was then punished by Isis for the death of her husband . . ." (1, 88, 4–5).

55. See branding discussion on p. 109.

56. See discussion of the *wabw* priests in Ghalioungui (1963, pp. 68, 105). Ire-Nakhty was one such "pure-priest" (*wab*), his name and titles appear in the tomb of Ptahhetep at Saqqara (fifth dynasty, reign of King Djed-Ka-Re (Isesi), *c.* 2500 B.C.), where he is shown smelling blood to certify its purity (Ghalioungui and Dawakhly, 1965, plate 5). As noted on p. 144, blood was not impure to the Ancient Egyptians. But Greek tradition held that bulls' blood, if drunk, caused death by choking or suffocation (*Her.*, III, 15). In Greek mythology, Aeson, father of Jason, leader of the Greek Argonauts, reportedly committed suicide by drinking bulls' blood (Graves, 1955, 155, A).

57. This Greek description of Egyptian sacrifice is in part substantiated by a papyrus dated to the second century A.D. ". . . articles for the sacrifice to the most sacred Nile on Pauni 30: 1 calf, 2 jars of sweet smelling wine, 16 wafers, 16 garlands, 16 pine-cones, 16 cakes, 16 green palm branches, 16 reeds, likewise oil, honey, milk, every spice except frankincense . . .' (*S.R.*, II, 403).

58. Corn as understood in the United States is *Zea mays* (see Chapter 12).

The historical significance of the confusion in relation to maize and pellagra is discussed by Patwardhan and Darby (1972, pp. 34–56).

59. Lake Tritonis figures prominently in the Greek legend of the Argonauts (Graves, 1955, 154, E). Graves situates it in the vast salt-marsh region of southeastern Tunisia.

60. After Barca, an ancient city in north central Libya.

61. Moses was prudent in his consideration for Ancient Egyptian beliefs. As reported by Diodorus (1, 83, 8–9) some foreigners who ignored or accidentally broke local Egyptian traditions relative to sacred animals, were occasionally stoned to death.

62. A text in the tomb of Meryet-Amun, wife (?) of King Amenhotep II listed 21 "steak cutlets", 3 beef hearts, and 1 duck-leg as preferred meats (Winlock, 1932, p. 28).

63. A mina was equal to approximately 16 ounces.

64. The Egyptian term depicted by (q) signified "roast-joint" (*F.*, 6; *G.*, 550).

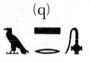

65. The Ancient Egyptian medical papyri bear the names of their finder, of their editor, or of the museums where they are now deposited. Among these documents are the *Ebers Papyrus, Berlin Papyrus, Hearst Papyrus, Edwin Smith Surgical Papyrus, Kahun Papyrus,* and several other documents. The longest and most useful is the *Ebers Papyrus* dated *c.* 1550 B.C. (Ebbell, 1937).

Since the successive translations of this papyrus are quite variable in accuracy and quality, and we shall often refer to it, a brief summary of the editions follows:

Joachim (1890) is outdated and many of his names for animals, plants, foods, and other ingredients are purely conjectural;

Wreszinski (1913) did not produce a translation, but an accurate transliteration of the original hieratic papyrus into hieroglyphic writing, that allowed widespread distribution of the content to scholars;

Bryan (1930) published an English translation based upon the Joachim edition, not upon the original document or its hieroglyphic transliteration. Much adverse comment directed towards this work is unwarranted since his primary aim was not to produce an exacting critical translation but to bring the medical facets of Egyptology to a wide interested audience. His jocularity, however, was received with little favour by Egyptologists;

Ebbell (1937) based his translation on the Wreszinski edition. His is perhaps the most readily available, although it too has received severe criticism of late because of his bold medical, zoological and botanical interpretations;

Von Deines and Grapow (1959, Vol. 6) correlated all known usage of specific Ancient Egyptian medical terms with translations known at present. Their compilation is the standard form for cross-reference to the Wreszinski working copy.

66. Unknown Egyptian products.

67. One should be interested in any historical medical traditions which utilized boiling. Did the Ancients observe that some preparations had a greater effect when boiled, or was this pure chance? Few contemplate the vast change in European public health after the return of Marco Polo from China and the establishment of a tea trade with the East— water had to be boiled in order to prepare tea.

68. See Chapter 4, and note 36, Chapter 4.

Chapter 4   *Meat: Pork*

Introduction

Pork is, in different cultures, the object of either the widest consumption, or of the most intense abhorrence. Examination of the basis of such divergent attitudes is of interest. The origin of pork avoidance in the Middle East, reflected in the Mosaic and Koranic bans, is attributed frequently to a collective historical experience that those who consumed pork contracted trichinosis, while those who abstained did not.

Trichinosis is an infestation with a microscopic parasitic worm, *Trichina* (*Trichinella*) *spiralis*, that may be found coiled in cysts in the muscles of man, rat or pig. When undercooked infected meat is eaten, the cyst is digested, viable parasites mature, reproduce, and deposit larvae in the intestinal mucosa. These are then disseminated by the lymphatics and blood to other tissues, especially skeletal muscle, where they again encyst. The patient experiences diarrhoea during the intestinal stage; then during migration, nausea, colic and fever; followed, in the tissular stage, by pain, stiffness, swelling (especially periorbital), sweating and insomnia.

Prohibition of pork may well have protected against this parasitic infection, but it is a naive over-simplification to attribute the establishment of Mosaic and Koranic food laws by the Ancients to their understanding of the aetiology of this disease. The cause and effect relationship between ingestion of undercooked pork and trichinosis was not established until the last century. Small calcified cysts, probably of *Trichina*, were first seen by Tiedemann (1821) according to Cobbold, Henle and others (see Cobbold, 1866), and later by Hilton (1833, p. 605) who thought they were small cysticerci. Not until Paget (1835), as a young first year medical student, investigated the contents of the cyst and found the "coiled worm," did the cysts attract more than a passing general comment. The organism was described and named by Owen (1835, pp. 315–325), who received sample material from Paget. Thus, prior to 1822, these cysts were regarded only as surgical nuisances, objects that blunted scalpels during dissection or operations and, as late as 1835, they were still considered benign, unrelated to general disease (Foster, 1965, pp. 68–79; Gould, 1945, pp. 3–17). Credit for first linking the disease with swine may be attributed to Leidy (1846, pp. 107–108), but Zenker (1860, pp. 561–572) presented the detailed information that established the relationship between ingestion of raw pork and intestinal and muscular infestation with trichinae (see Herbst, 1851; Davaine, 1860; Leuckart, 1866; Paget, 1866).

Both domestic and wild species of many animals, e.g. cattle, sheep, goats and various varieties of fish and fowl, serve as hosts for a multitude of diseases directly transmissible to man. In some of these the relationship between a disease and contact with, or consumption of the meat, is more readily apparent than in the case of swine; yet, for these species no dietary avoidance patterns are observed. Nor are there any taboos prescribed in ancient religions; Egyptian, Judaism, Christianity or Islam in regard to clearly recognizable toxic plants such as aconite, datura, or varieties of toxic mushroom, all of which are more acutely and manifestly lethal than trichina-infected meat. Consequently, one must search elsewhere in cultural history for the origins of pork avoidance. It is enlightening in this regard to examine the long history of swine in Egypt and the relevant facets of other eastern Mediterranean cultures.

Pork in Pre-Dynastic Egypt. The North and the South

During the late Paleolithic/Mesolithic Period, early peoples in Lower Egypt living in the vicinity of Helwan feasted on pork, as evidenced by finds of pig bones at this site[1] (Hayes, 1964, p. 71). Along the shores of Lake Moeris, Neolithic settlers hunted pig, as indicated by the archaeological investigations of Caton-Thompson and Gardner (1934, pp. 25 and 34) who found pig bones in the Fayoum "A" sequences. At neither of these sites, Fayoum or Helwan, however, were swine domesticated, and archaeologists have attributed these remains to wild forms (Caton-Thompson and Gardner, 1934, p. 89).

The date of the first appearance of domestic swine in Egypt is debatable.[2] It is known, however, that the early settlers (*c.* 5000 B.C.) at the western Delta site of El Merimda Beni Salama consumed great quantities of pork, as revealed by numerous remains of bones (Junker,

1929, p. 218). Indeed, several archaeologists have concluded that pork consumption was one of the characteristics of this culture[3]: but since a detailed study of these bones has not been made, it is debatable whether the Merimda remains came from hunted or domestic swine.

Subsequent investigations have unearthed pig bones from other Lower Egyptian Pre-Dynastic settlements such as El Omari (Debono, 1948, p. 567) and Maadi (Menghin and Amer, 1932, p. 52), a probable indication that, there, swine were raised and utilized as food. In Lower Egypt, therefore, the historical continuity of pork consumption is attested from *c.* 5000 B.C. until the period of unification, *c.* 3200 B.C.

Parallel information from Upper Egypt is more sketchy. That wild pigs were probably hunted[4] during the Late Paleolithic Sebilian horizon is indicated by the findings of bones of *Sus* sp. in strata correlated to this level (Sandford, 1934, p. 86; Gaillard, 1934, pp. 66–72). Pig bones have also been identified from Badarian sequences (Brunton and Caton-Thompson, 1928, p. 77). From later Pre-Dynastic settlements in Upper Egypt information is even more incomplete; but bones have been reported in excavations at Armant (Mond *et al.*, 1937, p. 258), Toukh (Ruffer, 1919, p. 22; Gaillard, 1934, pp. 66–72) and Abydos (Mond *et al.*, 1937, p. 258).

If all evidence known at present be considered, finds of pig bones in Pre-Dynastic levels in Upper Egypt appear to be rare, whereas they are a prominent feature in corresponding chronologic levels in Lower Egypt. So large is the difference between the two areas that the raising of pigs and consumption of pork appear to be a major distinguishing characteristic of the northern peoples (Menghin and Amer, 1932, p. 52; Kees, 1961, p. 91).

Evidence of Pork Avoidance during the Dynastic Period

After the conquest of the northern lands by the southerners, which ushered in the Dynastic Period of Egyptian history, the evidence for pork consumption in Lower Egypt nearly disappears, however, and a major shift in custom and tradition is immediately obvious. One possible explanation of this change is the assimilation by the northerners of the cultural and dietary traditions of the southern conquerors, that might have reflected some facets of southern religion and mythology.

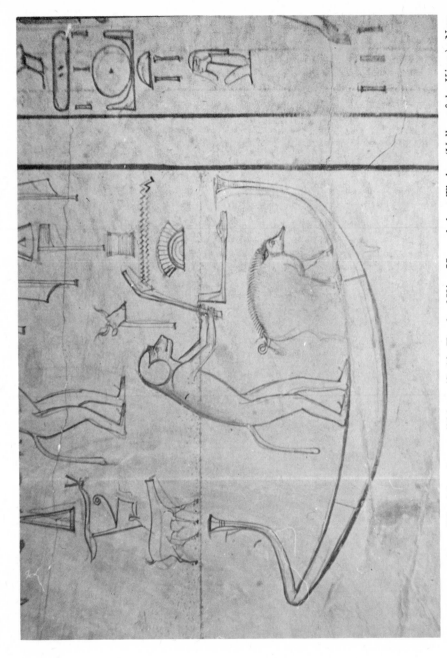

Fig. 4.1. The baboon (Thot) beating a wild boar (Seth). Tomb of King Horemheb at Thebes (Valley of the Kings); New Kingdom, nineteenth dynasty, c. 1320 B.C. Photographed 1969.

The conquest of the north might have thus ended the predominantly accepted position of swine in the Lower Egyptian dietaries. Although a complete ban on pork by the whole of Egyptian society did not result, it is apparent that swine were relegated to a position of religious disfavour. It may be concluded that the disappearance of any remains pertaining to the once flourishing "swine industry" is not simply a historical artifact, but that it represents dietary restrictions in practice near 2,000 years before codification of Mosaic pork traditions.

During the Middle Kingdom (2200–1580 B.C.) we know of no information that would indicate the existence of a codified or implied pork taboo. Under the New Kingdom (*c.* 1341 B.C.), however, evidence of such a taboo appears again. The tomb of Horemheb, the burial sarcophagus of Seti I, and the tomb of Rameses VI, all kings of the nineteenth dynasty, present inscriptions indicative of an Osirian oriented deprecation of the god Seth and of swine. One motif illustrates the god Osiris seated before a boat on which a boar, a manifestation of Seth, is beaten by the baboon-shaped Thot, god of knowledge and secret science. The accompanying text makes clear the unfavourable attitude towards Seth and his animal (Fig. 4.1).

This attitude is further confirmed by other texts from the *Book of the Dead*

". . . and he [the deceased] shall present as offerings oxen, and feathered fowl, and incense, and cakes, and ale, and garden herbs. And behold, thou shalt draw a presentation of this in colour upon a new tile moulded from earth upon which neither a pig nor any other animal hath trodden . . ." (*Papyrus of Nu: Book of the Dead*, Chapter 125, Rubric 47; Budge, 1949, p. 377; Barguet, 1967, p. 164.)

Although the silent voice argument is the weakest of the methods used in historical and archaeological interpretation (see Chapter 1, p. 29), it nevertheless offers an interesting relevant point during the New Kingdom. Dawson (1928, p. 599) believes it significant that the Harris Papyrus (*A.R.*, IV, 151–412) dated to the nineteenth dynasty, in a description of the religious and temple offerings made by King Rameses III (*c.* 1198–1166 B.C.), omits pork, although it includes extensive lists of animals, meats, plants, fruits, spices, minerals, and other goods deemed desirable offerings or sacrifices to the Egyptian gods. This extensive list possibly represents most of the desirable items found in Ancient Egypt and the conquered lands!

Late and Post-Dynastic Evidence

Evidence presented by Greek travellers overlaps in time the Dynastic
Period. During the first Persian occupation (twenty-seventh dynasty
522–404 B.C.) Herodotus visited Egypt and became acquainted through
priests and other informants with a wide variety of beliefs and attitudes
relative to swine

> ". . . the pig is regarded among them as an unclean animal, so much so
> that if a man in passing accidentally touch a pig, he instantly hurries to
> the river and plunges in with all his clothes on . . ." (II, 47)

Concerning the social position of swineherds during the twenty-
seventh dynasty Herodotus writes

> ". . . the swineherds, notwithstanding that they are of pure Egyptian
> blood, are forbidden to enter into any of the temples, which are open to
> all other Egyptians, and further, no one will give his daughter in marriage
> to a swineherd, or take a wife from among them, so that the swineherds
> are forced to intermarry among themselves . . ." (II, 47)

Discussing sacrificial offerings of pigs, Herodotus, who was familiar
with Persian methods of pig sacrifice as practiced at Babylon[6] (compare
Herodotus 1, 183 and Athenaeus 9, 396, C), stated

> ". . . they do not offer swine in sacrifice to any of their gods, excepting
> Bacchus [Osiris] and the Moon[7] [Horus] whom they honor in this way at
> the same time, sacrificing pigs to both of them at the same full moon, and
> afterwards eating of the flesh . . ." (II, 47)

According to Graves (1955, 2, 126, 1) boars were sacred to the moon
because of their crescentic tusks.

It is not certain from the text of Herodotus whether the event he
described was annual or monthly. Aelian, who wrote nearly six hundred
years later than Herodotus, believed it to be an annual festival

> ". . . and the Egyptians are convinced that the sow is an abomination to
> the sun and moon. Accordingly, when they hold the festival of the moon,
> they sacrifice pigs to her once a year, but at no other seasons are they
> willing to sacrifice them either to her or to any other god . . ." (10, 16)

Another consideration relative to religious sacrifice of swine is mentioned by Herodotus (II, 47)

". . . the remainder of the flesh is eaten on the same day that the sacrifice is offered, which is the day of the full moon; at any other time they would not so much as taste it . . ."

Herodotus then discussed the activities of the common man relative to this same feast, further revealing the relatively low status of the swineherd during this period

". . . to Bacchus [Osiris] on the eve of his feast, every Egyptian sacrifices a hog before the door of his house,[7] which is then given back to the swineherd by whom it was furnished and by him carried away . . ."

In his description, he inserts a puzzling passage

". . . there is a reason alleged by them [the Egyptians] for their detestation of swine at all other seasons, and their use of them at this festival; with which I am well acquainted, but which I do not think it proper to mention . . ." (II, 47)

This silent reason, perhaps his obligation to secrecy and his scrupulous respect to preserve the mysterious sacrificial rites at Eleusis,[8] if revealed, might have unlocked for twentieth century investigators the door to better understanding of the customs, manners, and taboos relative to swine as food and, thereby, provided clearer insight into present day dietary laws.[9]

Manetho (middle third century B.C.) is also known to have discussed swine. Aelian (10, 16) preserves a literary fragment, attributed to him, that describes one reason why pork was avoided in Egypt during his time

". . . and I learn that Manetho, the Egyptian, a man who attained the very summit of knowledge, says that one who has tasted of sow's milk becomes covered with leprosy and scaly diseases . . ."

As an example of parallel themes developed in different cultures, Plutarch (*I. and O.*, 353, 8) wrote

". . . the bodies of those who drink it [swine's milk] break out with leprosy and scabrous things."

Greek mythology offers a similar association between swine and leprosy. It relates that Teuthras, King of Teuthrania in Mysia, flushed a boar while hunting. The creature shouted

"Save me; I am the nurse of the goddess Artemis."

But the king ignored the plea and killed it; whereupon Artemis, enraged at this inconsiderate deed, inflicted leprous scabs on Teuthras (Graves, 1955, Vol. 2, 141, h).

From a historical viewpoint it is an extraordinary fact that the alleged relationship between swine and leprosy was accepted as common knowledge in Europe even into the nineteenth century. Nearly twenty-one centuries after the report of Manetho, Sonnini, a French traveller to Egypt during the late eighteenth century, wrote

". . . the vast quantity of fat with which this animal [pig] is loaded—renders the Egyptians more liable than elsewhere to the leprosy—Such a disposition as this was more than sufficient to inspire Egyptians with detestation at a species of animal—the Egyptians thought it was absolutely requisite to abstain altogether from this sort of food . . ." (1799, Vol. 3, pp. 254–255)

Even today, this belief persists in parts of Asia (see Gaster, 1959, p. 130).

Plutarch (*I. and O.*, 353, 8, F), however, offered an unusual reason for pork avoidance in Egypt

". . . in like manner they [the Egyptians] hold the pig to be an unclean animal, because it is reputed to be most inclined to mate at the waning of the moon . . ."

This explanation reflects on Egyptian mythologic belief concerning the attack and mutilation of the "Eye-of-Horus" (the Moon) by Seth; an event heralded as temporary dominance of the forces of evil over the forces of good. Any animal inclined to procreate at a time when "evil was upon the land" would be considered obscene and to be avoided. Plutarchus further stated that Egyptian priests absolutely avoided pork

". . . the priests feel such repugnance for things that are of a superfluous nature that they not only eschew most legumes, as well as mutton and pork, which leaves a large residuum, but they also use no salt . . ." (*I. and O.*, 353, 5, F)

Athenaeus (7, 299, F-7, 300, A), on the authority of Anaxandrides of Cameirus, reports a dialogue of a Greek with an Egyptian

"I couldn't bring myself to be an ally of yours, for neither our manners nor our customs agree . . . you eat no pork, but I like it very much . . ."

Literary references are not, however, the sole source of information pertaining to pork avoidance during the Post-Dynastic period in Egypt. The temple of Edfu (237–57 B.C.) contains battle scenes illustrating the conflict between Horus and Seth, where Seth is shown at times as a hippopotamus, and at other times as a pig (Fig. 4.2). The latter clearly

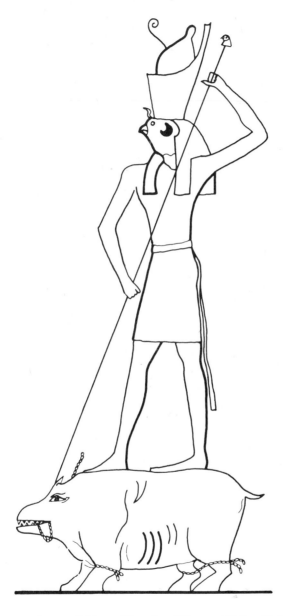

Fig. 4.2. Horus spearing a wild boar. Temple of Horus at Edfu; Ptolemaic-Roman Period. Redrawn after Budge.

illustrate that swine were abhorred during this late period, and at this geographic locality—the site of the traditional battle between the two religious adversaries.

The temple to the god Mandulis built at Kalabsha[10] in Nubia during the reign of Augustus (Octavianus) likewise contains an edict attributed to Aurelius Besarion, governor of Elephantine and Ombos dated to A.D. 248 wherein the governor ordered that pigs be kept away from the sanctuary of the nome of Talmis (Gauthier, 1911, Vol. 1, p. 193).

Evidence of Pork Tolerance in Egypt

Dynastic Period

Ruffer (1919, p. 21), one of the early authorities on food and diet in Ancient Egypt, did not believe that swine were universally condemned or considered abominable during the Old Kingdom. He cites as proof of acceptance examples of slate cosmetic palettes carved in the silhouette of a pig, and dated to the early dynasties of the Old Kingdom. He argues that had the pig been considered repulsive and an animal to be avoided, no Egyptian woman would wish to use paint from a palette in the shape of such an unpleasant creature.

Newberry (1928, p. 211), on the authority of Sethe (1932, 1, 3, 1), discusses the earliest known literary mention of swine in Egypt, a biographic record attributed to Methen, a noble of the third dynasty. The Breasted translation of this biography (*A.R.*, I, 171) tells that after the death of Methen's father, Anubisemonekh, the son was given people (servants) and small-cattle. These latter are considered to be swine since they appear with the hieroglyphic determinative of a pig. It may be assumed that since the two nobles participated in Egyptian religious rites and ceremonies, their association with swine would imply that pigs were raised in this instance without stigma.

Another important indication of a permissive attitude towards swine during parts of the Old Kingdom are the several porcelain pigs (Fig. 4.3) dated no later than the fourth dynasty, found *inside* the sacred compound of Osiris at Abydos, the burial place of the heart of the god and a seat of Osiris worship for all of Egypt (Petrie *et al.*, 1903, p. 25).

Furthermore, according to some traditions, the god Min, most commonly associated with the city of Coptos in Upper Egypt, but widely

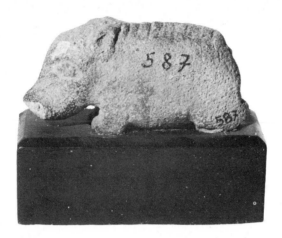

Fig. 4.3. Statuette of a sow. Abydos; Old Kingdom, date uncertain (pre-fourth dynasty). Photographed with permission of the Ministry of Agriculture and the officials of the Agricultural Museum, Dokki, ARE (1969).

accepted as a minor deity throughout much of Egypt, was born of a white sow (Newberry, 1928, p. 214), a genealogy that would have gained little acceptance had swine been held in contempt throughout all the country. There is a possibility, also, that Min might be linked to a region near Meidum, known during the fourth dynasty as (a), or "Domain-of-the-white-sow" (Jacquet-Gordon, 1962, p. 446), a region where evidence that swine were tolerated is seen in the third to fourth dynasty tomb of Nefemmaet (Nefermaat) at Meidum, in which swine figure as hieroglyphic determinatives (Petrie, 1892, plate 21).

(a)

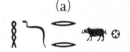

Slightly later, Seth, represented in the form of a pig, with erect bristles along his back, appears in the Annals of King Sahure (second king of the fifth dynasty), inscribed in the Palermo stone (Figs 1.20, 1.21), implying a permissive attitude towards swine at this time (Newberry, 1928, p. 214). All such evidence indicates that the cult of Osiris/Horus was not uniformly accepted throughout the land, nor by all kings of the Old Kingdom.

Pictorial evidence which would support a tolerant attitude toward swine in the Old Kingdom is confused. A controversial relief (Fig. 4.4) found in the sixth dynasty tomb of Ka-Gem-Ni at Saqqara (reign of King Teti, *c.* 2423 B.C.), was described by Firth and Gunn (1926, Vol. 1, p. 114) as that of a "young dog," while the earlier monographs by von Bissing and co-authors (1905–1911) did not elaborate on the relief.

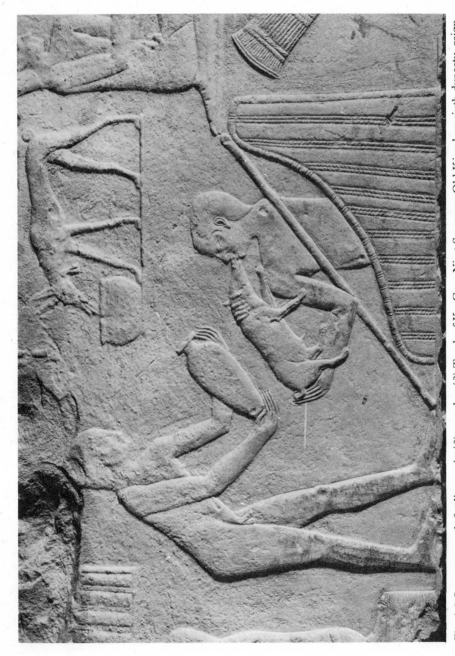

Fig. 4.4. Servant mouth-feeding a pig (?) or a dog (?) Tomb of Ka-Gem-Ni at Saqqara; Old Kingdom sixth dynasty, reign of King Teti, *c.* 2390 B.C. Photographed 1969.

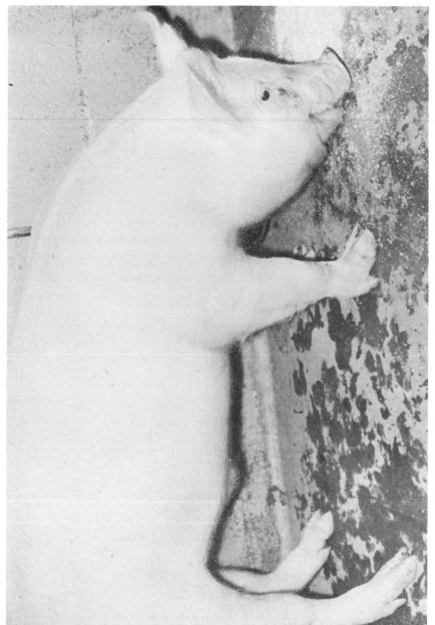

Fig. 4.5. Pig with weak or broken pasterns. Courtesy of Dr Richard Barnes.

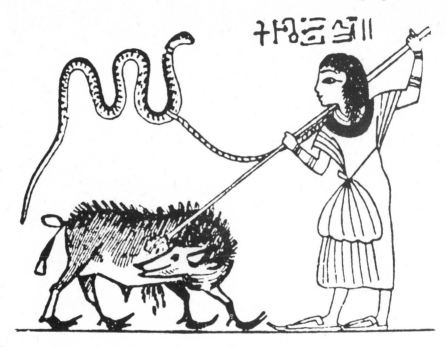

Fig. 4.6. The deceased spearing a pig. Note the pig's feet. Reproduced from Budge (1949) p. 162.

The question that archaeologists and zoologists have been unable to solve is whether the animal represented is a pig, a dog, or a composite creature, part dog and part pig. The upper portion of the relief[11] is now missing and the associated text is lost. Thus it is not certain whether the young animal was a part of the missing upper relief, or was intended to be related to the scenes to the left or right. Evidence against the animal being a pig seems convincing on examination of its feet where definite toes and claws are seen rather than sharp hoofs![12] The blunt tapering face of the young animal, coupled with its distinctive fat abdomen and short curly tail, would apparently disqualify it as the pup of the slim saluki dog feeding from the bowl, but would not rule out the possibility that it is the pup of another variety of canine. Another illustration is known, however, of an indisputable pig drawn with feet that would disqualify him as such (Budge, 1949, p. 162) (Fig. 4.6). The experts whom we consulted informed us, however, that this could be due to weak or broken pasterns, an appearance often seen in animals raised on hard floored sties (R. Barnes, H. Cole, M. Ronning, personal communication). We were shown several examples by Dr Barnes who kindly provided us with pictures illustrating these hooves (Fig. 4.5).

At the close of the Old Kingdom, several texts describe the unrest and anarchy of what historians call the First Intermediate Period (*c.* 2200–2060 B.C.). A desperate one, *The Admonitions of a Prophet*, describes both the condition of swine kept by the nobility and the feeding of man

> ". . . nay, but men fed on herbs and drink water. No fruit nor herbs are longer found for the birds, and the [food?] is robbed from the mouth of the swine, without it being said, as before, 'this is better for thee than for me,' for men are so hungry . . ." (Erman, 1966, p. 99)

Also from the First Intermediate Period is a text, *The Eloquent Peasant* (Gardiner, 1923), which supports the thesis that swine were not considered abhorrent, for they are listed among the favourable farm products

> ". . . his Upper Egyptian corn [wheat], his barley, [his] asses, [his] swine,[13] his small cattle . . ."

During the Middle Kingdom information on pork and swine is sketchy.[14] One noble, Menthuweser, who lived during the reign of King Senusret 1 (*c.* 1970–1936 B.C.) held the title "overseer-of-the-swine," (b) an indication that Menthuweser was not concerned about defilement by swine (Newberry, 1928, p. 211). In the Middle Kingdom tomb of Khety (number 17) at Beni Hassan there is a painting of ambiguous "marsh-animals" (Fig. 4.7), which bear a greater resemblance to swine than to hippopotami or other semi-aquatic forms. Unfortunately, the artistic representation of the feet of these animals is vague and inconclusive. Dawson (1928, p. 598) who knew of this painting remained

(b)

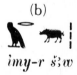

imy-r s̆3w

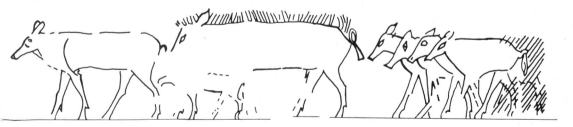

Fig. 4.7. "Marsh-animals" swine (note the bristles). Tomb of Khety (17) at Beni Hassan; Middle Kingdom, eleventh dynasty, date uncertain. Drawing used with permission of the Ministry of Agriculture and the Officials of the Agricultural Museum, Dokki, ARE (1969).

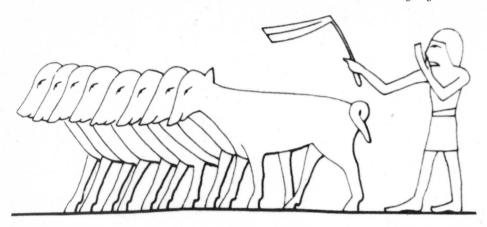

Fig. 4.8. Herds of swine. Redrawn from *The Tomb of Paheri at El Kab.* Tylor and Griffith (1895) plates III and IV.

unconvinced, and held to the belief that swine were not illustrated in Egyptian tomb art before the eighteenth dynasty. But the late Nazir, specialist in ancient agriculture at the Dokki Museum, believed as we do, that the paintings probably represent swine (personal communication, 1969).

One text, attributed to Khamose, who ruled Upper Egypt during the waning years of the Second Intermediate Period, describes the King's power over the southern and middle portions of the land and mentions the rearing of swine

> ". . . Elephantine is strong, and the middle part [of the land] belongeth to us as far [north] as Cusae.[15] The finest of their fields are ploughed for us, our oxen are in the Delta, wheat is sent for our swine, our oxen are not far away . . ." (Erman, 1966, p. 53)

In the early dynasties of the New Kingdom reports of acceptance and tolerance of swine are frequent. The rock tombs at El Kab may shed light on pig sacrifice[16] during this period. A record from the tomb of Reni describes a herd of swine numbering 1,500[17] (Sethe, 1906, 4, 75, 1). Paheri, another noble buried at El Kab, had artists portray scenes of swine under care of a herdsman (Fig. 4.8).

Newberry (1928, p. 212) believes that the tombs at this site represent the earliest known instances of swine in Egyptian tomb art.[18]

Most interesting, however, are the several New Kingdom tombs at Thebes that illustrate swine in agricultural scenes. At Drah Abu el

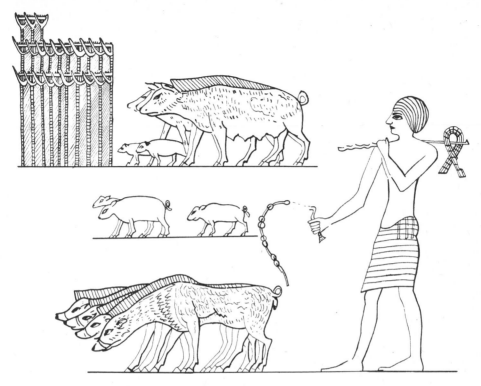

Fig. 4.9. Swine assisting farmer. Tomb of Inena (number 8) at Thebes (Upper Enclosure); New Kingdom, eighteenth dynasty, date uncertain. Redrawn from Wilkinson (1878) Vol. 2, p. 100, Fig. 360. This painting has been destroyed and was not visible during our visit to the tomb in 1969.

Naga the tomb of Neb-Amon (number 24) contains a painting depicting swine assisting farmers who are planting grain—exactly in the method described by Herodotus. Until excavations confirmed it, historians had doubted this Herodotian description

". . . but the husbandman waits till the river has of its own accord spread itself over the fields and withdrawn again to its bed, and then sows his plot of ground, and after sowing turns his swine into it[20]—the swine tread in the corn [wheat] after which he has only to await the harvest . . ." (II, 14)

Other scenes depicting swine assisting in this task are known but, unfortunately, have suffered from vandals[21] or have been destroyed completely. One, illustrated by Wilkinson (1854, Vol. 2, p. 18, and 1878,

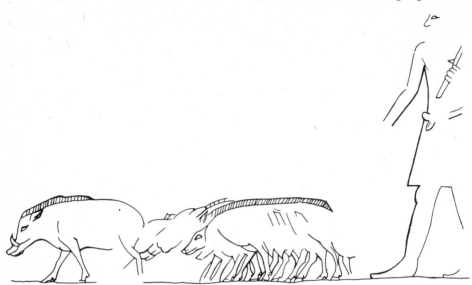

Fig. 4.10. Tomb of Amenemhat (number 123) at Thebes (Sheikh Abdel at Gourna); New Kingdom, eighteenth dynasty, reign of King Thutmose III, *c.* 1475 B.C. Redrawn from photograph taken in 1969.

Vol. 3, p. 100) (Fig. 4.9) was found in the tomb of Inena (number 811 at Thebes and greatly suffered damage as early as 1911 (Roushdy, 191), p. 63). Our examination of the tomb in 1969 revealed no trace of the painting. Another tomb (number 146) which belonged to a noble named Neb-Amon was described by Northampton *et al.* (1908, plate 13) as containing a painting showing swine treading grain. Unfortunately, this painting too was not visible in 1969. The tomb of Amenemhat (number 123) at Thebes shows swine with their swineherd (Fig. 4.10). The medium is high limestone relief instead of plaster and thus has better withstood damage, although it, too, has greatly suffered. It is justifiable to presume that, had all these personages felt repugnance towards swine during life, they would certainly not have included them in their tombs and hence be associated forever with an "unclean" animal.

Artists, moreover, would not have included swine in scenes of everyday life unless they were familiar with them. Swine were certainly known and eaten by workers and artisans of the Ramessid Period. Kees (1961, p. 92), who reported large numbers of bones in trash deposits around workers' houses at a Theban village dated to that era, most probably referred to the village of Deir-el-Medina where numerous skulls of swine have been found. These skulls are now on deposit in the collection of the Agricultural Museum, Dokki, ARE.

Additional New Kingdom records indicate that some kings looked with favour on swine. Amenhotep III (*c.* 1405–1370 B.C.) offered 100 pigs and 1,000 (young?) pigs to the temple of Ptah at Memphis and Seti I, father of Rameses II, (*c.* 1318–1298 B.C.) allowed pigs to be raised inside the temple consecrated to Osiris at Abydos (Newberry, 1928, p. 211); a sporadic custom with religious precedent dating earlier than the fourth dynasty.

Seti I, however, presents an interesting religious enigma; his name etymologically means "He who belongs to Seth," and it would thus be logical for him to present swine at Abydos. Yet his burial sarcophagus portrays the theme of swine in disgrace.[21]

The Medicinal Use of Products Derived from Pigs

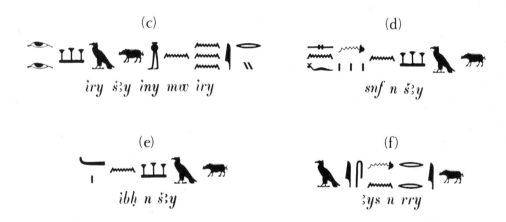

(c)

iry š'y iny mw iry

(d)

snf n š'y

(e)

ibḥ n š'y

(f)

'ys n rry

Practitioners of medicine in the New Kingdom did not hesitate to use products derived from swine in their prescriptions. The Ebers Papyrus lists humour of "pig's-eyes" (c) which was injected into the ear to cure blindness (*Eb.*, LVII = 356). Another ophthalmic prescription contained the blood of pigs (d) and kept "hair-from-growing-in-the-eye" (*Eb.*, LXIII, 425).[22]

Pig's tooth[23] (e) cat's dirt, dog's dung, and the fruit of the myrtle (?) were crushed and bandaged onto affected parts of the body to "expel exudation" (*Eb.*, LXXIV, 580). Pig's brain or pig's "viscera"[24] (f) was an ingredient in another cure to combat "eating", translated by Ebbell as cancer (*Eb.*, XCV, 814).

The latter prescription is interesting because of the manner of preparation. To leave the medicine overnight in the dew indicated a belief that night air and condensed moisture had magical curative powers— a belief still held in rural Egyptian folk medicine[25] and considered of therapeutic value in Europe and America into the last century. Pig's bile might also have been used (Dawson, 1929).

Late and Post-Dynastic Evidence

Pigs were found among the animals sacrificed and placed during the twenty-sixth dynasty inside the step-pyramid complex of King Sekhem-khet (third dynasty) at Saqqara. Although their inclusion is significant, the small number, relative to the total number of animals offered at this ancient structure, suggests that in the region of Memphis during this late period, swine, although tolerated, did not serve as a regular food source (Moustafa, 1964, p. 260). Additional possible evidence that swine were tolerated during the initial years of this dynasty is provided by the inclusion of a questionable wild boar/hedgehog within a hunting scene in the tomb of Ibi at Thebes (Fig. 4.11), dated to the reign of King Psammetik I, founder of the dynasty.

Writers of the Ptolemaic and Roman Periods reveal ambivalent feelings in regard to this controversial animal. Some maintained that it was abhorred, a view shared by Plutarch (*I. and O.*, 353, 5) and Aelian (10, 16). Sextus Empiricus writes

". . . no one would sacrifice a pig to Sarapis but they sacrifice it to Hercules and Asclepius . . ." (3, 220)

Elsewhere, he states

". . . for a Jew or an Egyptian priest would sooner die than eat swine's flesh . . ." (3, 223)

Other writers disagreed.

A papyrus dated to 118 B.C. reveals that swineherds enjoyed then a status equal to that of any other rural worker, in sharp contrast to the statements of Herodotus four centuries earlier (pp. 176)

". . . all wool-weavers and clothmakers, and swineherds and gooseherds, and makers of oil and castor oil, and beekeepers and brewers, who pay

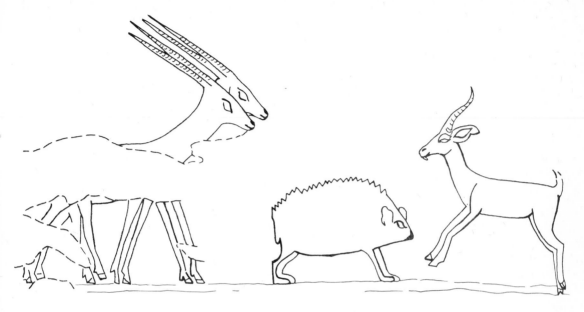

Fig. 4.11. Pig (?) or hedgehog (?). Tomb of Ibi (number 36) at Thebes (Asasif); New Kingdom, twenty-sixth dynasty, reign of King Psammeti I, *c.* 640 B.C. Redrawn from a photograph taken 1969.

to the Crown the sums due from them, shall not have anyone quartered in the individual houses in which they severally live . . ." (*S.P.*, II, 210)

Pliny (13, 9, 50) indirectly mentions large herds of swine, and the foods used in Egypt to fatten them, dates (*Phoenix dactylifera*) or the lotus stem (*Nelumbo nucifera*) that, according to him was

". . . more useful then any other fodder for fattening pigs. . . ." (13, 32, 110)

Athenaeus (4, 149, F), on the authority of Hermeias[26] of Methymne, in his description of the religious events held at Naucratis in the Delta suggests an equally permissive attitude

". . . thereupon each diner is served with a loaf of pure wheat bread moulded flat, upon which lies another loaf which they call oven-bread; also a piece of swine's flesh . . ."

He then continues to explain that pork consumption was not restricted to these annual rites

". . . but on all other days of the year, any diner who wishes may go up to the town-hall and eat, after preparing at home for his own use a green

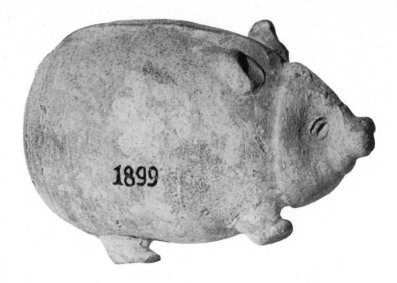

Fig. 4.12. Sow, Graeco-Roman Period, date uncertain. Photographed with permission of the Ministry of Agriculture and the officials of the Agricultural Museum, Dokki, ARE (1969).

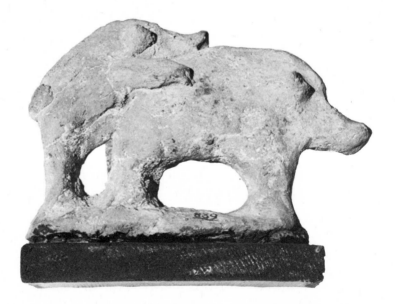

Fig. 4.13. Boar and sow mating; Roman Period, date uncertain. Photographed with permission of the Ministry of Agriculture and the officials of the Agricultural Museum, Dokki, ARE (1969).

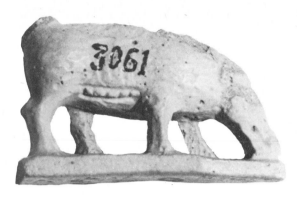

Fig. 4.14. Porcelain sow amulet; New Kingdom, date uncertain. Photographed with permission of the Ministry of Agriculture and the officials of the Agricultural Museum, Dokki, ARE (1969).

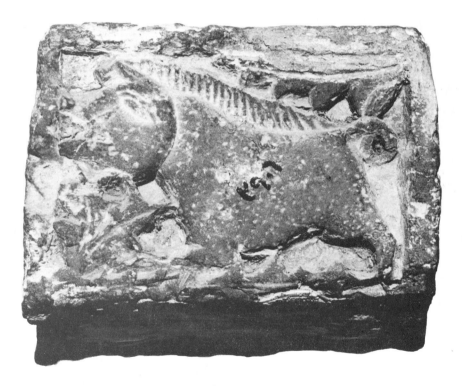

Fig. 4.15. Boar; Coptic Period, sixth to seventh century A.D. Photographed with permission of the Ministry of Culture and the officials of the Coptic Museum, Cairo, ARE (1969).

or leguminous vegetable, some salt-fish, or fresh fish, and a very small piece of pork; sharing these [he receives] a half-pint of wine . . ." (4, 150, A)

This description is, however, confined to Naucratis, that was nearly entirely Greek.

Of this period, too, there are abundant finds of amulets and terracotta statues of pigs and boars (Figs 4.12, 4.13, 4.14, 4.15) that further underline the continuing ambivalent attitudes, revealed also in a papyrus from the Ptolemaic Period (248 B.C.) that discusses the rent and leasing of sows and the associated value of piglets (*S.P.*, I, 72) in the statements of Polyaenus of Macedon *c.* A.D. 163 that during his time swine were raised near Memphis (*Strategems of War* 4, 19), and in the assertion of Heliodorus (fourth century A.D.) that swine were raised at Aswan (Underdowne, 1587, p. 130).

One obtains a somewhat humorous insight into the complexities of Roman life in Egypt then, particularly into the problems that faced a good host

". . . see, however, that we are provided with every attention, and above all with a good pig for our part, but again, let it be a good one, and not lean and unfit to eat like the last . . ." (*S.P.*, I, 140)

Boar hunting is mentioned as early as the fourth century B.C. as a pleasurable pastime in Egypt. It had played a prominent role in Greek Mythology, of which the famed Calydonian boar hunt is the most notable example: Denos, King of Calydon, having sent a plea to all Greece for help against a boar sent by the goddess Artemis to destroy his cattle and crops, the bravest heroes of the country responded and eventually slew the boar (Graves, 1955, Vol. I, 80, b-i). Theophrastus (4, 12, 4) described such hunts in the Delta region among islands of "floating plants" on which boars sought refuge. A papyrus dating from the Roman Period further discussed this subject

". . . take heed to supply the hunters whom I have sent to hunt wild boars with everything necessary for their many requirements, that is, everything that they and their animals are accustomed to receive, so that they hunt with all zeal . . ." (*S.P.*, I, 143)

It should be noted that wild swine are extinct in Egypt today. They had been nearly exterminated from the Delta by the early 1890s and the last boar known to have been shot was taken in Wadi Natrun during 1902[27] (Flower, 1932, p. 442).

Reconciliation of the Inconsistencies

A framework for consideration of the inconsistencies encountered in the preceding sections is that events in one locale cannot be viewed as indicative of behaviour throughout the whole of Egypt. The lingering Seth worship at Tanis, Ombos and elsewhere, during periods of Osirian dominance shows that Egypt was only rarely under the domination of a common religious thought.

If one accepts the thesis that the Osiris-Seth-Horus cycle represents a veiled history of the conquest and unification of Egypt by the southern followers of Horus who vanquished the northern followers of Seth,[28] some incidents of the legend that cast an interesting light on religious attitudes relative to pork may be relevant.

> ". . . Ra said to Horus, let me see what is coming to pass in thine eye, and forthwith he looked thereat. Then Ra said to Horus, look at that black pig and he looked and straightway an injury was done unto his eye—now the black pig was Seth who had transformed himself into a black pig and it was he who had caused the blow of fire which was in the eye of Horus. Then said Ra unto those gods, the pig is an abominable thing unto Horus; O but he shall do well although the pig is an abomination unto him . . ." *Papyrus of Nu* (*Book of the Dead*, Budge, 1949, p. 336)[29]

More than one thousand years after this description, and three thousand years after unification, Greek travellers to Egypt recorded variations of the myth that equally associated swine with Seth[30]

> ". . . the story which they relate at their only sacrifice and eating of a pig at the time of the full moon, how Typhon [Seth] while he was pursuing a boar by the light of the full moon, found the wooden coffin in which lay the body of Osiris, which he rent to pieces and scattered . . ." (Plutarch, *I. and O.*, 353, 8, F-354, 8, A)

However, if we except some periods of fanatic religious intolerance, like the one that characterized the Amarnian episode, a basic feature of Egyptian thought was the acceptance of local deities not universally worshipped elsewhere in the land. Thus when Ruffer (1919, p. 21) offers the slate cosmetic palettes shaped like pigs as proof that swine were not *universally* abhorred (italics ours), his generalization holds true, for although strict adherence to Horian and Osirian beliefs would have never accepted such representations followers of Seth would have found them pleasing.

One major difficulty in analysis of pork acceptance and avoidance is the existence of faience pig amulets at scattered localities throughout dynastic time. Egyptological literature contains conflicting information relative to these amulets.[31] Ruffer (1919, p. 21), using the authority of Maspero (1883), states that some swine amulets in the Egyptian museum collection bore the inscription

". . . may Isis give happiness to the owner of this sow . . ."

On the other hand, Reisner (1907, pp. 12286–12303), subsequent to Maspero, examined the amulet collection and made no comments as to any inscriptions on the swine amulets. This may have been an error or an oversight; or the amulets in question may have been lost. In any case, this paradoxical association of Isis with swine deserves examination.

Isis, wife/sister of Osiris and mother of Horus, could not be considered a close associate with swine, one of the chief animals of Seth; but she was often confused with the Sky-Goddess Nut by both worshippers and artists. Early in Egyptian cosmological representation, Nut was visualized as an enormously elongated woman, raised on her hands and feet and separated from Geb (Earth), her mate and twin brother. A secondary development equated her with swine. As she was imagined to give birth in the morning to the sun, that then travelled up to her mouth where it disappeared at night, she was compared to the mother sow who devoured her young (compare Aelian, 10, 16). It is not surprising, therefore, to find her imagined as a gigantic celestial sow (Helck and Otto, 1956, p. 251). Thus the faience sow amulets believed to be associated with Isis more likely represented Nut.

The action of King Seti I who raised swine inside the sacred compound of Osiris at Abydos may be interpreted as an instance of religious vindication, a break with tradition. Seti I, etymologically "the-one-belonging-to-Seth," could of course be expected to exercise certain powers to illustrate his devotion to the god Seth.

Hence, one may tentatively conclude that religious avoidance of swine and pork during the nineteenth dynasty was less severe than in other times of Horus/Osiris dominance.

The medicinal use of pork may be understood in terms of sympathetic magic, based on the Osirian myth that Horus had been blinded by a black pig. The treatment of "weeping eczema" with a pig's tooth (*Eb.*, LXXIV, 580)[32] is reminiscent of the statements of Manetho, Plutarch and Aelian, that exposure to swine's milk brought about leprosy. A confusion of eczema and leprosy, possible at the time, could therefore have brought a similar homeopathic concept to bear on their treatment.

The negative viewpoint towards pork at the time of the visit of Herodotus (II, 47) is clearly expressed, but it is likewise obvious that no few members of Egyptian society during this period kept swine. One logically inquires, if swine were so disgusting and impure, why were so many raised? Wilkinson (1878, Vol. 2, p. 394) tried to explain this contradiction by concluding that swine were not raised as food but for their assistance in agriculture, as illustrated in the eighteenth dynasty tombs at El Kab and Thebes (pp. 187, 188) and to forage the weed-strewn land following the flood. But did not the Egyptian barnyard offer several taboo-free varieties of animals, such as the goat, sheep and cattle, that could equally have performed this task? Indeed, if the point of Wilkinson is further developed, might it be that swine were held as useful and cooperative creatures and not as objects of contempt, as Aelian did in fact state (10, 16), on the authority of Eudoxus,[33] that Egyptians *refrained* from sacrifice of sows because of their helpfulness during the planting season, although he contradicted that statement by asserting that swine were sacrificed at festivals associated with the moon (Horus).

Porphyry (1, 14) adopted a different position, arguing on the relation between the availability of a particular animal and its sacrificial use

". . . neither is a hog sacrificed to the gods in Cyprus or Phoenicia, because it is not indigenous in those places and, for the same reason, neither do the Egyptians sacrifice this animal to the gods . . ."

It is, of course, logical to assume that an unknown animal cannot be sacrificed or, in fact, cannot be deified. It may be interesting to speculate here, on the possible deification of the horse in Egypt, as in some other ancient countries, had this animal been indigenous there in the legendary times when Egyptian religion was born. But as swine were known in the Nile Valley even in prehistory, Porphyry's explanation has no support in fact.

Aelian (10, 16), as we have seen, contradicts both Eudoxus and Porphyry, by stating that swine were sacrificed by the Egyptians at festivals associated with the Moon (Horus). In this regard it is interesting to note that El Kab, site of the tombs of Reni and Paheri which contain illustrations of swine, was known to the Greeks as Eileithyia,[34] a town where Selene, the moon goddess, was worshipped. One might suppose that Reni and Paheri raised swine for regular Moon sacrifice nearly two thousand years before Aelian's report!

The attitude of Greeks in Egypt presents similar problems of interpretation. The story of the centaur Chiron who raised the infant Achilles on the

". . . innards of lions and swine and the marrows of bears . . ." (Apollodorus, *The Library*, 3, 13, 6)

is only an example of sympathetic magic that claims the ability to acquire the qualities of a living being by ingesting its flesh, rather than an indication of dietary habits, for it is not at all certain that the Greeks ate lions and bears. It does suggest, however, that boars were not subjects of any taboo.

It is clear, from historical tradition that Greeks relished pork.[35] A spurious Hippocratic text says

". . . pork is the best of meat; it should not be too fat, nor too lean, and the animal not too old. It must be eaten rather cold without the skin . . ." (Hippocrates, *On the Regimen for Acute Diseases*, 18).

At the same time, some Greeks outside Egypt avoided pork

". . . in Crete they tell the story that the birth of Zeus occurred on Mount Dicte, where there is a secret rite. For it is said that a sow offered suck to Zeus, and as she roved about, she, by her own grunting, caused the infant's whimpering to be inaudible to the passers-by. Hence, this creature is universally regarded with great reverence, and no one would eat of its flesh . . ." (Athenaeus, 9, 375, F-9, 376, A, on authority of Agathocles of Babylon).

The same author states that

". . . the people of Praesus even offer sacrifices to the pig and this rite is regularly observed by them before the marriage ceremony . . ." (Athenaeus, 9, 375)

On the other hand, the worshippers of Adonis in Greece and Asia Minor (Table 3, Chapter 3) abstained from pork because a boar had killed their god (Frazer, 1959, p. 310).

It is probable that the Osiris-Seth-Horus myth represents the key to the first positive evidence of dietary pork avoidance in history. It far antedated the Mosaic codes against pork and, rather than being related to any observed cause-effect relationship between pork and disease,[36] it was a reflection of religious attitude towards the sacred animal of Seth.

There is no historical or archaeologic evidence of a religious or dietary imposition by one group of Egyptians upon other Egyptian subjects at any period. After the unification of the country, *c.* 3200 B.C., the religious attitudes of the southern conquerors, and a general avoidance of pork prevailed by gradual assimilation, rather than by compulsion. This affected mainly the nobility, priesthood, and royalty who had much to lose, in the religious sense, by breaking with established custom and tradition (see also Rawlinson, 1880, Vol. I, p. 89). The poorer classes probably did not change their dietary customs. One may further conclude that religious considerations were probably influential, but that pork avoidance rather than being universal in the country at any given time, was the result of the free choice of the individual.

There appear historically to have been two major periods of avoidance in Ancient Egypt; a first which originated in the south and was carried northward *c.* 3200 B.C.; a second, which started sometime after the Ramesside Period (*c.* 1085 B.C.) and before the first Persian conquest (525 B.C.) between the twenty-first and twenty-seventh dynasties. It is tempting therefore, to associate events and customs occurring in the twenty-sixth dynasty (Saite Period) with the contemporary archaistic revival of Old Kingdom customs, art, architecture and literature— sometimes explained as inward reflection on past grandeur before the final decline. Was the emergence of this second period of pork avoidance, just prior to the visit of Herodotus, a return to earlier Old Kingdom usage? Did it represent a rebellion against the tolerant attitudes toward swine exhibited during the "Ramessid Period" and an attempt to re-establish firmly orthodox Osirian beliefs?

Mosaic Pork Avoidance

". . . and the swine, though he divide the hoof, and be clovenfooted, yet he cheweth not the cud; he is unclean to you . . ." (Leviticus, 11, 17)

The tantalizing question of the origin of Mosaic pork taboos has been asked for centuries. As early as the third century A.D., Prophyry discussed this point

". . . the Phoenicians, however, and Jews, abstain from it [pork], because in short, it is not produced in those places . . ." (1, 14)

In the early part of the New Kingdom the Israelites resided near

Tanis (Zoan of the Bible) the nineteenth dynasty capital, and a former center of Seth worship where, by inference, swine would be sacred. Further, the ban on swine appears in the Bible only after Exodus, earlier prohibitions being restricted to blood

> ". . . every moving thing liveth shall be meat for you . . . but flesh with the life thereof, which is the blood thereof, shall ye not eat . . ." (Genesis, 9, 3–4)

The Mosaic pork ban might be interpreted, therefore, as expressing the desire to set the Israelites apart from their Egyptian masters, or as suggested by Newberry (1928, p. 215), as a rejection stemming from the association between swine and the false gods of agriculture.

A third view also suggests that pig abhorrence aimed at a discrimination from pig worshippers. This is based on an allusion of Isaiah to a dissident pork-eating Israelite sect

> ". . . I have spread out my hands all the day against a rebellious people, which walketh in a way that was not good . . . that provoketh me to anger continually to my face . . . which eat swine's flesh . . . which sayeth, Stand by thyself, come not near to me, for I am holier than you . . ." (Isaiah, 65, 2–5)

Coptic Pork Avoidance

Sethan worship and the concomitant veneration of pigs seem even to have persisted among an early Christian sect of gnostics that, according to St Epiphanus, identified the pig with Christ and hallowed it (Michailidis, 1962). This may be the significance of a small statue described by Keimer (1943b), that represented a pig lying on a rectangular socle bearing on each side the chrism or "crux monogrammatica." Keimer formulated two alternative hypotheses, either that the statue had belonged to the above mentioned sect, or that it was a caricature ridiculing Christians. Michailidis proposed a third explanation. In a period characterized by the interpenetration of all creeds and a recrudescence of all kinds of superstitions and rites, it would be natural for a neophyte from a pig-sacrificing religion (Sethian) to offer to his new god this animal rather than the traditional lamb. He quoted, as proof of the regard of Copts for pigs, several examples proving that St Menas, one of the main Coptic saints, kept pigs, and that some people who stole or killed his pigs were miraculously punished.

In fact, though paganism persisted long side by side with the new religion, and in spite of contact with the influential Jewish community which was very numerous especially in Alexandria and some great centres, like Elephantine, the Egyptian Christians or Copts saw no reason to avoid pork now that the old gods had fallen from grace (Simoons, 1961, p. 20).

The Arab conquest in A.D. 641, however, initiated new attitudes. Although no overt attempt was made by the conquerors to slaughter the herds of swine or to force pork avoidance upon the Christians, the herds decreased and pork became available only with difficulty. By the late eighteenth century, it had nearly completely disappeared

". . . nothing is more scarce in the Said[37] than this animal . . . upon my arrival at the convent of Neguade,[38] in which hospitality is so treacherous, some catholic Copts hastened to inform me that I might see a rare and singular animal there. I hastened, in my turn, to request them to shew it me. They conducted me to a corner of the yard, and I was surprised to find nothing in it but a pig which the monks were rearing, and which the Egyptians looked upon as a very curious animal . . ." (Sonnini, 1799, Vol. 3, pp. 255–256)

Acceptance of Islamic pork restrictions may have thus become ingrained in Coptic tradition, once interest in raising swine had disappeared. Moreover, most butchers were Moslems and would not slaughter swine, so as not to be defiled. Hence, availability of pork to rural Christians in Egypt has been severely limited since the Arab Conquest and conversion of the majority to Islam.[39] That few Copts eat pork today is a result of these influences, neither of which is inspired by Coptic religious instruction.

Roushdy (1911) studied instances of pork consumption among Copts living in Upper Egypt where pork was not usually eaten. In rural areas the Copts sometimes attribute to the meat a special medicinal value as a preventive against rheumatism and colds in winter, a tradition that it is tempting to see as an extension of Ancient Egyptian customs, seeing the antiquity of the lore associating swine with therapy. The use of these animals in planting has not been transmitted down through history, however, in spite of the persistence of traditional, alongside modern, agricultural techniques. In any case, the impact of Islam would have wiped it out. An interesting counterpart of the disappearance of pork from Egyptian tables and of swine from the countryside is the total absence of proverbs mentioning swine.

Islamic Pork Avoidance

". . . These things only has He forbidden you: carrion, blood, the flesh
of swine . . ." (Holy Koran, 2, 168)

The majority of Moslems simply abide by pork interdiction as an act
of faith. One person we interviewed stated this firmly

". . . swine are forbidden because of religion, not because they are dirty.
The chicken is the dirtiest of all animals, and is not forbidden . . ."

Few feel that there is any relationship between the Koranic and Biblical
laws, which is natural since it is the Moslem belief that the Koran was
directly dictated by God. Others rationalize the ban on one of the health
reasons discussed earlier (pp. 171, 177).

On the other hand, popular imagination has invented some most
fantastic explanations. One of these was recorded by Jean Palerne, a
Frenchman travelling in Egypt in the sixteenth century (Sauneron
1971, p. 57)

". . . the reason is that they find in their Alcoran that Noah . . . having
set the dung of all the animals on one side of the ark, found the ark leaning
on that side because of its weight. He consulted God who advised him to
turn the back of the elephant to the other side, whereupon the elephant
voided dung that brought forth a piglet, and the piglet ate up the droppings
of all the other animals . . ."

It is obvious that Palerne did not go to the trouble of reading the Koran,
for no such fanciful tale is told in it. But the curious idea that the pig is
derived from the elephant recurs in some old Arabian books of zoology.
Sauneron, who edited Jean Palerne's relation, quoted a few of these
parallel tales. In one of these, Noah is said to have smacked the elephant,
that consequently sneezed and threw out the piglet that ate all the dirt.

Some exegetes hold that the ban is directed only at pork meat not
at pork fat. Al-Demiry (I, 305) commented

". . . God Almighty forbade selling alcoholic drinks, dead flesh, and pork,
but there is a difference of opinion on whether the pig could be utilized
[i.e. for other purposes].

"Eating it is forbidden because of God's saying 'I find not in that which
hath been revealed unto me anything forbidden unto the eater . . .
except it be that which dieth by itself, or blood poured forth, or the flesh
of the pig for it is an abomination.'

"El Mawardy is of the opinion that the pronoun 'it' in 'it is an abomination' refers to 'the pig,' because it is the nearest word to it; but Abu Hayan opposed him, saying that it refers to 'the flesh' because if there occur a construct word and its genitive complement, the pronoun relates to the construct not to the complement, since the statement concerns the word, and the complement is only mentioned incidentally, to define the word and to specify it. El Qortoby says, in explaining the sourate of "The Cow," that there is no question but that the whole of the pig is forbidden, except its bristles, for they may be used in sewing.

"The pig is even worse [more impure] than the dog for, unlike the dog, killing it is desirable, and its utilization is forbidden. It was told that the Prophet, asked about sewing with its bristles, answered that there was no harm in it and he never forbade it; nor did any of the Imams after him.

"Possessing a pig is not permissible, whether it attacks man or not. If it does, killing it is obligatory; otherwise, there are two opinions: killing is considered obligatory or facultative."

It should be added here that Moslems may hunt boar without stigma. The Marsh Bedouins of South-East Iraq have to kill it to defend their crops; but whether they eat it is debatable, for they would not publicize the fact.

Known to few non-Moslems is the fact that Moslems may indeed eat pork and not transgress Koranic law, provided this is not habitual and is dictated by necessity, not by sinful desire[40]

". . . But unto him who shall be compelled by necessity to eat of these things, not lusting, nor wilfully transgressing, God will surely be graceful and merciful." (Holy Koran, The Bee, 115)

This permission, in itself, negates the alleged health motive and places prohibition on the religious plane. One Moslem we interviewed made a few points in favour of a naturalistic origin of the ban. He argued that, in early Islam, support from the Jewish and pagan inhabitants of Arabia, and their conversion to the new faith, would have been facilitated and made less of a break with tradition by the incorporation of some of their beliefs. To this we basically agree, for the history of Christianity offers several comparable instances of compliance with previous usage. Thus Christmas was made to coincide with the pagan mid-winter festival, and Easter with the spring feasts. Similarly, Peter, to avoid offending converted Jews by Gentile Christians, had to prohibit

". . . things strangled and blood . . ." (Acts, 15, 20)

even after his dream of

> ". . . a voice that spake unto him, what God hath cleansed, that call thou
> not common . . ." (Acts, 10, 9–15)

liberated Christians of all previous restrictions. The prohibition, however, was purely complimentary and was never applied.

Our interviewee further argued that swine are hardly desert creatures
and the wild boar is ferocious. The growth of domesticated herds would
have been most uneconomical and difficult; their skin bears no wool
for weaving; they cannot be used as beasts of burden; and they would
compete for the meagre water resources. Under such conditions, it
would be easy to forbid that which was dangerous or not readily available.

The last point, however, calls for some reservations. In Southern
Arabia, water is abundant and land is among the greenest and most
fertile. Pigs were numerous there; their bristles were used in sewing
clothes; and the mere measure of forbidding them presupposes their
existence and use in pre-Islam.

Conclusions

The "health" motives of the interdiction of pork, invoked by ancient
as well as recent observers (Manetho, Aelian, Sonnini, etc.) were
probably late rationalizations of the much earlier religious codes attested
in Egyptian texts and old chronicles. It is likely that the Israelite settlers
of Zoan in the northeastern Delta[41] could no more realize the relation of
pork to disease, discovered only in the nineteenth century, than their
Egyptian hosts. The Mosaic interdiction probably resulted from their
reactions to contact with the Egyptians and, later, with the pork-eating
Babylonians.

Nowadays, conditioning during early childhood is perhaps the
greatest factor that influences acceptance or rejection of food. We have
known intellectuals, persons who could challenge society as well as
Divine commandment, who became nauseated and ill at the mere
sight of pork. The imprint dating from their early education could not
be erased from their mind.

Unfavourable psychological images play still another role in acceptance or rejection of food. One cannot imagine, for example, a European eating a rat, a worm, or a dog. We know of a young woman born

and reared in Egypt among the Egypto-Greek community, who had eaten pork all her life and relished its taste and flavour. On a visit to the United States in 1967 she saw for the first time a pig-sty with all the accompanying odours, and the visual scene caused her such distress that for months she lost all desire for pork, a food she had previously enjoyed.

The ambivalent attitude throughout Egyptian history concerning pork is no more confusing nor strange than the attitudes and beliefs encountered in many parts of the world. Today in the United States pork is often illogically and without cause regarded as harmful in some manner. It is commonly considered as "difficult to digest," bad for one with renal disease, or bad for the heart or blood pressure. Such beliefs are found not only in folk medicine, but are often perpetuated by dietitians, physicians, and others, whose background should make them more critically objective.

The people of the eastern Mediterranean today consume or reject pork on the basis of religious and health concepts, or purely by personal choice. Moslems reject pork because of the Koran, Jews reject it because of the Mosaic codes, and Christians of the region rarely eat pork for various reasons, none of which stem from religious imposition. The complex factors influencing pork avoidance can be traced through processes of assimilation and acquired learning. From Koran to Torah, back to original contacts with early Egyptians and religious beliefs in remote antiquity, pork avoidance has a continuity through more than 5,000 years of recorded history.

Notes: Chapter 4

1. Of the contrary opinion is Montet (1958, p. 77) ". . . I know of no documentary evidence for the eating of pork, goat, or mutton, but this must remain an open question . . ."
2. One essential prerequisite for domestication of swine is a partially settled existence and an implied beginning of agriculture. The domestic pig is not a pastoral creature. Although the settlers at Helwan and Fayoum "A" had achieved such conditions there is no evidence that they domesticated swine. The cultural geographer, Carl Sauer, believes

that the pig was first domesticated in Southeast Asia (1969, p. 28). Reed (1959) would not rule out the possibility that swine could have been domesticated in Southwest Asia (even in Egypt) but argues that the decision must be based on osteological evidence instead of cultural guesses.

3. In view of the evidence presented by Junker during his excavations of Merimda Beni Salama it is difficult to agree with Roushdy (1911, p. 163), who sweepingly writes that Ancient Egyptians did not eat the flesh of swine.

4. Dunbar (1941, plate 20, Fig. 97) offers an unusual sketch from the Pre-Dynastic Period of Upper Egypt. It resembles a pig in the hindquarters, but from the front resembles an elephant. He remarks that it may be a composite of an aardvark or ant-eater, or of a pig eating a fish!

5. Frazer (1959, p. 451) discusses the duality of this point. He states that at Hierapolis on the Euphrates River, pigs were neither sacrificed nor eaten and that if a man touched one, he was unclean for the rest of the day. In analysis he considers that the unclean attitude reflects the idea that pigs were sacred.

6. See Smith (1928) p. 861.

7. Herodotus (II, 47) adds ". . . the poorer sort, who cannot afford live pigs, form pigs of dough which they bake and offer in sacrifice . . .". Badawi and Khafaga (1966, p. 247, 2) remark that dough pigs have been found in Egyptian tombs. They give, however, no authority for this statement. Our examination of museum material in Egypt during the summer of 1969 did not confirm the existence of such loaves.

8. The pig was an essential element in the Eleusian mysteries as evidenced by the fact that coins of the city were stamped with its image. The relation of swine, agriculture (Demeter), and Eleusis is told in a story connecting this site with the abduction of Persephone by Hades. Eubuleus, brother of Triptolemus, chanced to be herding swine at Eleusis when the ground opened and his pigs vanished (Pausanias, 1, 14, 3). The followers of Demeter stored the flesh of sacrificed pigs and sowed it in the soil with the seeds of grain to ensure a good crop (Frazer, 1959, p. 450; Aristophanes, *The Frogs*, 337–338). This custom is reflected today in the traditions of various agricultural peoples, particularly peasants living near Hesse and Neiningen in Germany. There, the flesh of pigs is eaten on Ash Wednesday and the bones kept until sowing, whereupon they are planted with grain (Frazer, 1959, p. 451). Grain, agriculture, resurrection, springtime, and pork, have been linked for thousands of years, giving cause for reflection on the high regard for roast ham as the traditional Easter meat among many Christians of the world today.

9. Herodotus (IV, 186) also states that some Libyan tribes to the west of Egypt abstained from pork, particularly the women inhabitants of Barcea.
10. The Kalabsha temple in Nubia was saved from flooding by the combined efforts of the German Federal Republic and the Arab Republic of Egypt. It has been re-erected at a safe and prominent position adjacent to Lake Nasser just south of the Aswan High Dam.
11. Even identification of the "mature dog" is controversial. According to Egyptian specialists at the Dokki Agriculture Museum, dogs are not known to have been portrayed eating from bowls, whereas wild desert game including ibex, antelope, and other forms are frequently depicted in this manner. Identification of the animal in the upper portion of the Ka-Gem-Ni relief as an antelope or as a feeding saluki is still open for debate (Nazir, personal communication, 1969).
12. The authors had been inside the tomb probably over 100 times and, until 1969, had never observed claws on the feet. Two men, one an artist and the other an uneducated tomb guard from the village of Saqqara, drew our attention to the feet. They had viewed the relief through eyes unencumbered by controversy and saw the relief at face value. The eyes of a guide or archaeologists can sometimes be unobjective.
13. Swine, in this instance is written as depicted by (g).

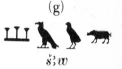

(g)

š3w

14. Dawson (1928) reports that swine are discussed in Middle Kingdom coffin texts.
15. Koussieh, located approximately 40 miles north of the modern city of Asyut.
16. Herodotus (II, 45) mentions that Egyptians sacrificed swine during his time (see above).
17. Ruffer (1919, p. 21) gives the number as 300.
18. Newberry (1928, p. 211) regards the Beni Hassan "marsh-animals" as questionable representations of swine and omits discussion of the Ka-Gem-Ni relief; presumably he believed it to be a dog.
19. Rawlinson (1885, Vol. 2, p. 17) who discusses Herodotus (II, 14) and cites the authority of Plutarch, Aelian and Pliny in regard to swine and agriculture in Egypt, believed the ancient writers to be in error ". . . but no instance occurs of it [swine] in the tombs; though goats are sometimes so represented in the painting . . ." Rawlinson believed that swine were used to root weeds and thus clear land for cultivation, but that they were not actually involved in the treading of grain.
20. Diodorus (1, 36, 4) also discusses a similar technique of planting utilizing herds and flocks. He does not, however, specify swine. Although swine were driven into fields to assist in planting, no tomb relief or painting known at present depicts swine threshing grain. Scenes of goats, donkeys and cattle performing this task are known from the Old, Middle and New Kingdoms.

21. This duality may reflect institutional variation during his reign. Seth worship was most probably officially condoned in the northern regions, while elsewhere in Egypt the king kept a more prudent outlook toward Osirian faith; indeed, he built a magnificent temple to Osiris at Abydos (see Gardiner, 1961).

22. This prescription parallels one found in the Hearst Medical Papyrus (*H.*, 20).

23. Though it is tempting to imagine the use of an actual tusk, one should certainly entertain the possibility that this ingredient was the Ancient Egyptian name for a herb or other medicinal plant (*Wb., Dr.* 78). A modern example of similar usage is "fox-glove" (*Digitalis purpurea*).

24. Another use in Egyptian medicine for pig's brain or pig's viscera was for "worm-in-the-finger" (*Ber.*, 19).

25. Fruits, usually dates, are placed inside a brass "fright" cup, called by the Arabs "Taset el Khadda." The inner and outer portions of the cup are inscribed with magical spells which are sometimes true texts but more often nonsense syllables or mystic code. The fruit, softened by the night air and dew, is eaten at morning, and the fright incurred the day before reportedly vanishes.

26. Nothing is known of his life.

27. According to Strekalovsky (1949, p. 6), the last boar was shot in Wadi Natrun in 1892.

28. See Huzayyin (1941, p. 373) for full discussion and philosophy in support of this thesis.

29. This Budge translation is essentially followed by Barguet (1967, p. 149) who further attests that this myth is found in Pyramid Text 1268 where Horus is "blinded by a pig."

30. Some animals, because they exhibit characteristics that parallel those traditionally associated with a god, become associated and equated with the deity. For example, the destructive hippopotamus and crocodile, in the minds of Horus worshippers, were equated with Seth. The crop-destroying boar may have been, likewise, assimilated to him. The origins of the association of swine and Seth are unclear, but one part of the Osiris cycle explains it thus: when Seth fled in defeat from Horus, he and his followers threw themselves in the Nile and were changed into pigs and hippopotami.

31. Compare, for example, statements on swine amulets by Dawson (1928) and Petrie (1914).

32. Possibly a plant.

33. The identification of this Eudoxus is uncertain. Scholfield (1959, Vol. 3, p. 443) suggests it was Eudoxus of Rhodes who flourished in the late third century B.C.

34. Named for the Greek goddess, Eileithia, who presided over childbirth.

35. For pork "foie gras" see p. 273 and note 12.

36. Since antiquity, Middle Eastern peoples have been infected with parasites including, not only trichinae, but the round worm, Ascaris, beef tapeworm, hookworm and a wide variety of parasitic protozoa and helminths that may cause diarrheal and general diseases. It is difficult to believe that the Ancients would have singled out trichinosis from the rest of their parasitic diseases and perceived any relationship to the ingestion of pork.
37. The Egyptian term for Upper Egypt.
38. More commonly spelled Naqada.
39. Large herds of swine are raised today in Upper Egypt in the vicinity of the Fayoum, Minya, and Naqada. They are exported to Cairo and Alexandria where consumption is generally restricted to Christians, foreign residents, and tourists.
40. Such a situation was encountered by Moslem Turkish troops during United Nations involvement in Korea when they were faced with "GI" rations that sometimes contained pork-and-beans.
41. The Biblical form of Tanis = Ancient Egyptian *dja'net* = modern San-el-Hagar.

Chapter 5

Other Mammals: Ovines, Wild Species, Equids, Cervinae, Canidae, Miscellaneous

Divided sheep are led by a scabious goat
(Popular maxim)

Ovines

Terminology

Sheep: *sr, ʿwt ḥdt*
Ram: *ba, sr*
Kid: *ib*
Goat: *wʿty, ʿr*
Ibex: *nꜣw, nrꜣw, niꜣ*

Domestication of Ovines

Kees (1961, p. 90), in his discussion of the geographic origins of various domesticated animals in Egypt, concluded that "cattle" (meaning large cattle) were first tamed and raised in the Delta area, while "small-cattle" (the term applied to sheep and goats by the Ancient Egyptians) probably first appeared in the southern region where the arid conditions and the type of soil, beyond the restrictive valley cliffs, favoured the stubby coarse pasture sought by small grazing animals.

211

In support of this view is the predominance of ram worship in the south, but exactly when domesticated goats and sheep first appeared in Egypt is difficult to determine. The earliest drawings of ibex and Barbary sheep are the Mesolithic/Neolithic or Early Pre-Dynastic Amratian drawings on the cliffs edging the Nile Valley, and along the trails between southern Egypt and Nubia (*MAE*, p. 73). Drawings of ibex are also found among the Neolithic desert rock drawings east of Dakhla attributed to the "Early Oasis Dwellers" (*MAE*, p. 102), although these can hardly represent an attempt at domestication.

That domestication occurred before the Maadian period, is suggested by the abundant finds of bones of goats and sheep at Maadi among remains of many other animals (*MAE*, 122). Bones of wild sheep and goats have also been found in the Fayoum "A" sequence (*MAE*, 93); bones of sheep and goats in Merimda (*MAE*, p. 112); and of goats in Omarian deposits (*MAE*, 119).

Sheep, Ram

Two races of sheep are illustrated by Ancient Egyptian artifacts.

Ovis longipes palaeo-aegyptiacus

This species has horns growing perpendicularly outwards from the head in the shape of two corkscrew-like spirals; the legs and tail are rather long and the males have an abundant mane which covers the neck. In drawings, males are well differentiated from females by the genitals, the mane, and the much larger size of the horns. This species was a poor wool producer and disappeared from Egypt at the end of the Middle Kingdom, but it apparently persisted for a while in Nubia. This is the ram whose shape was assumed by Khnum, Harsaphes and other gods (Fig. 5.1).

Ovis platya aegyptiaca

From the Middle Kingdom on, another species, *Ovis platyra aegyptiaca*, was increasingly depicted until it entirely replaced the first species.

Probably of Asian origin, it is recognizable by its aquiline forehead, dangling ears, horns directed downwards, thick at their base, tapering, crescentic with the concavity forwards, and keeping close to the head; a long tail, broad at its base, although not so thick as present day's fat-tailed sheep. This ram was the incarnation of the god Khnum-Amon who, in some illustrations (Fig. 5.1), presented to archaeologists a curious problem, in that it possessed characteristics of both of the mentioned types, as well as some of a goat: outward spiral, in addition to crescentic horns, and often a small beard. Although four-horned sheep are known (Fig. 5.2) Keimer thought that this was not the case in Egypt. The explanation of this curious chimera, according to many authors, is that the lateral-horned ram was originally widely worshipped in Egypt but that, at the time when this curious synthetic animal was drawn, it had already disappeared and had been replaced by the curved-horn ram. The artist, however, drew it in the conventional way although he added, "to be on the safe side," the curved horns of the ram he knew (Keimer, 1938). This is proved by the discovery at Elephantine, a known place of Khnum worship, of mummies of curved-horned rams fitted with wooden models of lateral horns, possibly as parts of the composite crowns ꜣtf or ꜥnd̲-ty that, since prehistoric times, included that animal ornament (Figs 1.1, 5.3). In addition, these rams often were fitted with wigs and false beards, like royal personages. The latter ornament, mistaken for a natural beard, led to the erroneous identification of this animal with a goat.

Nevertheless, it is likely that if a four-horned specimen like the one illustrated in Fig. 5.2 was ever born in Egypt and brought to the attention of the priests, it would have been doubly hallowed, first as all freaks were in antiquity and, secondly, as bearing the attributes of two deities of the first order, Khnum and Amon. Conceivably, its memory might have lingered in the memory and records of Egyptian priests as a historical divine manifestation.

Ram Worship

The virility and aggressiveness of the ram made it an obvious symbol of fertility and power. It is tempting to find a cognate relationship between the Arabic word for sheep, *ghanam*, and a series of ram gods, all called *Khnum*, who were early worshipped in Egypt, especially in Upper Egypt

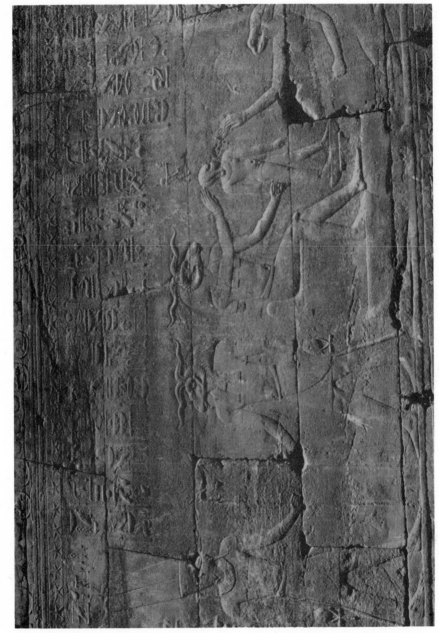

Fig. 5.1. The god Khnum creating mankind at the potter's wheel. Dendera. Notice the presence of both horizontal and crescentic horns. Photographed 1969.

where they were an object of adoration in six of the twenty-two nomes (first: Elephantine; fourth: Thebes; tenth: Aphroditopolis; eleventh: Hypselis; twentieth: Herakleopolis Magna; and twenty-first: Nilopolis), in contrast with Lower Egypt's two out of twenty nomes (fourteenth: Tanis; sixteenth: Mendes). This is part of the evidence that deification of sheep had a southern origin.

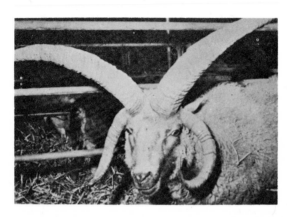

Fig. 5.2. Prized rare ram that boasts four horns, a choice example of the nearly extinct Manx Loghtan breed. Reproduced from MD Magazine, New York, March 1974, Vol. 18, No. 3, p. 85.

One of the earliest and major centres of ram worship was Elephantine Island, near the first cataract of the Nile that was considered to be the source of the river. Khnum was regarded as the Nile god. He had two wives, Sati and Anukis, and although childless with them, his fertility had Cosmic dimensions; for he was the "great potter," the "moulder of men," who continuously fashioned mankind out of clay at the potter's wheel (Fig. 5.1.) Because of this aspect he was besought by the sterile, and by pregnant women (Ames, 1965, p. 106).

From Elephantine, Khnum's worship spread south to Nubia where he was assimilated to local ram gods, like Dedun and others (Ames, 1965, p. 106). In the north, Khnum was incorporated with Amon at Thebes where the ram statues lining the mile-long sacred way between the temple of Luxor and Karnak still excite visitors' admiration (Fig. 5.4).

In Lower Egypt the ram was also identified with Osiris in Mendes (Ames, 1965, p. 130) where it was treated albeit on a lesser scale, with

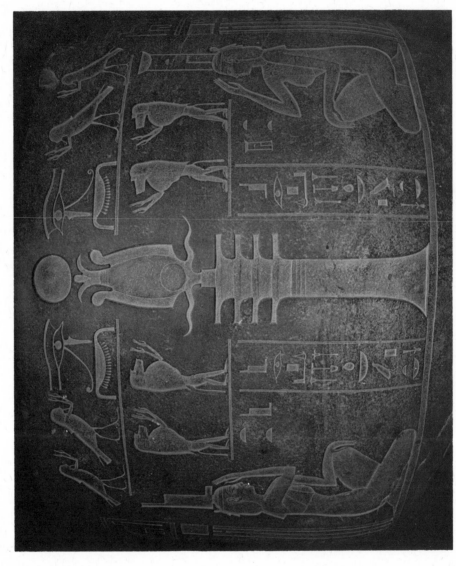

Fig. 5.3. Composite crown with the lateral horns of the ram, on the "Tet" of Osiris. Cairo Museum. To the left, Isis, to the right, Nephthys.

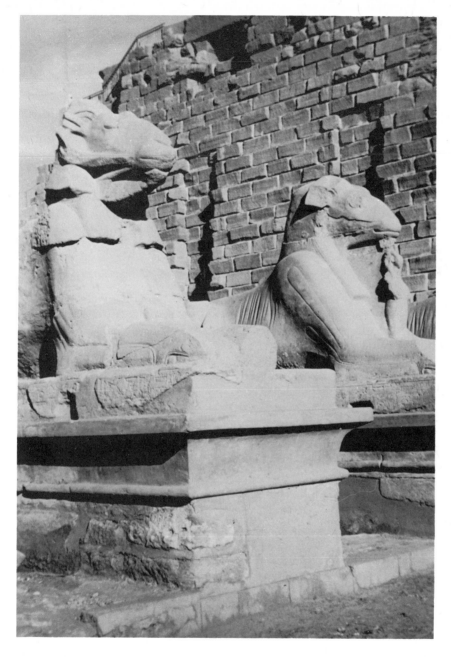

Fig. 5.4. Part of the sacred way lined by ram-headed sphinxes, leading from the Luxor Temple to Karnak. Photographed 1969.

the same pomp as the Apis bull, another incarnation of Osiris, was in Memphis. Like Apis, Khnum was buried in huge sarcophagi. At certain religious anniversaries, the death of Osiris was commemorated by sacrificing a ram

> ". . . upon one day in the year, however, at the festival of Jupiter [Amon], they slay a single ram, and stripping off the fleece, cover with it the statue of that god, as he once covered himself, and then bring up the statue of Jupiter an image of Hercules. When this is done, the whole assembly beat their breasts in mourning for the ram, and afterwards bury him in holy sepulchre . . ." (*Her.*, II, 42)

This was a reference to a tale where Herodotus, as was his wont, Hellenized ram worship

> ". . . Hercules,[1] they say wished of all things to see Jove [Amon], but Jove did not choose to be seen of him.[2] At length, when Hercules persisted, Jove hit on a device . . . to flay a ram, and cutting off his head, hold the head before him and cover himself with the fleece. In this guise he showed himself to Hercules. Therefore the Egyptians give their statues of Jove the face of a ram . . . such then is the reason why the Thebans do not sacrifice rams but consider them sacred animals . . ." (*Her.*, II, 42)

In Siwa, too, the ram was worshipped. Flavius Cresconius Coryppus, a poet of the sixth century A.D. writing on Africa, mentioned a Libyan god named Gurzil who was represented with a ram's head and was thought to be the descendent of the original Siwan god (Belgrave, 1923, pp. 75–76). An easy association was thereby established between him and the Theban ram Khnum, considered then a manifestation of Amon. It was during these contacts that the oracular powers of the Siwan god were revealed, although these were mainly consulted by foreigners and had almost no influence on Egypt (Fakhry, 1944).

As the story was allegedly told to Herodotus by Egyptian priests, one of two women, kidnapped from Thebes by the Phoenicians, was sold to the Libyans and founded the oracle; the other of the two women was sold to the Greeks and founded the oracle of Dodona. But the Greeks preferred to believe that these two oracles had been founded by two black doves (*Her.*, II, 54, 55).

On occasions, Zeus (Fig. 5.5) and Dionysus (or Osiris, depending on the point of view) are represented as having horns. In the case of Dionysus this is a reference to his encounter while lost in the Libyan desert, with a ram that led him safely to water. Some believed this ram to be his father (Lemprière, 1963, pp. 100, 101). The god then built a temple

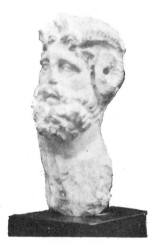

Fig. 5.5. Zeus-Amon. Personal collection of the authors.

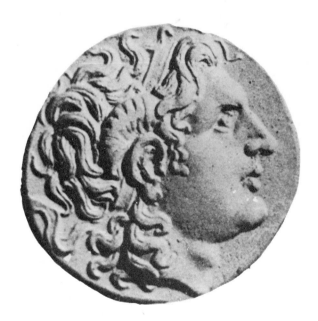

Fig. 5.6. Coin made to the effigy of Alexander the Great with the rounded horn of Khnum-Amon. Reproduced from Carson (1963).

commemorating the ram, the cult object having a ram-head (Belgrave, 1923, 78).

The fame of the oracle of Siwan Jupiter-Amon was spread, however, through the visit of Alexander the Great in 332 B.C. There, the conqueror learned that he was the "son of Zeus." The other messages revealed to Alexander have not been preserved, for the king was sworn to silence until after his return to Greece. Fate willed it that the young general died of fever at Babylon and the oracular secrets were never revealed.

Behind him in Egypt, Alexander left a legacy of tolerance and the city he created bore his name and later became the major centre of philosophy, research and medicine. Its fine silver coins (Fig. 5.6) depicted the flayed ram's fleece and its sacred horns.[3] Thus, in death, Alexander truly became equated with the god-like heroes of Ancient Greece. The coins of his city persist as tangible evidence of history, while the massive Hercules, who had once requested to see Amon but was allowed to gaze only at the flayed ram's fleece, took second place behind the Macedonian King of Egypt.

Taboo on Sheep

Because the ram was worshipped at Thebes and elsewhere, the sacrifice of sheep was relatively rare through much of Dynastic time. Rawlinson (1881, Vol. I, p. 88) writes that mutton was not held in esteem as a food and that, due to religious veneration, sheep were seldom killed. Yet Herodotus (II, 42) informs us that, on occasion, rams were sacrificed to Amon at Thebes. Plutarch (*I. and O.*, 352, 5) reported that priests eschewed mutton, and added that the inhabitants of Lycopolis (Asyut) were the only people to eat mutton because the wolf, whom they held to be a god, ate it.

Sextus Empiricus (*Outlines of Pyrrhonism*, III, 220) added that to sacrifice a sheep to Isis is forbidden, but it is offered up in honour of the so-called Mother of the gods, while it is regarded by a Libyan as a most impious thing to taste of the meat of a sheep (III, 223). The fact is that mutton is nowhere mentioned in the long ritual menus of the gods.

There is yet another facet to this taboo. Plutarch (*I. and O.*, 352, 4) reported that the Egyptian priests did not wear woollen garments

". . . priests, because they revere the sheep, abstain from using its wool, as well as its flesh . . ."

Writing nearly 500 years earlier, Herodotus (II, 37) recorded

". . . they wear linen garments, . . . their dress is entirely of linen, and their shoes of the papyrus plant: it is not lawful for them to wear either dress or shoes of any other material . . ."

He then discusses the dress of the *common man* in Egypt

". . . they wear a linen tunic fringed about the legs, and called *calasiris*: over this they have a white woollen garment thrown on afterwards. Nothing of woollen, however, is taken into their temples or buried with them, as their religion forbids it . . ." (II, 81)

The use of wool by commoners may be the reason for keeping the huge flocks of sheep recorded in Ancient Egyptian documents ". . . plus 5,800 sheep . . ." (Edgerton and Wilson, 1936, Vol. II, plate 75).

The garments of the lower classes, who had little to lose by breaking taboos since they seldom participated in temple worship, therefore could be made of wool, while linen was the primary material of the nobility's clothing. Thus we see by the wealthy a general trend of avoidance of sheep, and possibly goat products.

Did this affect the practices of the Hebrews who, for centuries, lived in the "country of Goshen" near an era of ram worship? The problem is to reconciliate this cult with the Passover tradition of sacrificing a lamb that would have certainly aroused the Egyptians' anger, unless the Egyptians did, themselves, consume these ovines and find nothing wrong with it.

Utilization

The sacred position of sheep was attributed by Diodoris (I, 87) to their utility in providing wool, butter, cheese and milk. They do not appear to have been destroyed in great numbers by sacrifice since only under the few circumstances related above were they so used. The large herds that were, according to Ruffer (1919, p. 14), kept under the New Kingdom at El Kab probably served, therefore, as a source of wool and dairy products. On the other hand in the twenty-sixth dynasty Sekhet-khem pyramid cemetery, Moustapha (1969) found bones of scores of hundreds of a species of sheep, *Ovis aries*, showing some differences from the three varieties common in Egypt at the present time; and he suggests that *Ovis aries* disappeared and was replaced later by imported species.

Goats

Goat Cult: Possible Confusion with the Ram

One commonly encounters references to a goat-cult during the Late Dynastic Period, principally practiced at Mendes in the Delta. Herodotus (II, 46) was the first to describe it

". . . some of the Egyptians abstain from sacrificing goats, either male or female . . . these Egyptians, who are the Mendesians, consider Pan[4] to be one of the eight gods who existed before the twelve,[5] and Pan is represented in Egypt by the painters and sculptors, just as he is in Greece, with the face and legs of a goat . . . the Mendesian hold all goats in veneration, but the male more than the female, giving the goatherds of the males especial honour . . . in Egyptian [language], the goat and Pan are both called Mendes."[6]

And he added

". . . They represent him thus for a reason which I prefer not to relate."

Strabo, who believed that both male and female goats were venerated in Mendes (*Geo.*, 17, 1, 40) quoted from Pindar the reason that presumably Herodotus prudely chose to hide (*Geo.*, 17, 1, 19)

". . . Mendes . . . where the goat-mounting he-goats have intercourse with women . . ."

This astounding story, probably a fertility-rite in which a priest performed in the guise of a goat, seems to be confirmed by the discovery of a mould illustrating this particular ritual (Michailidis, 1965).

Manetho, too (Waddell, Frag. 8, p. 35), reported a most ancient history of goat-worship at Mendes, which he dated initially to the second dynasty. All this evidence strongly confirms the goat as a Mendesian cult animal. Nevertheless, no archaeological evidence supports this view. Quite to the contrary, many texts assert that the worshipped animal was originally a ram. An alabaster vase of Abydos bears the inscription

". . . King of Upper and Lower Egypt [Teti] of Djedet [i.e. Mendes], beloved of the Ram god." (Mariette, 1880)

The "stele of Mendes" (Cairo Museum Guide, 1910, p. 206, No. 666)

expressly mentions "The Ram Lord of Mendes"—and Ptah, speaking of the birth of Rameses, addressed the King thus

". . . I assumed my form as the Ram, Lord of Mendes, and begot thee in thy august mother . . ." (*A.R.*, III, 400)

It is quite probable, therefore, that this ram was later changed into a goat, either through the process of pictorial confusion alluded to above in the section on rams, or to accommodate it to the source of the goat-Pan-concept of late Greek residents.

Utilization

Although the Biblical ordinance to cover the tabernacles with curtains of goat hair (Exodus, 26, 7) suggests that the goats taken out of Egypt were long-haired, tomb illustrations depict only short-haired varieties that could provide little for wearing. This, in itself, indicates that goats were raised for food, for there would seem to be no other justification to keep the huge herds recorded

". . . 3609 cattle . . . 9,136 goats, and 23,120 [? species of] goats . . ." (Edgerton, 1936, Vol. II, plate 75)

or for their exaction as tribute by Meneptah (*A.R.*, III, 584), Thutmose III (*A.R.*, II, 139), and Rameses III (*A.R.*, IV, 298–347). This again attests to their economic value.

Pictures of goats adorn tombs at Beni Hassan (Fig. 3.18a) and the walls of the funerary chapel of Ra-n-wser (fifth dynasty); but they are seldom shown being sacrificed or cooked. A rare example is seen at Deir el Gebrawi (Fig. 3.45).

Similarly, goats were apparently sacrificed at certain festivals

". . . 1089 goats offered in sacrifice to the Nile god . . ." (*A.R.*, IV, 298)

and this, preferably to sheep

". . . Such Egyptians as possess a temple of the Theban Jove [Amon] or live in the Thebaic canton offer no sheep in sacrifice, but only goats . . ." (II, 42)

This again shows that goats were eaten (Fig. 3.45).

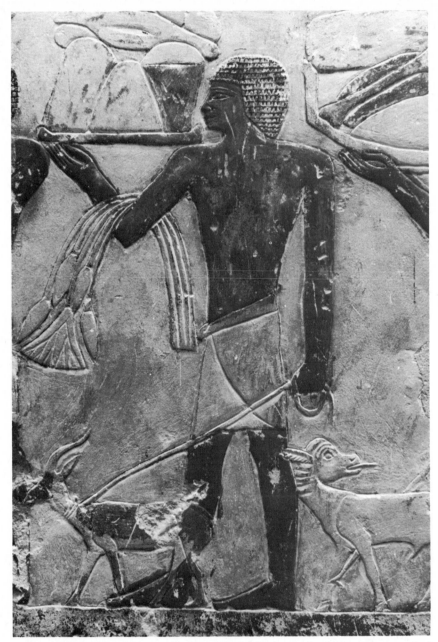

Fig. 5.7. Goat and ram (?) as offering, depicted in the tomb of Idut. Photographed 1969. Inclusion of these animals among the food offered in the procession supports the position that they were eaten (see p. 223).

Ibex

Ibex, wild goats or Nubian goats, have been illustrated since very early times in graffiti (Fig. 5.8) or in tombs as being hunted or led into captivity, e.g. in the Old Kingdom tombs of Ptahhetep and Mereruka at Saqqara (Fig. 5.9) and in Middle Kingdom tombs (Figs 5.13 and 5.24). They are also seen in slaughter scenes, but less commonly than bovines (Montet, 1910, p. 42). Similarly, Sinouhe in his narration said that he ate wild goats (ibex) (*A.R.*, I, 496). These were hunted and trapped, a practice that gave a metaphor to the Libyans, telling of their discomfiture in the second Libyan war against Rameses III

". . . The Lord has taken us as a prey like wild goats creeping into a snare . . ." (*A.R.*, IV, 91)

Medical Uses of Sheep, Goats and Ibex

Burnt dung of "small cattle" was applied to burns (*Eb.*, LXVII, 482). Certainly, a more effective treatment was ibex fat (*Eb.*, LXVIII, 490). A salve for a septic wound was made with goat fat, honey, writing fluid, and vermilion (*Eb.*, LXX, 522); and another with goat fat and wax (*Eb.*, LXX, 525) was prescribed to dry wounds.

Ibex fat was rubbed, with the fat of other animals into the scalp to promote hair growth (*Eb.*, LXVI, 465) and was anointed into the limbs to "soften them" (*Eb.*, LXXIX, 634).

Goat blood was included in a composition that was to prevent the re-growth of a removed eyelash (*Eb.*, LXIII, 425); and goat bile in the dressing of human bites (*Eb.*, LXIV, 433).

By far the most fascinating, however, was a picturesque therapy of burns, that evoked, in one of the rare spells in the Ebers papyrus, a dialogue between Isis and a messenger come to announce that her son Horus was ablaze in the desert.

"*The Messenger:* Your son is burning in the desert
Isis: Is there any water there?
The Messenger: There is no water there

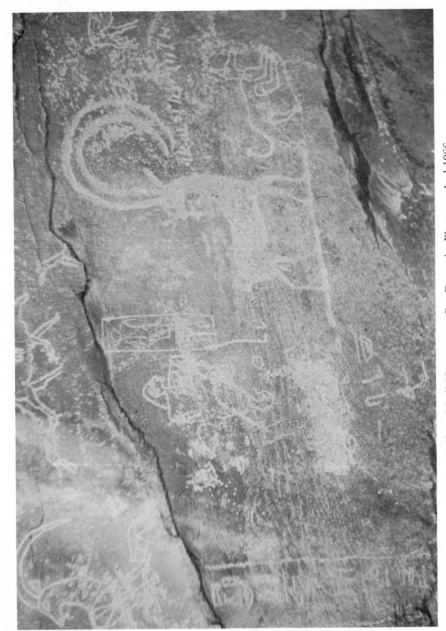

Fig. 5.8. Ibex. Wadi Hammamat. Pre-Dynastic. Photographed 1966.

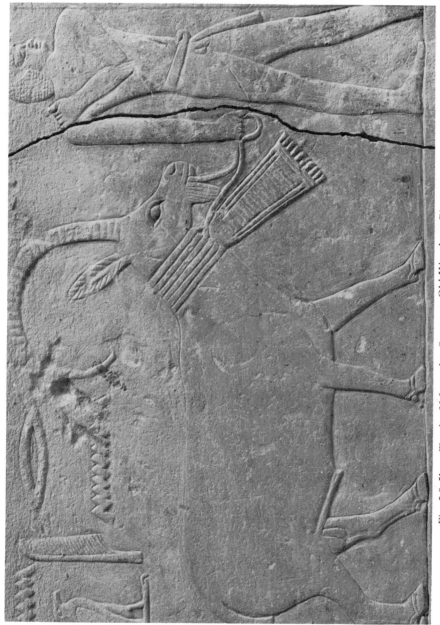

Fig. 5.9. Ibex. Tomb of Mereruka. Saqqara. Old Kingdom. Photographed 1969.

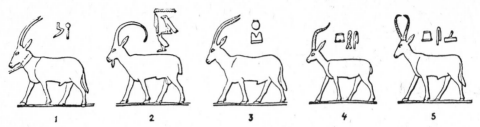

Fig. 5.10. A number of "horned" animals from the tomb of Idout at Saqqara, together with their names written in hieroglyphics—1: oryx; 2: ibex; 3: addax; 4: gazelle; 5: bubal or hartebeast.

Isis: There is water in my mouth and a Nile between my thighs. I came to extinguish the fire.

To be recited over the milk of a woman who had a male child, gum, and a ram's hair. To be placed on the burn" (*Eb.*, LXIX, 499)

A magic writing, the London papyrus (*L.*, 47) repeats this same prescription, but replaces ram's hair with a cat's hair.

Wild Species *(Fig. 5.10)*

Before the appearance of man in Africa, large herds of animals of many sorts roamed through the whole of that continent; its now desolate north was covered with a vegetation as rich and lush as that of its tropical and southern regions, and it teemed with wildlife such as is displayed today in the splendid game preserves of East and Central Africa.

As testimony to the fact that the modern deserts were not always lifeless areas of blight, heat and drought, stands the silent witness of the rock carvings. Here, either under the urge of a precocious creative impulse or, more probably, to conjure up abundant quarries, early men left magnificent records of the beasts they hunted (Fig. 5.11). Under the shelter of cliff sites throughout the northern and central Sahara, along the desert routes that lead from the oases to the Sudan, and along the former migratory routes of the herds, records of varying style tell of a land that teemed with antelope, gazelle, zebra, hartebeest, elephant, giraffe, cattle, canidae and even lions and rhinoceros. Examples of these are to be seen scattered between the Hogar (Ahagar), in Algeria, and Uwainat, at the meeting point of the three frontiers of modern Egypt, Sudan, and Libya.

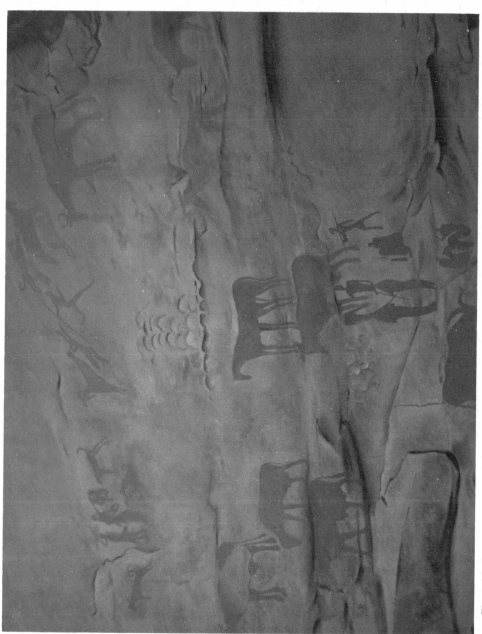

Fig. 5.11. Cattle herders. South Central Sahara. 10,000–8,000 B.C. Location uncertain. *Source*: Algiers Museum.

Today, most of these animals have vanished from Egypt and similar desert areas. The lingering exceptions are a few sturdy gazelle (*Gazella dorcus*) and ibex, often called Nubian goats (*Ovis lervis*).

"African" fauna is first encountered some 300 miles south of Khartoum, about a thousand miles, as the crow flies, from the present southern frontier of Egypt. This desolation was partly brought about during the Pleistocene by a progressive desiccation that drove the immense herds which inhabited these broad plains and forests towards the remaining watering and feeding areas along the Nile and in and around the oases of Siwa, Bahariya, Dakhla, Kharga and Uwainat. Man, however, is not entirely innocent, for he has contributed, especially in the last two millenia, to the extermination of several species that had found partial sanctuaries in and around the oases.

But, prior to the establishment of agriculture in Pre-Dynastic Egypt, hunting was not a sport in the modern sense, a mere satisfaction of a killing instinct, or a feat of skill and endurance. It was a vital search for food, clothing, and utensils; and these wild species remained a major source of meat until, in relatively late Pre-Dynastic times, cattle, sheep and goats were domesticated.

After the unification of Upper and Lower Egypt and the growth of a leisurely nobility, hunts provided an occasional "different" meat, but it was the chase and capture that were sought, not the mere killing. Montet (1958, pp. 76–77) is certainly right in his evaluation of these desert hunts, not as major sources of food, but as a pastime for the wealthy, and a sacrifice of wild animals as a reminder of the past.

Many records tell of kings who offered desert species to their gods

". . . I appointed for thee hunting archers to capture white oryxes, in order to offer them to thy *ka* at all thy feasts . . ." (*A.R.*, IV, 266)

Important men, like the high priest Osorkon (reign of Sheshonk III, twenty-second dynasty, *c.* 800 B.C.), made similar offerings:

". . . then he made a great oblation, bulls, gazelles, antelopes, oryxes, fatted geese, in tens of thousands . . ." (*A.R.*, IV, 768)

In the gardens surrounding their vast estates, such potentates raised and tamed the young of wild species as pets, and as witnesses of their manliness in braving the rigours of desert life to capture them; and throughout history, their tombs were covered with pictures of oryx, ibex, gazelle, bubal, hare and deer, either being hunted or tamed.

The principal wild animals thus hunted for food or for sport were the equids; but other forms like some rodents and, at times, the wallowing hippopotamus were not scorned. Before World War II, there still were vast herds of gazelle and similar species around Siwa, the Wadi Natrun, and water spots in the Eastern desert; and Bedouins and campers occasionally feasted on one. But modern hunters, euphemistically calling themselves sportsmen, mounted on automobiles, nearly brought them to extinction. Tall tales of thousands of kills in a single day are still narrated in the Cairo bars, as the participants from various nations recall their experiences of desert warfare in 1942–1943; and these unbelievable yarns seem to be corroborated by Bedouin and Siwan witnesses of this wanton slaughter.

Concern for wildlife led the Egyptian authorities to establish a gazelle farm in the Eastern desert, and to forbid hunting any kinds of "gazelle." A comparable situation has arisen in Jordan, and a similar concern led King Hussein to authorize an expedition to study the problem of disappearing wildlife in his country, as part of the International Biological Programme. The conclusions of the expedition, in the most instructive and remarkable *Portrait of a Desert* by Guy Mountfort (1965) confirmed the report of a past Director of Forests of the country, that the country had decreased its production level from one which could support eight times the present population to one that could hardly support it at all (p. 169).

During World War I, gazelle and bustard still could be easily shot anywhere. There were plenty of oryx and ostrich. In 1950, there were still about one thousand or more oryx in Arabia, but the slaughter there was even more ruthless than in Africa as hunters, armed with sub-machine guns and automatic rifles, and mounted at times in helicopters, came into action from neighbouring countries. In 1962, only eleven were believed to remain. The wild ass was killed off by 1920, the fallow deer by 1922, the Syrian bear in 1930; and the last ostrich was seen in 1932. Only a few gazelle survive in miserable condition, and a few ibex hide in the more inaccessible mountains. In Israel, the expedition reported that army officers are credited with having killed one thousand *dorcas* gazelles in less than five years in the Negev region alone (Mountfort, 1965, p. 58).

Equids

Bones of antelope, hartebeest, gazelle, oryx, addax, deer, horse and donkey have been found in Pre-Dynastic sites throughout Egypt, and there is abundant evidence that many of these have been serving for food in Egypt right to this century. By modern taxonomical criteria, they are distinct, but it is not clear how finely the Ancient Egyptians differentiated between some of them (Fig. 5.10). Nowadays, throughout North Africa the names for deer, gazelle, bubal, addax, oryx and ibex, are as confused in local dialects as they were in old chronicles (Joleaud, 1935, pp. 59, 61). Even modern writers often interchange their names. The present account may, therefore, reflect some of the confusion of the authorities from whom our information was drawn.

Antelopes *šs3w; Addax nwdw*

Rock drawings of antelopes in an ancient depression east of Dakhla have been attributed by Winkler (1939, Vol. II, pp. 27–30 and 33–36) to a Neolithic population, the so-called "early oasis dwellers," who are possibly identical with the "peasant Neolithic cultivators of Kharga" (Caton Thompson, 1952, pp. VI, VII; *MAE*, pp. 101, 102). Bones, identified as antelope bones, were found in Palaeolithic sites at Kom Ombo, and southwest of Wadi Halfa (*MAE*, pp. 67, 68); and bones of a large antelope with bovine characteristics have been discovered in a Middle Palaeolithic site in Egypt's western plateau (*MAE*, p. 58).

Ruffer (1919, p. 19) mentions paintings of antelope on prehistoric pottery at Neqada and Ballas (Petrie and Quibbell, 1896, plates LI, LII), and evidence from prehistoric Hierakonpolis (Quibbell and Green, 1900–1902, Hierakonplis, II, plate LXXV) indicates that they were kept in enclosures to be fattened. The animals painted on the Pre-Dynastic vases of the family called "decorated" by Petrie, were also identified as the antelope (*Addax nasomaculatus*) by Keimer (1943a). The same author also recognized a horse-antelope (*Hippotragus equinus*) on a bas-relief of the Unas ramp in Saqqara. In the opinion of this experienced archaeological naturalist, the accuracy of the drawing proves familiarity of the artist with this animal, although it must have been rare at the time (Keimer, 1943c). Other illustrations are also known, at Saqqara (Fig. 5.10), Beni Hassan (Newberry and Fraser, 1893–1894, Vol. II, plate XIV), and elsewhere (Montet, 1910, p. 43); and these animals are mentioned in the lists of offerings of the eighteenth (*A.R.*, II, 553) and twenty-second dynasties (*A.R.*, IV, 768).

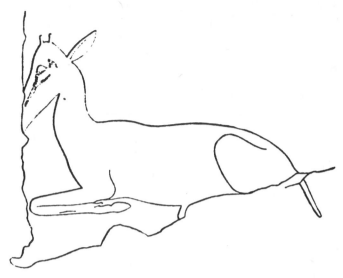

Fig. 5.12. The *iw* hieroglyph of a bubal kid. Southern obelisk of Hatshepsut at Karnak (from Keimer, 1943a).

Hartebeest

The Hartebeest *šsȝw* (*Bubalus* or *Alcelaphus buselaphus*), a large antelope characterized by lyriform horns set upon a sharp prominence on top of the head and by a pointed elongated maw, played, according to Keimer (1943a), a great role in Ancient Egyptian life. Bones of this animal were found in a Late Palaeolithic deposit at Kom Ombo (*MAE*, p. 67), at Saqqara (Gaillard and Daressy, 1905), and in Fayoum "A" deposits (*MAE*, p. 93), and it has been recognized on a prehistoric palette from Hierakonpolis (Quibbell and Green, 1900–1902, Vol. II, plate LXXV).

According to Loret (1892a), its female was known as *hbn*, a name different from that of the male (*cf.* horse and mare, buck and doe, etc.) while Keimer (1943a) identified the hieroglyph *iw* (Fig. 5.12) as the kid of the hartebeest. *Alcephalus buselaphus* (Northern or Bubal hartebeest), a species now extinct, but that he considered was typical of Ancient Egypt. He pointed to the error of Gaillard and Daressy who stated that illustrations of the hartebeest are rare, and asserted that the Ancient Egyptian artists clearly illustrated several of its varieties. This is confirmed by perusal of the published reproductions of paintings of all periods (Figs 5.14, 6.42). Paton (1925, p. 14) mentions several illustrations from the tombs of Sahure at Abusir, Baqt III and Amenhotep at Abusir, tombs at Deir el Gabrawi, and there are countless others.

Gazelle

Gazelle, *ghs*, is recognizable with certainty in carvings of the Paleolithic/ Mesolithic boundary, and in Neolithic or Early Pre-Dynastic Amratian drawings (*MAE*, p. 73).

Bones of that animal were found in Kom Ombo Sebilian deposits (*MAE*, pp. 8, 67) and in other prehistoric sites, in the temenos of Osiris at Abydos (Petrie *et al.*, 1903, Vol. I, p. 16), in the mummy tombs of Dendera, that were used from the eighteenth dynasty to Ptolemaic times (Petrie, 1900: *Dendera*, p. 29), in the twenty-sixth dynasty animal cemetery of the Sekhemkhet Pyramid (Moustafa, 1964) and elsewhere (Ruffer, 1919, pp. 19, 20), and mummified bodies were found in numerous sites (Lortet and Gaillard, 1909, Vol. I, p. 78).

Throughout the Dynastic Period, they appear in most hunting scenes, and are often shown captive or being led to be sacrificed (Figs 5.16, 5.24 and 6.37) (Montet, 1910, p. 42).

Fondness for this graceful animal manifested itself in artful objects carved in its shape, in the many offerings to the gods, and in the tales of wonder woven around them. An inscription in the Wadi Hammamat relates the miracle that happened on the first *Sed* Jubilee of King Mentu-hotep IV, when a gazelle came forth, offering herself for sacrifice on the uncut stone meant to be the lid of the king's sarcophagus (*A.R.*, 1, 436). Gazelles must have been common in that region, for a second marvel happened while work was in progress on the sarcophagus lid. Rain poured, the form of the god appeared, and a well surged in the midst of the valley, filled with fresh water, undefiled . . . and cleansed from gazelles (*A.R.*, I, 451). Records of tributes of gazelle (*A.R.*, IV, 724) and offerings by later kings are numerous (*A.R.*, IV, 190, 242, 392, 768).

Oryx *m ꜣ or mꜣhd*

The oryx, standing on the emblem-stand before a bundle of fresh food, was the emblem of the sixteenth nome of Upper Egypt (the Hermopolite).

Apparently, two kinds inhabited Egypt, *O. beisa* and *O. leucoryx*. Early illustrations of this animal on a cylinder from Neqada, on an ivory plate probably prehistoric, on the prehistoric Hierakonpolis palette, on Neqada and Ballas vases, and on an ivory lid, have been reviewed by Ruffer (1919, p. 17). The animal is depicted in numerous scenes (Figs 4.11, 5.10, 6.42) of all epochs, and a sacrificed specimen is being dressed in the tomb of Sahure, with the caption

"Seizing stable-bred oryx, choosing the choice joints. (Borchardt, 1910, II, plate 28, p. 43)

It was deemed a valued offering to be made by kings to the gods, witness the numerous offerings of Rameses III (*A.R.*, IV, 190, 242, 293, 392, 768); and, in one of his records, he

". . . sent hunters to capture oryxes to offer them to the *ka* of the god." (*A.R.*, IV, 266)

Donkeys

Bones of donkeys, apparently of undomesticated forms, not unlike the onager, have been found in Sebilian deposits. By the time of the first dynasty, donkeys were well known, and sometimes appeared on cosmetic palettes. The time of the first domestication of the donkey, however, is not clear. It was certainly one of the main pack animals used, but it does not appear to have been ridden by Egyptians. There is no evidence that it was ever eaten, even though it might have been with the other sumpter-beasts that the army of Cambyses ate during its ill-fated Ethiopian adventure (*Her.*, III, 25).

In spite of its usefulness and of the numerous pictures that show it patiently performing its usual chore—though at times under threat of the stick—the donkey was at later times considered an essentially evil animal except in a single formula of *The Book of the Dead*, by which the deceased had to drive away a snake called "the eater of the ass." It was a manifestation of Seth. The people of Busiris and Lycopolis were said not to use trumpets because they made a sound like an ass (*I. and O.*, 362–30), and eventually it became the supreme scapegoat, its image being destroyed in magic rituals. When the bantering Egyptians wanted to ridicule the cruel Ochus, they nicknamed him "the ass," an insult to which the Persian retorted by slaughtering Apis and feasting upon it (*I. and O.*, 363, 31).

Medicinally, several parts of the donkey were used; but one wonders whether these, like the English "toadstool" or "foxglove," were not imaged names of plants, e.g. donkey's tooth (*Eb.*, LXVI, 470); leg (*Eb.*, XXV, 108); hoof (*Eb.*, LXV, LXVI, 460, 468); ear (*Eb.*, XCII, 770); phallus (*Ber.*, 124); dung (*Eb.*, LXV, 460, *Ber.*, 64, etc.); hair (*Ber.*, 69); or head (*Eb.*, XXV, 106). On the other hand, it is probable that some parts really meant their names, e.g. donkey's fat (*Eb.*, XLVII, 249, *H.*, 121, etc.); liver (*Eb.*, LXVI, 463; *K.*, 1); blood (*Eb.*, LXIII, 425); bone-marrow (*Eb.*, LVIII, 362); and gonads (*Eb.*, XC, 756).

These were used for various conditions, but they do indicate that, at least at the time when the prescriptions were written, the donkey was acceptable to patients and physicians alike.

The magic part of this animal's status is evident in the utilization of its hair as a magic component of knotted amulettes (*L.*, 40, 13, 11 and 13, 12).

Horses

One of the most interesting problems of Ancient Egypt concerns the existence of the horse in Pre-Dynastic times, its "extinction" during the Old Kingdom, and its "reintroduction" during the Second Intermediate Period. Bones that could be positively assigned zoologically to *Equus caballus* and *Equus sivalensis*, the horse of modern nomenclature, have been uncovered in the Sebilian levels of Upper Egypt (*MAE*, 67–68). But there is no evidence of that animal, thereafter, until its reappearance in texts and artifacts under the eighteenth dynasty. It has been asserted that it was reintroduced by the Hyksos invasion, *c.* 1730 B.C. It seems likely, however, that the first Hyksos came on foot. The horse and chariot were diffused by the Aryans in the seventeenth century in the Near East and it is probable that Egypt received the horse towards the end of the Hyksos episode. Its late arrival, after the age of the gods, explains its absence from the Egyptian Pantheon.

Some believe it unlikely that the horse completely disappeared during Late Pre-Dynastic/Early Dynastic times, and had to be reintroduced (a problem similar to that of the camel and several plants and fruits in Egyptian antiquity). But such a sequence is not beyond credibility. In North America the horse was one of the most common Pleistocene animals, as evidenced by numerous fossil deposits; but it was unknown to the Indians of North, Central, and South America before the Spanish reintroduced it in the sixteenth century A.D.

There is no indication, however, that the horse ever served as a food source in Egypt.

Zebra

Zebra, described by Arab writers as "striped black and white donkeys that no one could ride," were still to be seen at Siwa long after the Arab invasion (Belgrave, 1923, pp. 91–92), but there is no indication that they were known to the Ancient Egyptians, even as an exotic animal.

Cervinae

Members of the deer family, collectively called by the name, *hnn*, and characterized by their branching horns, seem to have early disappeared from Egypt. Aelian (XIII, 10) was positive

"In Libya there is an absence of wild swine and stags."

Several artifacts, however, prove their persistence until the historical period. Joleaud (1935) came to the conclusion that these were represented by the fallow deer (*Cervis dama*) and that the statements of ancient authors, like Herodotus, Aristotle and Pliny, who denied the existence of deer in Africa, were the result of a religious ban forbidding the uttering of its name by the indigenes, since Aristotle and Pliny when speaking of the Barbary fauna, mentioned a branched horned Bubal quite similar to deer, a fact that suggests that the word "bubal" was used by their informers for deer to avoid pronouncing the latter's name.

Fallow deer were sacrificed by the Hebrews. King Solomon's provisions for the day included harts, sheep, roebucks and fallow deer (1, Kings, 4, 22); and it was similarly offered by Parthians and Phoenicians (Porphyry, *De abstinentiae*, 11, 25). Bones of cervicorns were found among Late Palaeolithic deposits of Upper Egypt and Nubia at Wadi Halfa (*MAE*, p. 68), Kom Ombo (*MAE*, p. 67), and possibly in the neolithic settlement of Merimda Beni Salama (*MAE*, 112).

The oldest Pre-Dynastic artifact showing a deer (a fallow deer) is the

Carnarvon ivory knife handle that depicts it with elephant, lion, oxen and other animals (Benedite, 1918). Another well-known prehistoric artifact, the Hunter's palette (Legge, 1900), half of which is in the British Museum and the other half in the Louvre, shows the capture of hare, bubal, gazelle, oxen and deer, and has been interpreted by Joleaud as a late evocation of the religious character of domestication in the East (1935). In addition, from Coptos (Petrie, 1896), a drawing hammered on a first dynasty statue of the god Min is that of a deer head; and a rock protohistoric drawing in Wadi Sabah Regala of the Djebel Silsileh, is witness to its existence (Joleaud, 1935).

Illustrations of Cervinae, however, are few. From the Old Kingdom, the deer is illustrated in the famous hunting scene of Sahure (Borchardt, 1910), in tombs at Meidum (Petrie, 1892, plate XXVII) in Ti's tomb (Steindorff, 1913, plate CXXVIII), and in Ka-Gem-Ni's tomb at Saqqara (von Bissing, 1905, Vol. 1, plate XXV; and 1911, Vol. II, plate XXIII, etc.). In most of these scenes it appears as a tamed animal.

From the Middle Kingdom illustrations are known from several tombs at Beni Hassan (Newberry and Fraser, 1894, Vol. II, plate IV), at Meir (Fig. 5.13) and at Thebes (Fig. 5.14), etc. Joleaud (1935)noted, however, that none of these deer are free, all being enclosed in parks or enclosures where they could be hunted at leisure. He further pointed to the clumsiness of some of these drawings indicating that the artists were unfamiliar with their models at that time.

Illustrations of deer became extremely rare under the New Kingdom, a period during which artists showed an even greater ignorance of this animal's characteristics, depicting, for example, horned females (Fig. 5.15), or males with horns of quite unrealistic shape.

No illustration of deer for the Saitic Period is known; but they reappear during the Ptolemaic Period in the tomb of Petosiris (Lefebvre, 1924, Vol. III, plates XXXV, XLVI, XLVII, XLIX) (Fig. 5.16). Errors of drawing, then, were even more pronounced, however.

The majority of authors agree that deer seem to have disappeared from Egypt at an early period (Bissing, 1905; Benedite, 1918; Hilzheimer *in* Borchardt, 1910, p. 172, No. 32) and that, after the New Kingdom, it could be ranked only as an exotic, imported animal (Davies, 1913, p. 8; Borchardt, 1910, p. 169, No. 27).

Relatively recent authors (Alpino, 1735; Hartman, 1864) noted, however, its existence in Egypt in their time. A graphic witness to this is a painting in the Louvre[7] that represents the reception by Sultan El-Ghoury in 1512 of a Venetian Embassy in Cairo (Fig. 5.17). In this picture a branching horned animal is let free in the Court, a custom attested by the French traveller Pierre Belon du Mans (Sauneron, 1970, p. 119b), who related, in 1547, seeing an animal in the same circumstances. This animal he at first thought to be a fallow deer, but he later identified it by some of its features, notably by the absence of horns, to be the animal called by Pliny *axis* (*N.H.*, VIII, 31). The credibility of the Louvre painting is increased by the extreme accuracy of the details of clothing, architecture, weapons, and crest of El-Ghoury on the citadel wall, which imply personal observation by the artist.

Medically, stag horn was prescribed by Ancient Egyptian physicians in an external application to cure headaches (*Eb.*, XLVIII, 259). This is the earliest therapeutic mention of hartshorn which, after having been used by the Copts, Greeks, Syrians and Arabs, became frequent in the medical works of Western Europe. "Spirits of hartshorn," as a solution of ammonia has been called, was originally the name of the ammoniacal distillate of horn shavings (Dawson, 1929, p. 111). Even later than the Ebers papyrus, the magic London-Leyden papyrus (Griffith and Thompson, 1904–1909) applied an obvious example of sympathetic magic by binding the hide of this agile animal to gouty legs (XXXII, vs. 10).

Canidae

Dog (Canis familiaris), Egyptian "Jackal" (Canis lupaster)
z꜍ b (F., 209)

It is generally accepted that the dog was one of the earliest, if not actually the first, among the animals man domesticated; although the statement that it was initially kept for its flesh seems highly controversial (Lang-Kavel, 1899–1900).

One may even postulate that the dog attached itself to man, rather than the reverse. Konrad Lorenz (1952) in a delightful and loving analysis of pet mentality, carefully distinguished between the "aureus" and "lupus" varieties of dogs, and the resulting different man-dog relationship contrasting the infantile, servile attitude of the "aureus," with the proud sworn one-man allegiance of the "lupus."

Some time or other, he postulated, this age-old covenant was "signed"

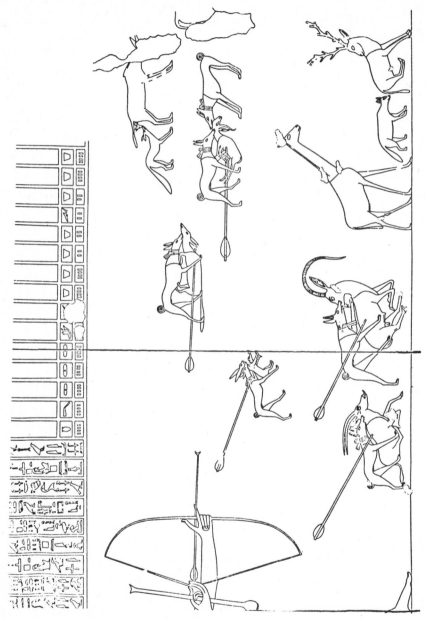

Fig. 5.13. A hunting scene with, below: deer, giraffe, ibex, oryx; in the centre: a dog catching a rabbit (Blackman, 1915a 2, Tomb Chapel B, No. 2, plate VIII).

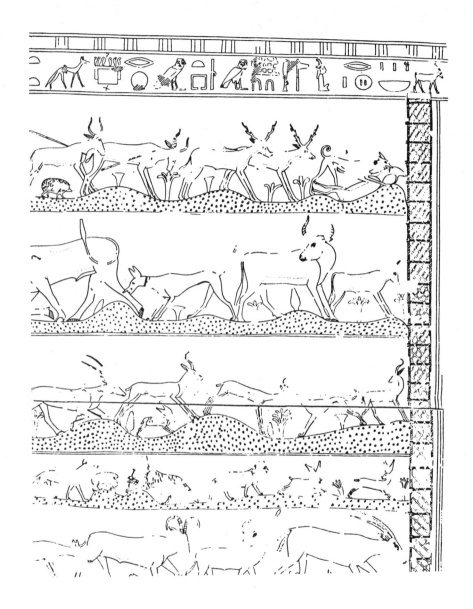

Fig. 5.14. Upper row; Two deer and two bubal. Tomb of Antfeoker (Davies, 1920, plate VI).

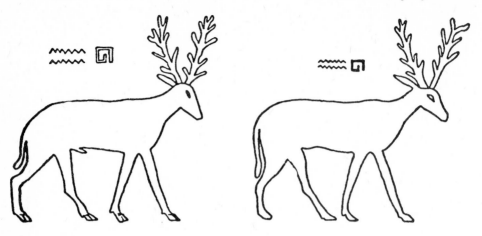

Fig. 5.15. Deer. Left a male, Right, a doe: note the masculine horns with the absence of male genitals (Beni Hassan, redrawn from Joleaud, 1935, Figs 18, 19).

voluntarily between the parties. The pack of jackals, accustomed to a good meal of entrails or refuse after the passage of the hunter, was naturally induced to follow the trails, of animals which, by their scent, were promising and took to running before instead of behind the hunter; even to track game, to call the hunter's attention to it, and to bring it to bay. The rest was the result of the ability of the dog to "feel" the moods of its master, and to understand a considerable number of words. Lorenz added, and one cannot disagree,

> ". . . there is no faith which has never yet been broken, except that of a truly faithful dog."

Several varieties of dogs can be recognized in Ancient Egyptian tomb walls, but zoologists believe that the indigenous variety approximated the "saluki" in appearance. All these illustrations portray the closest relation to their masters. One of the most moving is the tombstone of Prince Antef on which his four dogs, belonging to four different breeds, and each bearing a different name, are carved. But everywhere, dogs are seen assisting their masters in the hunt or in the keep of guardians.

The attitude to canidae in Ancient Egypt and, in fact, in the whole of the ancient world, was, however, a very complex one.

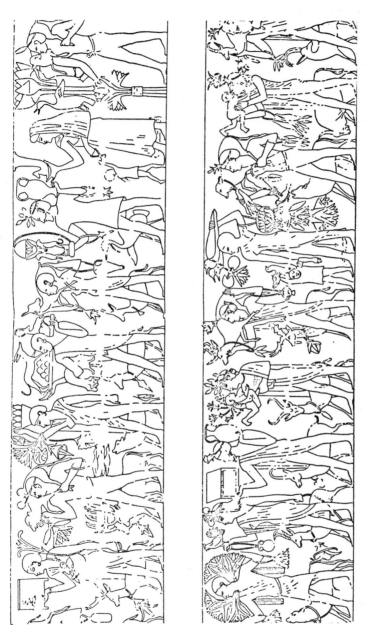

Fig. 5.16. Offering bearers with deer and gazelle. Tomb of Petosiris (from Lefebvre, 1924, plate XLVI).

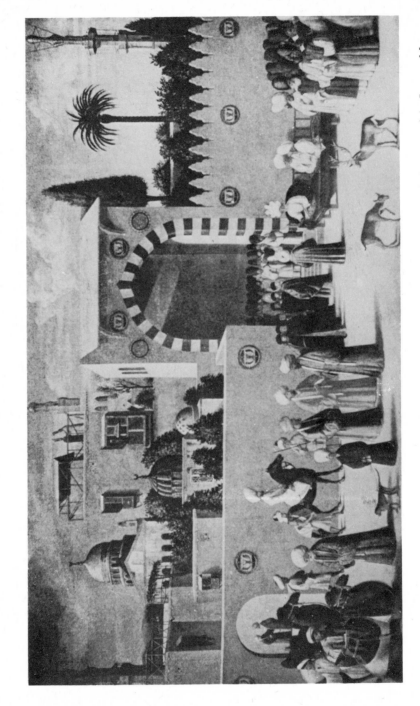

Fig. 5.17. Sultan el-Ghuri receiving a delegation from Venice in A.D. 1512. School of Gentile Bellini. Courtesy of the Louvre Museum and M. Mustafa (1969–1970).

Deification

Several canines were gods. These are commonly said to have been jackals; but true jackals do not exist in Egypt. Under this name are described roving dogs, a more or less pure strain of *Canis lupaster*, with large pointed ears, long muzzles, lithe bodies, and long bushy tails. The ritual writings decreed the shape and markings of the animals to be worshipped, but ordinary people in Assiut and Cynopolis were less discriminatory and artists' renditions that often resembled dogs or wolves, added to the confusion of the Greeks who thus called Assiut, where *Wp-wȝwt* was worshipped, Lycopolis, "the city of the wolf." Plutarch, mistaking the god Anubis for an ordinary dog, stated that originally the dog had held a place of primacy that it had lost in his time. This whole passage of Plutarch deserves to be quoted for the light it sheds on the way theological symbolisms are created and developed into most elaborate confabulations. Playing on the birth of Anubis from an extramarital relationship between Osiris and his sister and sister-in-law, Nephthys, he said

"When Nephthys gave birth to Anubis, Isis treated the child as if it were her own; for Nephthys is that which is beneath the Earth and invisible, Isis that which is above the earth and visible; and the circle which touches these, called the horizon, being common to both, has received the name Anubis, and is represented in form like a dog; for the dog can see with his eyes both by night and by day alike. And among the Egyptians Anubis is thought to possess this faculty, which is similar to that which Hecate is thought to possess among the Greeks, for Anubis is a deity of the lower world as well as a god of Olympus."

Then, punning on *Kyon* and *Kyo*, the Greek words for "dog" and for "to be pregnant," he added

"Some are of the opinion that Anubis is Cronus. For this reason, inasmuch as he generates all things out of himself and conceives all things within himself, he has gained the appellation of 'Dog.' There is, therefore, a certain mystery observed by those who revere Anubis; in ancient times the dog obtained the highest honours in Egypt; but, when Cambyses had slain the Apis and cast him forth, nothing came near the body or ate of it save only the dog; and thereby the dog lost his primacy and his place of honour above that of all the other animals." (*I. and O.*, 368, 44, E, f)

Three important deities had canine hypostases *Wp-wȝwt*, Khenti-amentu, and Anubis (Inepw).

Wp-w3wt "the Opener of the Way," was worshipped at Assiut. Its emblems preceded kings, and guided divine boats. Though closely connected with Khentiamentu and Anubis, it never became, like them, a god of the dead or of cemeteries. Under the Middle Kingdom it started to play a role at Abydos in the Osirean festivals where it represented the young kingship of Horus, as heir to the older generation (Helck and Otto, 1956, p. 388).

Khentiamentu (*Hnty-'imntyw*), "The First in the West," i.e. in the World of the Dead, was the local god of Abydos, the cemetery of the Thinite kings of the formative first two dynasties, where he had a temple dating to the first dynasty. During the fifth dynasty, Osiris absorbed and entirely superseded him as Lord of the Dead.

Anubis (*'Inpw*). The most famous of these canine gods, however, was Anubis who, at late epochs, was said to the be son of Isis and Osiris, although Plutarch asserted that Osiris begat him from his other sister Nephthys whom he mistook for Isis (*I. and O.*, XIV, 366B). More generally, he was given as mother Hesat, a sky-cow, which may account for his being called "Lord of the Milch Cows," besides his other titles that designated him as the past embalmer of Osiris, the patron of embalmers, and the leader of the deceased in the other world

> "The One of the Mummy wrappings, Chief of the Divine Pavilion, Lord of the Necropolis, He who is set on his Mountain."

In addition, he was one of the judges of the dead, and he verified the beam of the scales on which souls were weighed.

Anubis was thus one of the most important gods of the Egyptian Pantheon. Of his many sanctuaries the most famous was in the city the Greeks called Cynopolis, "The City of the Dog." He was represented either as a "jackal" sitting on all fours, black, the colour of the dead and of embalming resin (Fig. 5.18); ar as a human with a jackal head. The embalming priests identified themselves with him during the embalming rituals by wearing a jackal-head mask of which several examples are known (Fig. 1.6*a*).

He was further connected with the creation-god Khnum in the well-known scene of the divine birth of Queen Hatshepsut at Deir el-Bahari; and his interchangeability with *Wp-w3wt* gave him also the aspect of a king herald and protector, and of a fighter who, in Roman times, was shown in armour for, as the Osirean religion with its attendant dogmas of resurrection and immortality spread throughout the Hellenistic world, this god's cult became a general one in antiquity.

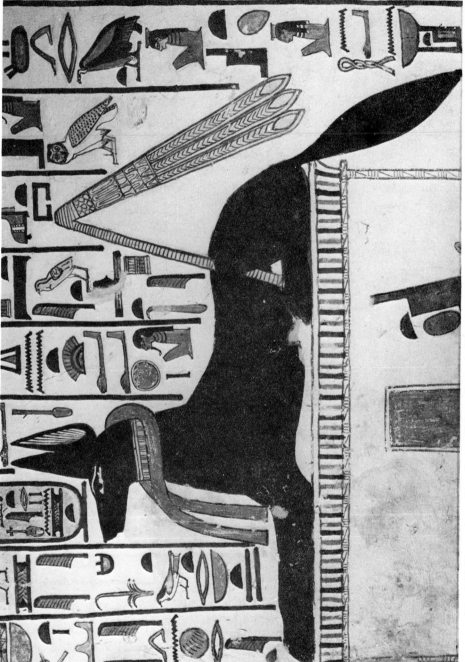

Fig. 5.18. The god Anubis. Queen Neferatri's tomb. Thebes. Courtesy of the Egyptian Documentation Centre.

The Dog in the Graeco-Roman Period

In the Graeco-Roman Period, dogs were, at times, despised; at others, venerated. Pliny (*N.H.*, XXIX, 14) described the conflicting attitudes

> "I have spoken of the fame won by the geese which detected the ascent of the Capitoline hill by the Gauls. For the same reason dogs are punished with death every year, being crucified alive on a cross of elder between the temple of Juventas and that of Summanus. But the customs of the ancients compel me to say several other things about the dog. Sucking puppies were thought to be such pure food that they even took the place of sacrificed victims to placate the divinities. Genita Mana[8] is worshipped with the sacrifice of a puppy and at dinners in honour of the gods even now puppy flesh is put on the table . . . Dog's blood is supposed to be the best remedy for arrow poison and this animal seems also to have shown mankind the use of emetics."

Pliny also asserted elsewhere that no dogs were admitted in the Island of Sygaros (*N.H.*, VI, 32) and was the author of the story of the Ptoem-phani of Sudan

> ". . . who have a dog for a king, and divine his commandments by his movements . . ." (*N.H.*, VI, 35)

Plutarch, in his "Roman Questions" (Moralia, IV, 263 C), attempted to answer the question why, although there were many shrines to Diana in Rome, the only one into which men may not enter is the shrine called Vicus Patricius. He asked

> "Is it because of the current legend? For a man attempted to violate a woman who was here worshipping the goddess, and was torn to pieces by the dogs; and men do not enter because of the superstitious fear that arose from this occurrence?"

Sextus Empiricus (*Outlines of Pyrrhonism*, III, 218–227), in his discussion of God, had several things to say of this animal. He first stated that ordinary people differ on the number and shapes of gods, even sharing the notions of the Egyptians who believe in gods that are dog faced, or hawk-shaped . . . etc. He continued his discussion by arguing that if the holy and unholy existed by nature, religious observances with regard to human diet would not be so diverse

> "Eating dog's flesh is thought by us to be sinful, but some of the Thracians are reported to be dog-eaters. Possibly this practice was customary also

amongst the Greeks, and on this account Diocles[9] too, starting from the practices of the Asclepiadae, prescribes that hounds' flesh should be given to certain patients."

Pursuing the argument he added

"The Hyrcanians[10] expose them [the dead] as a prey to dogs, and some of the Indians to vultures . . ."

These widely different aspects of dog-man relationships in different parts of the world have been well reviewed by Simoons (1961). According to this author, in Zoroastrian Persia, the dog was regarded as the most holy of animals, being associated with the god Ahura-Mazda. It was an offence to mistreat it, or kill it, or even to fail to feed it.

As further summarized by Simoons, in Haran, of Mesopotamia, a deity was referred to as "The Lord with the Dogs". In the Sudan, the Kuku are said to believe that civilization was taught to them by dogs. In Dahomey, dogs are sacred to the god Legba and, in Madagascar, the Sakalava nearly worship them. In Southeast Asia many groups believe that the dog is their ancestor, or regard it as a totemic animal and in the Nicobar Islands men wear ornaments typical of dogs.

Avoidance and Acceptance of Dogflesh

> *He was told 'Come to the kennel*
> *and take thee a dog'. He asked*
> *'A white or a black', and was*
> *told 'They all are dogs, sons*
> *of dogs'.*
> (Popular Egyptian saying)

These conflicting attitudes have not been limited to the worlds of the Mediterranean and Near East, for they are manifest in differences in customs all over the world.

Avoidance of dogflesh, which appears quite natural to Westerners, has not been—and still is not—so universal as one might think, although it has been spreading under pressure of dogflesh-avoiding groups, especially Christians and Moslems, and the areas of consumption are rapidly dwindling.

The avoidance attitudes of these two groups are quite different. The Westerner's attitude stems from a sentimental attachment to a beloved pet, a hunting companion, or a guardian of the household; the avoidance by the Moslem is an ingrained regard of the dog as an "unclean" or impure beast to be avoided. The basis of this Moslem view is obscure, as it is not revealed in the Koran. The depth of it is indicated by the fact that some bigots would consider their prayer valueless if the shadow of a dog fell upon them while praying.

An attempt at rationalization attributes this attitude to a realization of the relation between dogs and hydatid disease; but we have expressed our doubts elsewhere in these volumes on the sanitary reasons of animal taboos in general.

The abhorrence of dogs, the impurity of which is to be cleansed only by "seven lustrations, of which one with sand", is, however, tempered by the faithfulness of this traditional companion of man. A proverb says "If you eat with a man, he will betray you, but if you feed a dog with your waste, it will love you". As a result, contact is generally permitted with hunting and watch dogs.

In India, rejection is part of the general prohibition of killing or eating any animal flesh. In Zoroastrian Persia, in Horan, in areas where the dog is the totem of the clan, and in Cynopolis (see Chapter 7, p. 388) because of the assimilation of the dog to other canine deities, rejection rested on religious mythological grounds.

In some areas of southern Africa, the ban is not absolute. Whereas dogflesh is usually prohibited, it is eaten on some ceremonial occasions, like weddings and funerals; elsewhere, it is eaten only by men, not by women.

On the other hand, there are extensive centres of dog-eating. The most important, as mapped by Simoons (1961), extends in eastern Asia from eastern Siberia down to Assam, south, and to the Hawaii Islands east. In China, a special bread, the chow, was developed for the table. In Formosa, the delicacy is called "Fragrant meats" in restaurants (Simoons, 1961, p. 96).

Another centre is the region of rain forests and adjoining savannah in western Africa and the Congo Basin where, at one time, dog was prized so much that it was bartered for slaves.

The third centre, now restricted to rural Mexico, was Pre-Columbian America. Paradoxically, it is also stated that dogs are eaten by the Mohammedan Siwans, who are of a Berber stock, although we always heard this denied in the course of our many visits to this oasis.

Change is, however, slowly happening. Moslems and Christians have had a great influence on the people they conquered or converted and acceptance is rapidly declining.

Dog-eating in Ancient Egypt

In Ancient Egypt, evidence of the eating of dogflesh is confined to the single incident we related of Cynopolis (see Chapter 7, p. 388) that bespake, however, of religious vengeance, not of set custom.

The Dog in Therapeutics

We have seen Hippocrates describing the qualities of dogflesh and the physician Diocles prescribing it to his patients. Simoons (1961, p. 97) stated, after Hutton, that the Angami Nagas pluck out the eye of a living dog as an antidote for poison. It has also been said that Siwans roast puppies to treat tuberculosis, but we cannot vouch for this assertion.

The Ancient Egyptians, who used hound legs (*Eb.*, LXVI, 468), dung (*Eb.*, LXXIV, 578, 580; *Eb.*, LXXV, 584; *H.*, 41), or blood (*Eb.*, LXIII, 425) restricted their use to external applications for pains in the limbs, eczema (?), or purulency (?). Some of these prescriptions are particularly curious. One proposes for baldness

". . . a remedy prepared for the mother of His Majesty the King of Upper, and Lower Egypt, made of the leg of a hound, the hoof of an ass, etc."

Another, to remove hair, prescribes the genital (? menstrual) blood of a bitch (*H.*, 156), and a third purports to prevent the whitening of hair with the genitals of a bitch (*Eb.*, LXV, 460)—really early precursors of organotherapy.

The most curious prescription came, unexpectedly, from Dioscorides (II, 49)

"The liver of a mad dog being eaten roasted by those which have been bitten by him, is thought to keep them safe from the fear of water. For a precaution they also use the dog tooth of that dog which did bite, putting it into a bag and so tying it to the arm."

Hyena

Bones of hyena were reported in Sebilian assemblages (*MAE*, 67). Although these could have belonged to an animal accidentally killed during a general hunt of more usual species, several Old Kingdom tombs at Saqqara either depict them as fat, tame animals or illustrate their capture, domestication, and hand-feeding, reminiscent of the so-called "hyena-men" found today in Ethiopia.

In these feeding scenes, hyenas, unlike domestic animals, are always fed with their four legs tied (Fig. 5.19). No sacrificial slaughtering of any of them is depicted, save for the suggestive evidence of hyenas carved on the handle of a prehistoric sacrificial knife (Petrie and Quibbell, 1896, plate LXXVII).

A school of Egyptologists would credit all these scenes with religious meanings, namely, the repetition of the primaeval taming of wildlife, and the dramatization of the continuing victory of the gods and of their incarnation, Royalty, over Chaos.

Some observers reported having seen hyena-eating in Upper Egypt, although they probably witnessed an exceptional instance of folklore therapeutics. Hyena flesh still may be prescribed against rheumatism by healers in remote rural areas. The eyes and teeth may be credited with apotropaic powers as talismans, and the Bisharin may eat their boiled genitals to cure infertility; but these are obvious examples of sympathetic magic.

It would seem strange that this repulsive animal would appeal to a people living in plenty and known for their refinement. Gaillard (1912) thought that these tamed animals were used in the hunt and that, in the above-mentioned scenes, they were fed beforehand to remove any temptation to eat their prey. Montet, however, basing himself on their appearance in a sixth dynasty veterinary scene where they are fed, stated that they were originally eaten but that, thereafter, Egyptians desisted from feeding even the dead with such an unappetizing meat (1910, p. 43).

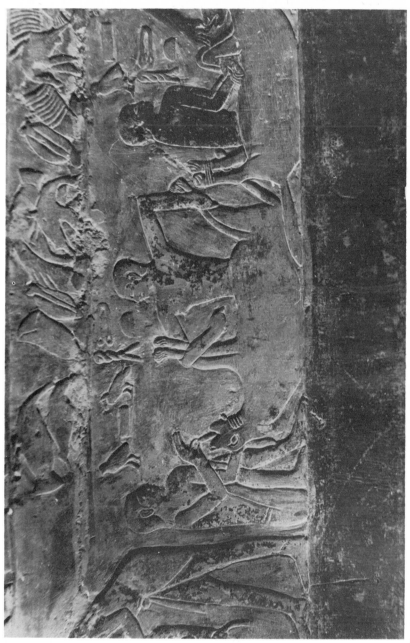

Fig. 5.19. Hyena being hand-fed with all four legs tied or secured. Mereruka's tomb. Saqqara. Old Kingdom. Photographed 1969.

Miscellaneous Mammals

Camel (Camelus sp.)

It is difficult to imagine Egypt or even North Africa or the Near East
without the camel that serves such a variety of functions. But the history
of the animal in Ancient Egypt is as perplexing as is that of the horse.

Camel bones were found in the Sebilian assemblage (*MAE*, p. 68).
A camel was found buried in the early historic Helwan cemetery (Saad,
1951, p. 38); a camel-shaped vase from Abu Sir el-Melek is known
(Scharff, 1957, plate 24, No. 209); and Caton-Thompson and Gardner
found camel-hair rope at Fayoum (1934). There is, therefore, no ques-
tioning the fact that the Early Egyptians were familiar with the animal
(Figs 5.20, 5.21).

Literary evidence, however, places the introduction of the camel in
the Persian Period and, in the interval, pictorial and archaeologic
evidence of its existence is utterly absent. The Bible cities it among
Pharaoh's animals

". . . and he [pharaoh] entreated Abram well for her sake; and he had
sheep and camels . . ." (Genesis, 12, 16)

Prior to the Exodus, the camel is again listed among the herds of the
king

". . . behold the hand of the Lord is upon thy cattle which is in the field,
upon the horses, upon the asses, upon the camels, upon the oxen, and upon
the sheep . . ." (Exodus, 9, 3)

Is it possible that the camel was "overlooked" by the artists of Dynastic
Egypt, and by the Greek and Roman traveller historians, because it was
too common to report? Or was the camel so usual in the Near East when
Genesis was written, that the writers of this Book thought it equally
common in Egypt at the time of Abraham's sojourn and of the Exodus,
and automatically included it in Pharaoh's animal park?

Whatever be the case, this animal seems never to have been eaten in
Egypt before the Arab invasion.

In Pre-Islamic Arabia, several taboos protected this most useful
animal, although exegetes are not in entire agreement on the qualifica-
tions that gained it affranchisement. Their general nature is, however,

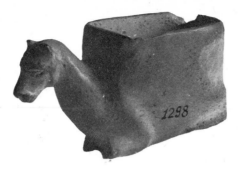

Fig. 5.20. Camel. Copy of vase excavated at Abusir el-Melek. Pre-Dynastic. Dokki Agricultural Museum. Photographed 1969. Used with permission.

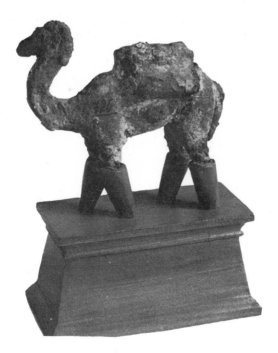

Fig. 5.21. Bronze camel. Roman Period. Dokki Museum. Photographed 1969. Used with permission.

understood. If a she-camel had borne ten times; when a male had a young that had begotten another young; when an ewe had yeaned seven times twins, and the seventh were a male and a female; if a stallion had sired ten times; or if a man had vowed to free a camel if he were cured of an illness, its ear was slit and none might drive it away from pasture, or water, or ride it, or eat of its flesh—all these bans were raised by the Koran.

Hippopotamus

This great lumbering water beast, so clumsy in its appearance that its head was used as a hieroglyph for heaviness, was once common throughout the length of the Nile, but now has disappeared from Egypt. In the thirteenth century it was still seen as far north as the Nile estuary at Damietta. But it must have been a rare sight, for Abdul Latif al-Baghdady, who reported the event, told that the local inhabitants did not know how to hunt it, and had Sudanese, trained in its capture, brought to overcome them (1965, pp. 99, 101). Its bones have been found in Sebilian strata (*MAE*, 1, 67) and in several sequences through the Maadian occupation (*MAE*, p. 130). Most important, however, was the extremely rare find, dated to the Fayoum "A" sequence, of a flint projectile tip embedded in a hippopotamus bone; a certain indication that early man in Egypt hunted it. The question of whether the Ancient Egyptians ate this animal, as do some of the southern Sudanese tribes today, must, however, be left open.

The gluttonous and destructive foraging habits of the hippopotamus must have appeared the picture of devastation to an early agricultural society. Hence, it is not surprising to find that it was considered a destructive god, and an embodiment of Seth.

Achilles Tatius (4, 4, 2–3) records this reason for concern by the farmers

". . . [the hippopotamus] is the greediest of all animals, sometimes taking a whole field of corn [wheat] at a meal . . ."

Diodorus Siculus (1, 35, 9–10) also commented on the harm wrought by the beast

". . . being a river and land animal, it spends the day in the streams exercising in the deep water, while at night it forages about the country-side on the grain and hay, so that, if this animal were prolific and reproduced each year, it would entirely destroy the farms of Egypt . . ."[11]

The destructive attributes of the hippopotamus were counterbalanced by those of a protective hippopotamus goddess, Ta-urt who oversaw childbirth and pregnancy (Fig. 5.22). Herodotus (II, 71) even writes that the hippopotamus was sacred in the province of Papremis, a further possible indication of Seth worship in that town. In locations where Ta-urt was revered, tiny faience statues have been found (Fig. 5.23). These may not have been cult objects, however, but "charms" to ward off the destructive effects of these creatures.

The numerous representations in the Egyptian tombs showing hippopotamus hunts, and the details of these almost ritual scenes (Fig. 7.19) possibly indicate that these may have been mere religious similes. Diodorus (1, 35, 10–11) wrote of such a hunt

". . . but even it is caught by the united work of many men who strike it with iron spears; for whenever it appears they converge their boats upon it, and gathering about it wound it repeatedly with a kind of chisel fitted with iron barbs, and then, fastening the end of a rope of tow to one of them which has become imbedded in the animal, they let it go until it dies from loss of blood. Its meat is tough and hard to digest and none of its inward parts is edible, neither the viscera nor the intestines . . ."

The last portion of this descriptive passage does indicate that the hunters at least knew the taste of the flesh of their victim; or perhaps shared in a ritualistic feast.

Medicinally, the fat of hippopotamus leg was used with other ingredients to prevent the fall of hair caused by a hated woman's concoction (*Eb.*, LXVII, 476); its fat, with other animal fats, made the hair of bald persons grow (*Eb.*, LXVI, 465); and the effects of vaginal fumigation with its excreta helped to diagnose sterility: if the woman vomited she was sterile; if she passed wind, she was fertile (*Carlsb.*, 5).

Elephant

Hayes (*MAE*, p. 48) reports bones of the elephant from Middle Paleolithic sites in Egypt. Rock carvings of elephants and elephant hunts are not uncommon along the eastern bank of the Nile. These are usually

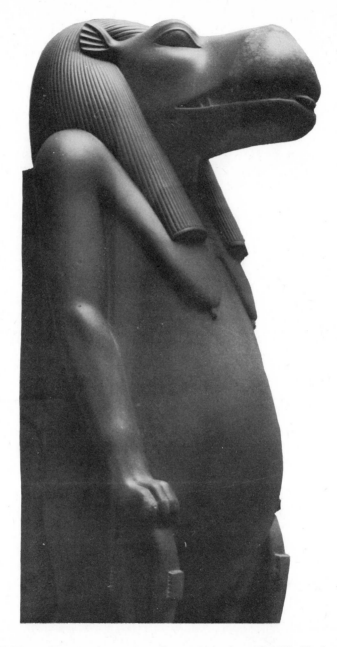

Fig. 5.22. The goddess Ta-urt. Cairo Museum. Photographed 1969. Used with permission.

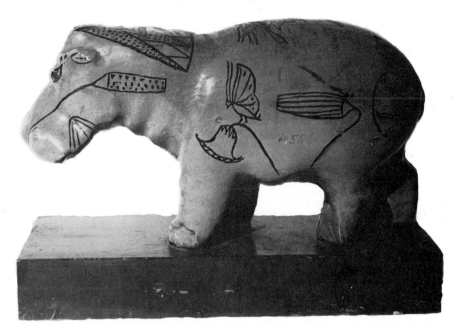

Fig. 5.23. Hippopotamus. Faience Amulet. Cairo Museum. Photographed 1969.
Used with permission.

dated to the Late Palaeolithic/Mesolithic time boundary (*MAE*, 73).
Elephant bones have, likewise, been found in the Fayoum "A" sequence
(*MAE*, p. 93), but have not further been reported in the Dynastic Period
except as imported "exotic" specimens from southern and central
Africa. It is evident that they were of no significant importance as a
source of food in ancient times.

Giraffe

Numerous carvings of giraffes in the western desert of Egypt have been
reported, particularly at the oasis of Khargah (*MAE*, 73, 102). Several
New Kingdom tombs at Luxor show the giraffe as an "exotic" specimen
received as a present or a tribute (Fig. 5.13); but there is no evidence to
support a claim that they were eaten.

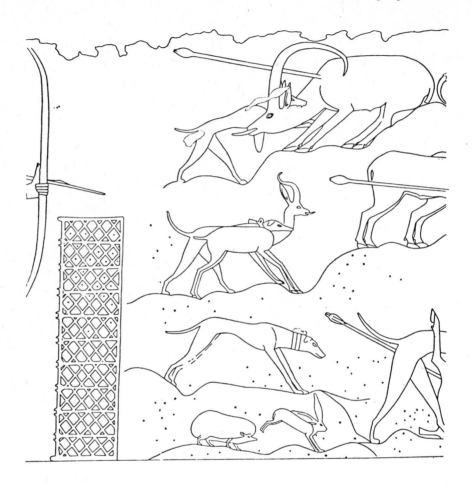

Fig. 5.24. Tomb of Senbi, Meir (Blackman, 1914, plate VII). Part of a hunting scene showing ibex and a running rabbit.

Hares and Rabbits   *śḫ't*

The hare was the nome sign of the sixteenth nome of Upper Egypt (Hermopolis Magna). Bones of this animal were found at Toukh as reported by Ruffer (1919, pp. 24–25). It is not mentioned in offering lists and has not been represented in pens or in captivity; but it is often a feature of hunting scenes, either wounded or running away and hiding (Figs 5.13, 5.24, 6.42). An occasional bearer is also illustrated holding a hare to offer it as a present. There is little doubt that it was eaten, but it is probable that the domestic rabbit had not been evolved yet, and that these animals were either hare or wild rabbits.

Mice   *pnw*

Abdullatif al-Baghdady, in his relation of Egypt (1965, p. 197), mentioned that in his time (thirteenth century A.D.), some people ate the field mice found in the deserts and low parts after the retreat of the Nile waters, and that they called them "the quail of the low countries".

Medically, physicians used mice in ointments. For example, *H.*, 149 recommended frying (or macerating) a mouse in fat and using it as a hair salve. Another prescription was mouse fat mixed with the fat of seven other animals (*Ram.*, V, no. III); and what seems, according to Grapow (*Wb. Dr.*, 198), an abbreviated version was content with only three other kinds of fat (*Eb.*, 658, LXXXII).

Magicians were even more weird. They fed a sick child or its mother a cooked mouse[12] and had them wear its bones, wrapped in a linen cloth knotted with seven knots (*Zaub.*, vs 8, 2–3).

But there is no evidence that indicates that mice were eaten in Ancient Egypt.

Notes: Chapter 5

1. It is interesting that the Greek Hercules, perhaps because of this initial confrontation with Amon at Thebes, was equated in Late Dynastic and Post-Dynastic times with the Egyptian god, Hershef, the Harsaphes of the Greeks; a ram-headed god of great antiquity worshipped at the town of Heracleopolis Magna in the Fayoum (Ames, 1965). In hieroglyphic writing a ram's head was added as a determinative of words meaning "power, prestige."

2. A reference to the "hidden" aspect of Amon, a pun on his name and *imn* "hidden."

3. A Koranic personage, called Alexander of the Two Horns, is believed by some to commemorate the memory of Alexander of Macedonia.

4. Born of various parentage according to several legends, this god of shepherds appeared as a monster with horns; his legs and feet were goat-like, while the rest of his body, with the exception of a tail, was human in appearance. Though a Greek god, Pan is closely connected in Greek mythology with Egypt; it was claimed that he appeared as a goat because when the gods (of Greece) fled into Egypt during their war against the Giants, Pan transformed himself into this animal, an example soon followed by the other Gods. (Summarized from Lemprière, 1963, pp. 439–440.)

5. Could refer to the twelve major gods of the Greeks, the *Dii consentes* of the Romans, or to the eleven major gods of the Egyptians (plus Pan): Nun, Atum, Ra, Shu, Tefnut, Geb, Nut, Osiris, Isis, Seth, Nephthys.

6. In the Late Dynastic Period the chief of the sacred ram gods was Ba-neb-djedet that easily degenerated in vernacular into "Banaded," from which the unfamiliar Greek ear might have developed "Mendes" (Ames 1965, p. 130).

7. According to a note from the Documentary Centre of the Louvre, kindly communicated to us by Mr S. Sauneron, the painting was brought to France in 1660 and formed part of the collection of Louis XIV. It was at first thought to illustrate a reception by Mohamet II in Constantinople, but its real subject was later recognized by Ch. Scheffer who quoted a relation of Zaccaria Pagani who described it as the reception, on May 10th, 1512, of Domenico Trevisano and five companions in the yard of the Cairo Citadel, by Sultan Qansouh al-Ghoury, whose crest figures on the wall.

  The painting had been attributed to Bellini, but Scheffer argued that Bellini, having died in 1507, could not have painted a ceremony that took place in 1512, although the painting had been definitely inspired by his sketches. In fact, it has been attributed to one of Bellini's pupils, Mansuetti, Belliniano, or Catena. Speaking of this painting, Sauvageon stated that it represented a corpus of European traders in Damascus, with their consul at their head, visiting the Governor of the city. He attributed it to Bellini, comparing it to a painting in Milano, and he suggested that Bellini had in fact sojourned in Damascus. The painting was copied in England, and inspired a tapestry at Bowis castle, of which Wace and Clayton wrote in 1938 that it was clearly related to a picture in the Louvre, and that it is probable that the picture in the Louvre was painted by an artist who had personal knowledge of the Cairene Court.

8. An old divinity supposed to have presided over childbirth.

9. A famous physician of the fourth century B.C.

10. South of the Caspian Sea.

11. Pliny (VIII, XXXVIII, 95) gave a fanciful description of the hippopotamus "A monster which has cloven hoofs like those of oxen, a horse's back, mane and neigh, a snub snout, a boar's tail. . . It feeds on the crops marking out a definite proportion beforehand for each day, so it is said, and making its footprints lead out of the field, so that no traps may be laid for it when it returns."

12. A similar usage has been observed by one of us (L.G.) among the Tlokwa of Botswana.

Chapter 6   Fowl and Eggs

Introduction

Egypt lies midway along the migratory route of the Palaearctic bird fauna. Twice yearly, migratory birds pass through it on their journey between central and southern Africa and northern Europe. On their way northward, many pause along the shores of the Delta lakes, or rest near the southern Mediterranean coastline before continuing their flight across the sea (Mackworth-Praed and Grant, 1957; Moreau, 1966; Etchécopar and Hüe, 1967; Williams, 1967). With the change of seasons the same coastal areas are filled once again with the birds returning to Africa (Lynes, 1909–1910; Moreau, 1953). In either case after their trans-Saharan or trans-Mediterranean flight, the birds reach Egypt in an exhausted state and, from the beginning of historical record, have been captured with relative ease, forming a substantial part of the seasonal diet of Egyptians.

Non-migratory indigenous birds were, likewise, well known to the early settlers in the Nile Valley. During the Pre-Dynastic and Dynastic Periods the goose, hawk/falcon, ibis, and vulture were adopted by Egyptian society into its religion, either as regional totems or as visual emblems or incarnations of specific gods (Figs 1.3, 1.7, 1.14). Gardiner (1950) lists 24 birds used as hieroglyphic signs, either determinatives because of distinctive characteristics; or phonetic, on the principle of homonymy; or based on acrophony, i.e., giving a picture the value of its first consonant.

There are many Ancient Egyptian, Greek, Roman and Arabic texts that describe the characteristics, behaviour, and culinary use of birds, and contemporary naturalists have added descriptive details and attempted their zoological classification (Whymper, 1909; Meinertzhagen, 1922, 1930, 1954; Thompson, 1966; Keimer, 1930; Lortet and Hugounenq, 1902, p. 18; Loret, 1892a).

It is difficult, however, to define the exact taxonomic identity of many of the birds illustrated in tombs or discussed in the literature of Ancient Egypt. There are, for example, several general terms that, at present, can be translated only as "bird" (*apd*)[1]; "wildfowl" (*ḳbḥw*,[2]

$h\ni w,^3$); "water fowl" ($msyt,^4$ $šdw^5$); or "poultry" ($wšnw,^6$ $ḫt^{c_37}$). These were undoubtedly used by the Ancients with more distinctive meanings, but at present their wide scope creates difficulties of identification. During the later periods, Ptolemaic and Roman, the general grouping of fowl better conformed to modern classification, and information is thus less ambiguous.

In a study of antiquity that attempts to understand retrospectively not only the varieties existant at a certain period but also their significance to culture and society, one may be forced to speculate on whether a particular variety was captured or raised primarily for food, religious use such as sacrifice, egg production, social status or as pets.

In this chapter no attempt is made to list all known instances where specific varieties of birds were used as food in Egypt. Such a presentation would merely catalogue most of the known Egyptian fowl. Instead, we have concentrated on the major fowl consumed by Egyptians in antiquity, but we have included some information on less common but especially interesting species.

Fowling Techniques

". . . it is good, however, when the net is drawn in and the birds are made fast . . ." (*Admonitions of a Prophet*, First Intermediate Period: Erman, 1966, p. 106)

The principal tool used by the Ancient Egyptians of all times to capture fowl was the field net. The commonest method of use involved a team supervised by a "signaler" or "look-out" man posted with a cloth in hand (Fig. 6.1) to watch for the prey. Rhomboidal double-sided clap-traps were spread on the ground, possibly baited with grain or immobilized live birds, as is sometimes practiced now in Port-Said. A tripping rope was played out some distance from the net, and the fowlers hid behind foliage or blinds of aquatic plants. On a silent sign the "signaler" made with his cloth, the rope was pulled and the net snapped shut on the birds. These nets were usually operated by servants but, in some instances, at Beni Hassan and Thebes, nobility participated (Fig. 6.2). No specialization was involved since the same word *šḫty* meant equally peasant, fowler and fisherman.[9]

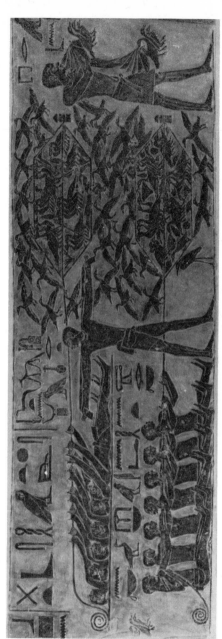

Fig. 6.1. A team of fowlers pulling the rope of a net under supervision of a "look-out" man. Tomb of Ptahhetep at Saqqara; Old Kingdom, fifth dynasty, reign of King Djed-Ka-Re, *c.* 2450 B.C. Rubbing by Ward Patterson; used with permission (1969).

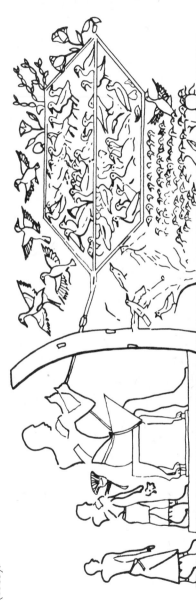

Fig. 6.2. A nobleman pulling at a fowl net. Tomb of Khnumhotep at Beni Hassan; Middle Kingdom, eleventh dynasty, date uncertain. Redrawn from Newberry and Fraser (1893b) Vol. 2, plate 33.

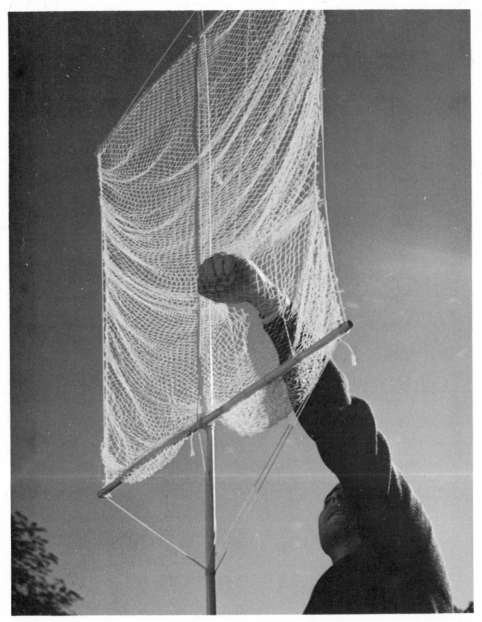

Fig. 6.3. Modern field net used in portions of the northeastern Delta to capture "song-birds". Compare construction with Figs 6.1 and 6.2. Photographed at NAMRU-3; used with permission (1969).

The continuity of culture is illustrated by the use, near the Mediterranean today, of traps similar to these (Fig. 6.3) to capture humming birds sold as pets (see also Dunham, 1937, pp. 52–54), or small birds for the table (beccaficos and other passerines), or hawks to be trained and sold in Arabia to hawk hunters.

A smaller type of net is known from the tomb of Mereruka at Saqqara (reign of King Teti, sixth dynasty, *c.* 2423 B.C.), where artists have depicted a flock of "quail-like" birds infesting a grain field, and a team of men using the smaller field net to catch them (Fig. 6.4).

Small "spring traps" were used during the Middle Kingdom in the region of Beni Hassan where artists portrayed the capture of fowl in two stages—the birds first diving towards the open net, and then ensnared within the traps (Fig. 6.5a, b). The traps and snares were baited with worms. One can nearly hear the amorous maiden, singing to her beloved

". . . I have come and catch with my trap in mine hand . . . All birds . . . settle upon Egypt . . . The one that cometh first, it taketh my worm . . . The voice of the goose, caught on its worm, crieth out, but love for thee holdeth me back and I cannot loose it . . ." (Erman, 1927, pp. 246, 247)

Bird traps constructed in Egypt today closely resemble those illustrated at Beni Hassan (Figs 6.6, 6.7, 6.8 and 6.9).

Another variety of trap not hitherto known from Ancient Egyptian illustrations may have been known in antiquity, considering its ease of construction and its wide use today in Egypt. A shallow pit is dug in the sand. Over this is balanced a heavy lid, most commonly a discarded tray, supported by a trigger mechanism made from split palm fronds. Grain is sprinkled inside the pit to attract birds. These trip the mechanism, and the heavy lid falls preventing their escape (Fig. 6.10).

As a sport, fowling is illustrated in numerous paintings and reliefs; and sufficiently large numbers of birds could occasionally be obtained by these procedures to be used as food. At all periods nobles are shown standing in their shallow marsh boats hurling "throw sticks" (*'m'm$t*), commonly but erroneously described as "boomerangs."[10] This technique, almost certainly a sporting survival of an earlier regular hunting tradition, is best illustrated in the New Kingdom paintings at Thebes. Its preponderance at that period may be a reflection of the expansion of leisurely activities among the nobility. But these "throw stick" paintings are so stereotyped that their near identity suggests a ritualistic significance to the act (Figs 6.11, 6.12, and 6.13). Only rarely did the artist imbue

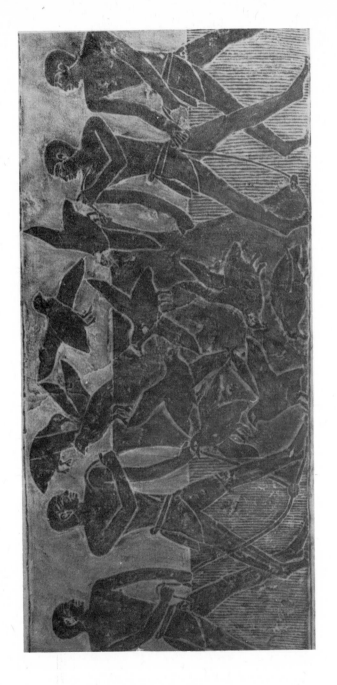

Fig. 6.4. Small quail net. Tomb of Mereruka at Saqqara; Old Kingdom, sixth dynasty, reign of King Teti, *c.* 2390 B.C. Rubbing by Ward Patterson; used with permission (1969).

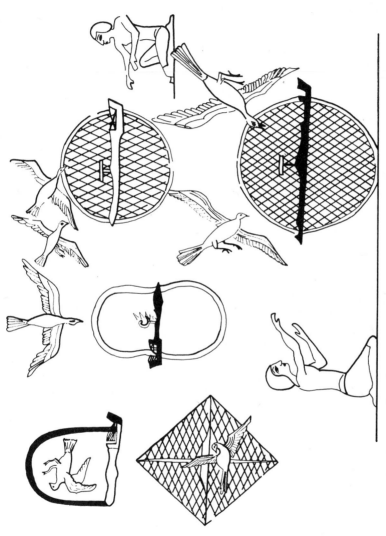

Fig. 6.5a. Egyptian bird traps. Several varieties depicted in the tomb of Khety (number 17) and Baqt III (number 15) at Beni Hassan; Middle Kingdom, eleventh dynasty, date uncertain. Redrawn from Wilkinson (1878) Vol. 2, p. 103, Fig. 362.

his nobleman with sufficient originality to confer upon him an individuality. Some interesting variations are seen, however, where decoy ducks[11] are held in the hand of the thrower, or placed prominently on the prow of the papyrus boat. In several instances pet cats seem to assist in retrieval.

Hunting marsh fowl with bow and arrow was also apparently a sporting event. From the earliest times, birds such as the ostrich were hunted in this manner. Although we know of no Old Kingdom tombs that show ostrich hunts, Pre-Dynastic rock carvings and vase ornamentation witness to the practice. Tomb paintings from Beni Hassan (eleventh dynasty) and Thebes (eighteenth dynasty), incised gold plates, and ivory and wood chests from Tut-ankh-Amon's treasure (Desroches-Noblecourt 1963, Fig. 41) confirm that far into the Dynastic Period the ostrich was shot by bow and arrow either for sport or for its feathers. Dogs were also used by the Pre-Dynastic and Dynastic Egyptians to bring down these large birds (Fig. 6.42). Excellent summaries on fowling in antiquity with contemporary attitudes and techniques used in the eastern Mediterranean and Egypt may be found in the writings of MacPherson (1897) and Clark (1948).

Raising Fowl in Ancient Egypt

Poultry yards are commonly depicted in Old Kingdom reliefs, especially at Deir el Gabrawi and Saqqara (Figs 6.14a, b) but, the first attempts to raise or domesticate fowl were plausibly not completely successful, and the number of birds produced in "pens" would presumably have to be supplemented with specimens freshly collected during the yearly migrations (Moreau, 1930, Vol. 1, p. 68).

Captured fowl were removed from the field nets or "spring traps" and placed in basket cages, but they were sometimes carried by hand, or strung by the wings or feet across poles carried by servants (Figs 6.15, 6.16a, b).

Fig. 6.5b. Birds diving towards a trap. From a painting by Cailliaud (1831), Darby Collection. Scenes from Beni Hassan, Middle Kingdom.

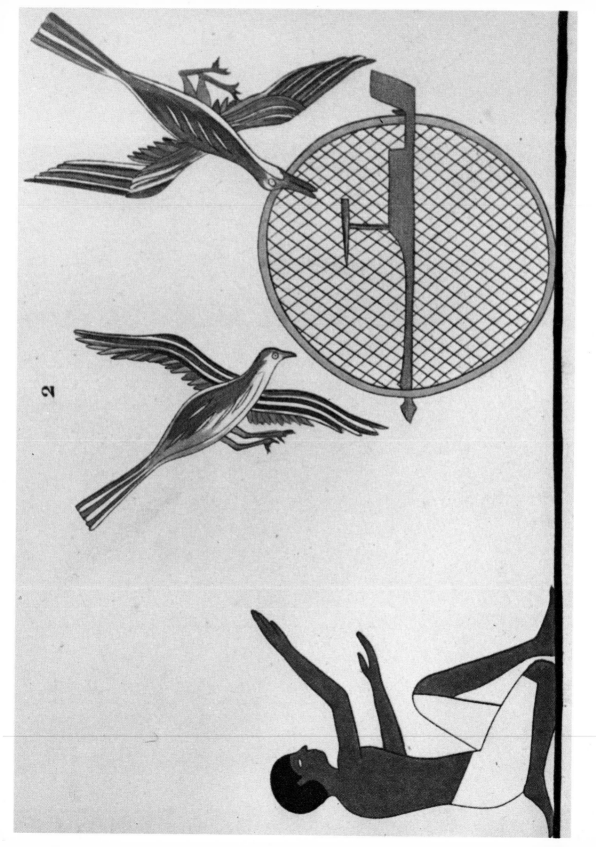

Poultry cages are illustrated as large structures filled with cranes, ducks, geese, or pigeons, each species being apparently isolated in an individual case. Their behaviour, fighting, pecking and preening is often shown with an accuracy not devoid of humour.

Servants fed the penned birds by scattering grain inside the enclosure. Forced feeding was used for fattening certain varieties, particularly cranes, ducks and geese. Grain was roasted, shaped into pellets, and stuffed down the gullet of the bird (Figs 6.17 and 6.18). Some geese were hand-fed, possibly because they were sick, but more probably in order to fatten them, or to enlarge their livers as in the production of *foie gras* (which has been documented since the Roman Period).[12]

Fowl as Offerings, Sacrifice and Food

One of the most common motifs of funerary art shows servants carrying various foods, domestic animals and birds, as offerings to the deceased (Figs 6.19a, b). The birds are carried by a variety of ways; by the wings, in baskets, or suspended on poles. Untamed large birds, such as geese and cranes, were immobilized to prevent possible danger to the eyes of the bearer. Tame fowl were herded or carried without restraint.

Fowl depicted as offerings were most usually live birds. In some instances, however, servants are shown wringing the necks of the fowl (Fig. 6.20) or even offering dressed birds (Fig. 6.21a).

Little is known concerning the purification and dedication of these offerings of fowl, but New Kingdom tombs at Thebes sometimes show them purified with oils, then laid upon special stands and singed (Fig. 6.21b).

Birds for human and, in rare Old Kingdom illustrations, for animal consumption, were killed by wringing the neck or by cutting the throat (Fig. 3.36). It may be significant that the same word *wšn*, but with a different determinative, means either to wring the neck of poultry or to make an offering.[13] Numerous paintings from Thebes show servants plucking feathers, as drab a task in antiquity as today (Figs 6.22 and 6.23); or illustrate cooked (?) or pickled (?) fowl hanging from the ceiling of meat shops (Figs 6.22, 6.23).

Dressed birds were sometimes preserved by pickling (Fig. 6.23). Herodotus (II, 77), writing from a period long removed from early

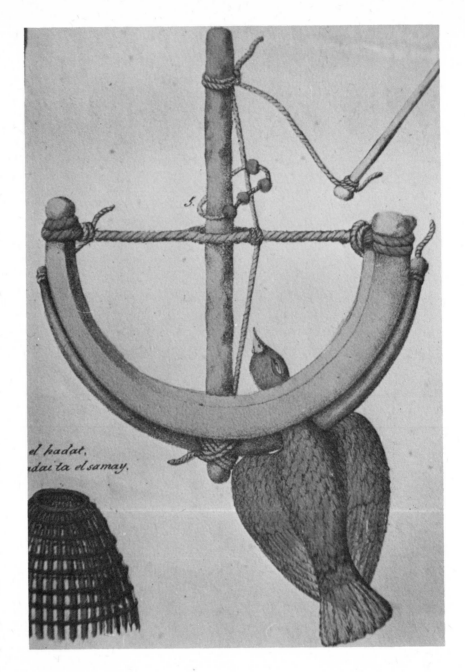

Fig. 6.6. Spring-operated bird trap used in parts of Egypt during the early nineteenth century. From a drawing by M. J. Rifaud (1830). Darby Collection.

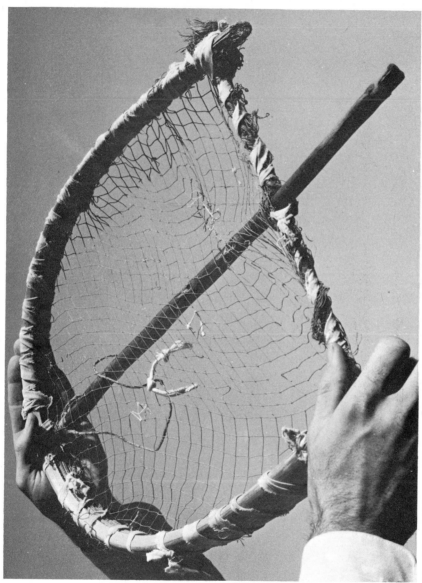

Fig. 6.7. Small spring-operated bird trap used today in parts of the northeastern Delta. (See Figs 6.8 and 6.9 showing trap in use.) Photographed at NAMRU-3; used with permission (1969).

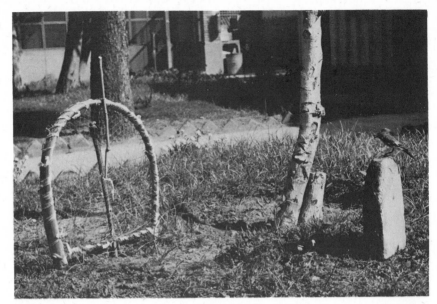

Fig. 6.8. Spring-operated bird trap detailed in Fig. 6.7 here shown in set position. Bird perched at right has been attracted to the bait. Photographed at NAMRU-3; used with permission (1969).

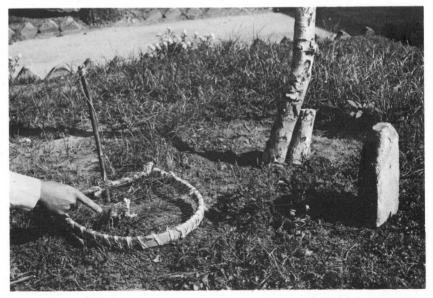

Fig. 6.9. Closed position of trap. Bird has been captured. Photographed at NAMRU-3; used with permission (1969).

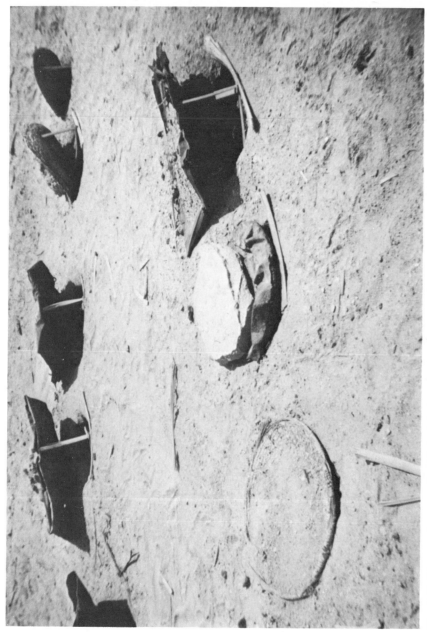

Fig. 6.10. Pit-traps for capturing birds. Split palm leaves form the trigger mechanism. Lids are discarded household trays or flattened "jerry-cans" from the Second World War. Qara oasis (Western Desert); photographed 1966.

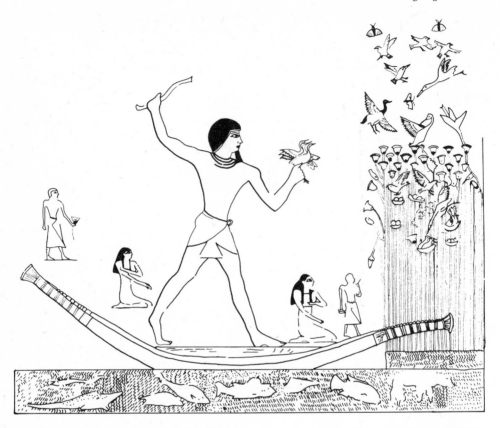

Fig. 6.11. Fowling by throwstick. Tomb of Khnum-hotep (number 3) at Beni Hassan; Middle Kingdom, eleventh dynasty, date uncertain, Redrawn from Newberry and Fraser (1893b), Vol. 2, plate 32.

New Kingdom art, offered the first Greek literary reference to pickled or salted fowl as a component of Egyptian diet

". . . quails also, and ducks, and small birds, they eat uncooked, merely first salting them . . ."

Usually, however, plucked fowl were skewered from end to end and roasted over a fire; less commonly, they were boiled (Fig. 6.24). In regard to both these methods of cooking, Herodotus (II, 77) observed

". . . all other birds and fishes excepting those which are set apart as sacred are eaten roasted or boiled . . ."[14]

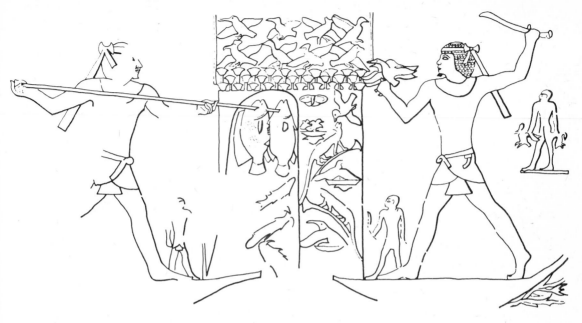

Fig. 6.12. Fowling by throwstick. Tomb of Akhet-hotep at Saqqara; Old Kingdom, fifth dynasty, reign of King Djed-Ka-Re, *c.* 2450 B.C. Redrawn from Petrie *et al.* (1952), plate 6.

Varieties of Fowl Eaten in Ancient Egypt

Egyptian texts are often vague as to the varieties of birds used. A record attributed to Senbi, a military officer under Pepi II (sixth dynasty, *c.* 2200 B.C.) says

". . . there was given to me the gold of praise; there were given to me rations, meat, and fowl . . ." (*A.R.*, I, 373)

It is likewise frustrating to learn that King Rameses III (nineteenth dynasty, *c.* 1198–1166 B.C.) offered to the gods of Egypt during a 31-year period more than 326,000 birds, only few of which can be identified (*A.R.*, IV, 168).

Usually, however, the problem does not lie with Egyptian neglect at classification, but with the inability of modern workers to assign scientific names to the varieties mentioned in antiquity. The Egyptians

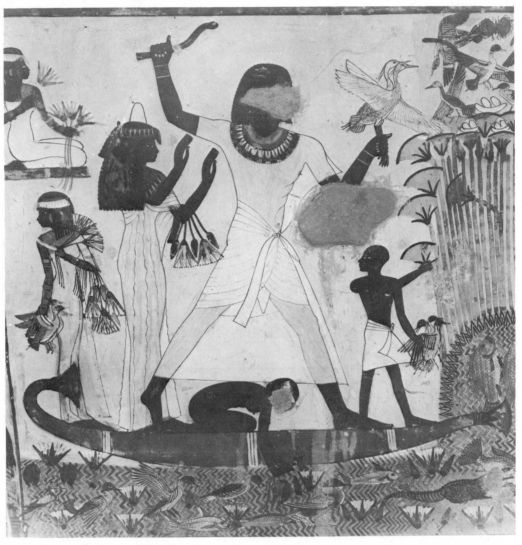

Fig. 6.13. Tomb of Mena (number 69) at Thebes (Upper Enclosure); New Kingdom, eighteenth dynasty, reign of King Thutmose IV, *c.* 1420 B.C. Photograph used with permission of the Ministry of Culture and the officials of the Centre for Documentation, Cairo ARE (1969).

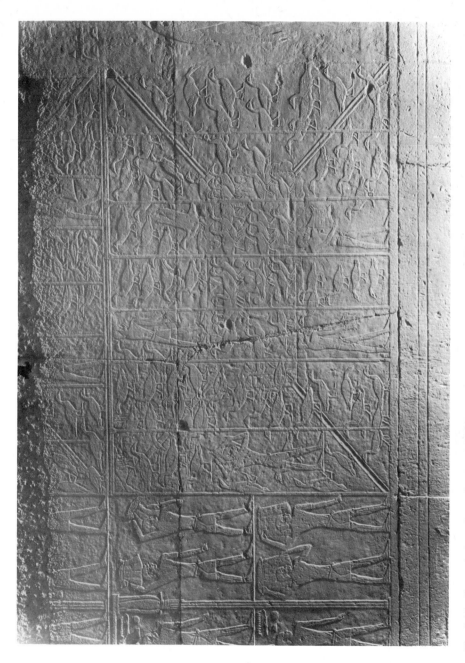

Fig. 6.14a. General view of a poultry yard, Saqqara Old Kingdom, fifth dynasty, reign of King Nefer-ir-ka-Re and Ne-Woser, Re, *c.* 2500 B.C. Photograph used with permission of the Ministry of Culture and the officials of the Centre for Documentation-Cairo, ARE (1969).

differentiated many kinds of fowl, as evidenced by their large vocabulary. There is even a long ornithological list at Beni Hassan in the tomb
of Baqt III (number 15), that gives nearly thirty individual names for
birds, with an accompanying portrait of each species. But the progress
of Egyptologists, classicists, and ornithologists in equating modern
names with ancient counterparts is slow, and much confusion remains
(see Capart, 1941; Davies, 1949; Thompson, 1966; Schuz, 1966).

Complicating the taxonomic problem is the possibility of a change
having taken place in the avian fauna of Egypt. Hence, the individual
varieties consumed in modern Egypt may or may not be identical with
the ones consumed in antiquity. As stated earlier, the varieties of fowl
listed in the following section form the core of those eaten in Ancient
Egypt.

Family Anatidae

Duck (*Anas and Related Genera*)

Bones, tentatively identified as belonging to duck, found in excavations
at the Pre-Dynastic settlement of El Omari, permit one to assume that,
early in this region, man captured migratory marsh birds for food
(Debono, 1948). At Saqqara, Old Kingdom sequences frequently
portrayed the capture, feeding, and presentation of duck as food for the
deceased. Paintings from the Middle and New Kingdoms in various
parts of Egypt confirm the regard in which duck was held as food. Many
paintings at Thebes, dated to the New Kingdom, depict their brilliant
plumage with such faithful accuracy that ready identification of the
species is possible.

Two words, *zt* or *st*[15] and *apd*[16] have been proposed as equivalent to
duck and "pintail duck" (*Anas acuta*), but additional research is needed
to determine other specific varieties of "water fowl." Ancient Egyptian
literature does not precisely identify "duck" as an article of diet, but
an artist's sketch, dated to the reign of King Amenhotep IV (Akhenaten)
late eighteenth dynasty depicts the enjoyment of a meal of "duck"
(Fig. 6.25).

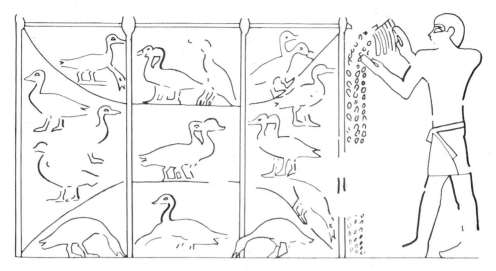

Fig. 6.14b. Poultry yard; Tomb of Aba. Redrawn from Davies, 1902.

Family Anatidae

Goose (Anser and Related Genera)

> *A thrifty wife serves a whole wedding party with one goose*
> Egyptian Proverb

Reverence of the goose dates to the beginnings of Egyptian cosmological thought. It was imagined that the "great cackler" or "cosmic goose," fathered the primordial egg from which the sun was born (Ames, 1965, pp. 27, 35, 52). As such, the goose was commonly associated with several Egyptian divinities such as, Amon (Fig. 1.1) and Geb (Fig. 1.3).

Some geese were dedicated to the Egyptian gods and left to flock in various temple pools (*A.R.*, II, 559). Such temple flocks are mentioned in the *Papyrus of Nu* (*Book of the Dead*) where the deceased, questioned by various gods, spirits, and genii, was required to swear

". . . I have not snared the geese in the pens of the gods . . ."

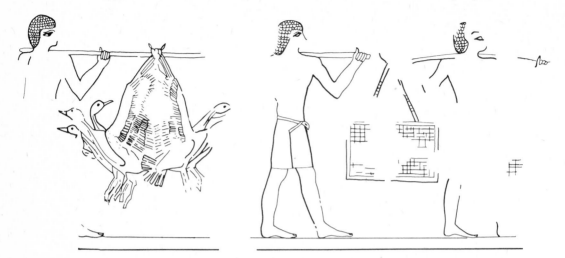

Fig. 6.15. Birds strung by their wings to poles carried by servants. Tomb of Thut-Hotpe (number 2) at El Bersheh; Middle Kingdom, twelfth dynasty, date uncertain. Redrawn from Griffith *et al.* (1894), plate 23.

(a)

smn

(b)

r

(c)

srw

(Budge, 1960, p. 575). It is highly probable, however, that they were later sacrificed.

The Ancient Egyptians distinguished several varieties of geese, but ornithologists cannot equate with certainty these names with modern species. Five words from Egyptian records are usually translated as "geese". These are depicted by (a),[17] (b),[18] (c)[19] (d)[20] and (?) (e).[21] An illustrated list of offerings (Fig. 6.26) in the tomb of Ptahhetep at Saqqara (fifth dynasty, reign of King Djed-Ka-Re) mentions three of these varieties among a larger list of fowl

". . . 121,200 *r}*-geese, 121,200 *trp*-geese, and 11,110 *smn*-geese. . ."

(Davies, 1900, p. 11). Piankoff (1968, pp. 136–137), using a different vocalization, also reported that *ra*-geese and *therep*-geese were offered to King Unas (fifth dynasty, *c.* 2423 B.C.).

One is, however, struck by the vivid representation of geese in art of Ancient Egypt. In the tomb of Itet at Meidum (third dynasty, reign of King Snefru, *c.* 2700 B.C.), that contained perhaps the best of all known geese paintings, these are so accurate that one forgets that they were painted nearly 5,000 years ago (Riddell, 1943). Unfortunately, the hieroglyphic names for these birds were not included.

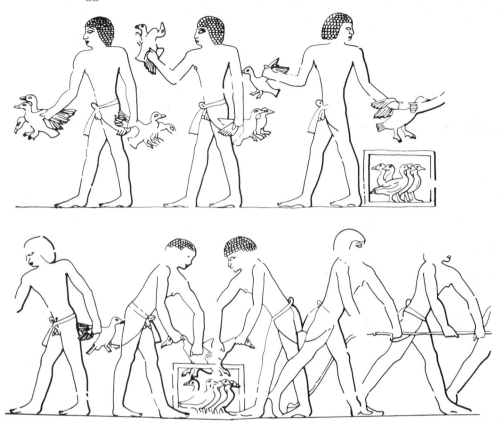

Fig. 6.16a. Fowls transported by hand or in cages. Tomb of Ptahhetep at Saqqara; Old Kingdom, fifth dynasty, reign of King Djed-Ka-Re, *c.* 2450 B.C. Redrawn from Davies (1901), plate 5.

Roasted goose was a common food throughout the Dynastic Period. Not only were dressed geese frequently included in funerary offerings to the deceased, but examples of preserved remains are known. A specially prepared goose, wrapped with strips of fine linen (Fig. 6.27), was found among the meat and food offerings to King Amenhotep II (eighteenth dynasty, *c.* 1425 B.C.). But these are relatively rare in comparison with the numerous instances of stone images of geese (Fig. 6.28), that were placed in the tombs as substitutes for the actual birds.

This position of the goose may be contrasted with that of the ibis, another sacred bird, that was strictly prohibited as food (pp. 323–326). One wonders whether the reason of the ban on ibis was its disagreeable

(d)

Gb

(e)

ṯrp

taste compared to that of the goose. It is interesting to find the goose, so important in Egyptian religion and mythology, among the major varieties sacrificed on temple altars and commonly eaten throughout the land. This inconsistency in regard to sacred animals perplexed the early Greek visitors to Egypt, in particular Herodotus, who was amazed that the goose that was sacred to the Nile god (II, 72), was also a major component in the diet of Egyptian priests (II, 37).

During the Ptolemaic and Roman Periods roast goose continued to be a favourite article of diet. Theopompus of Chios noted that the Egyptians served "fatted geese" and calves to their special guests (Athenaeus, 9, 384, A).

Family Columbidae

Doves and Pigeons (Columba and Related Genera)

Aristotle (*History of Animals*, 544, 13) divided his "pigeon family" into five categories: *Peristera*, the common pigeon; *Pelias*, the rock pigeon; *Phatta* or *Phassa*, the ring dove; *Oenas*, the stock dove; and *Trighon*, the turtle dove. Others, e.g. Sophronius, made a different usage of these words (Liddell and Scott, 1966) but, in general, ancient naturalists did not distinguish clearly between doves and pigeons and confused and misidentified them throughout antiquity.

Both were used for food, and were raised in similar structures, being considered in Egyptian, Greek, and Roman minds, basically the same. Their names are often interchanged. That references to "doves" are less frequent is most probably an artifact of confused etymology rather than an indication of predominence of "pigeons" in Egyptian history. Thus, we are considering them here as one group.

(f)

mnwt

Although the evidence is sketchy, doves/pigeons seem to have been a favourite table fowl throughout most of Egyptian history. In Ancient Egyptian vocabulary the term depicted by (f)[22] signified pigeon, and that signified by (g)[23] questionably meant dove. These birds are depicted in tombs of all periods either as offerings to the deceased, or as one of the main population of "poultry yards" (Abu-Bakr and Badawy, 1953, pp. 54–55; Davies, 1900, p. 11).

(g)

In addition to this pictorial evidence is the finding by Emery (1962,

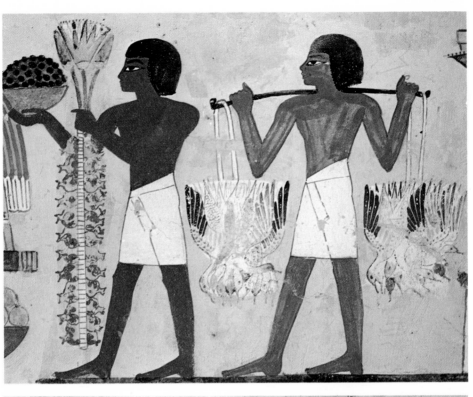

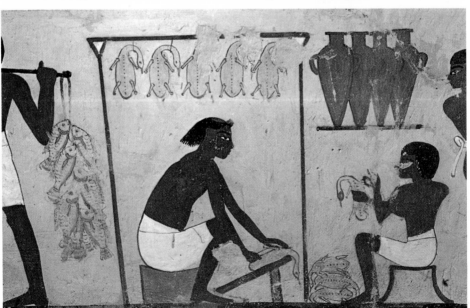

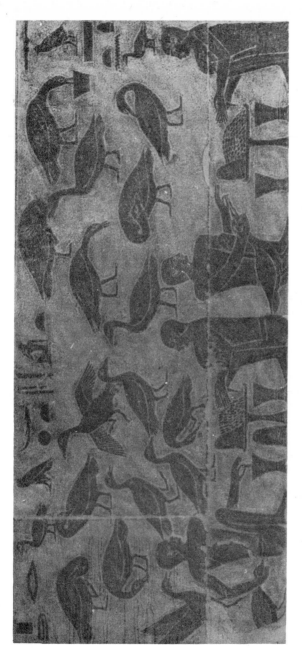

Fig. 6.16b (Facing page, upper) Transport of wild marsh fowl. Tomb of Nakht (number 52) at Thebes (Lower Enclosure); New Kingdom, eighteenth dynasty, reign of King Thutmose IV, *c.* 1420 B.C. Photographed 1969.

Fig. 6.16c. (Facing page, lower). Plucking and dressing fowl. Note pickling jars. Tomb of Nakht (number 52) at Thebes (Lower Enclosure); New Kingdom, eighteenth dynasty, reign of King Thutmose IV, *c.* 1420 B.C. Photographed 1969.

Fig. 6.17 (This page). Care and feeding of poultry. Preparation of feeding pellets. Tomb of Mereruka at Saqqara; Old Kingdom, sixth dynasty, reign of King Teti, *c.* 2390 B.C. Rubbing by Ward Patterson; used with permission (1969).

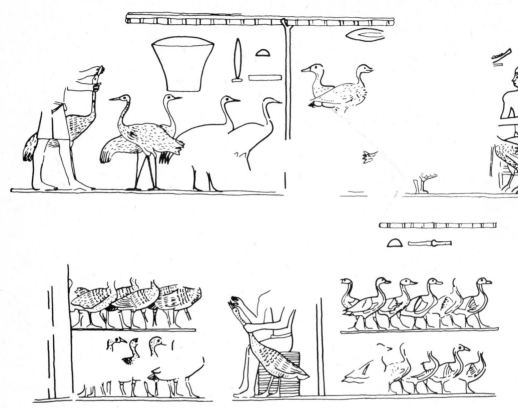

Fig. 6.18. Force feeding of cranes and geese. Tomb of Thut-Hotpe (number 2) at El Bersheh; Middle Kingdom, twelfth dynasty, date uncertain. Redrawn from Griffith *et al.* (1894), plate 22.

pp. 6–7) of a "pigeon" stew among the remains of a funerary meal in a second dynasty tomb at Saqqara. Nearly two thousand years later King Rameses III (nineteenth dynasty, *c.* 1198–1166 B.C.) offered 57,810 pigeons to the god Amon at Thebes (*A.R.*, IV, 242). Continuity of dietary use in the interval has not been documented, but seems likely.

Most information relative to doves/pigeons in Egypt dates to the Ptolemaic and Roman Periods. One description by Callixeinus of Rhodes tells of a Dionysiac procession held in Alexandria under Ptolemy, Philadelphus (285–247 B.C.)

". . . from this, pigeons, ring doves, and turtle doves flew forth along the

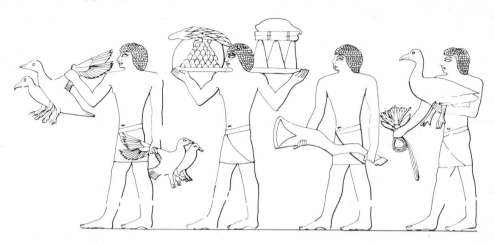

Fig. 6.19a. Food offerings of various desirable fowl. Tomb of Akhet-hotep at Saqqara; Old Kingdom, fifth dynasty, reign of King Djed-Ka-Re, *c.* 2450 B.C. Redrawn from Davies (1901), plate 26.

whole route, with nooses tied to their feet so that they could be easily caught by the spectators . . ." (Athenaeus, 5, 200, C)

A papyrus dated to 224 B.C. shows that, in addition to domesticated pigeons, wild pigeons were available to be hunted for food and sport

". . . we have got ready for the visit of Chrysippus the chief of the body-guard and dioecetes ten whiteheads, five domestic geese, fifty fowls; of wild birds there are fifty geese, two hundred fowls and a hundred pigeons..." (*S.P.*, II, 1934, 414)

Columella of Gades (8, 8, 7–8) noted two varieties of doves/pigeons in Egypt and advised that they should be kept separately

". . . Alexandrine and the Campanian[24] varieties should not be mated for they feel less affection for hen-birds unlike themselves . . . and do not often produce offspring . . ."

By that token, the five-fold classification of Aristotle (see p. 287) would have caused havoc in any ordinary poultry yard or pigeon tower.

The commonest method of raising doves/pigeons was in cotes, the architecture of which differed little from that of the pigeon towers that dominate modern villages (Hornell, 1947) (Fig. 6.29). One of these is listed in the bequest (126 B.C.) made by a soldier, Dryton, of his Egyptian property and land holdings (*S.P.*, 1932, 83).

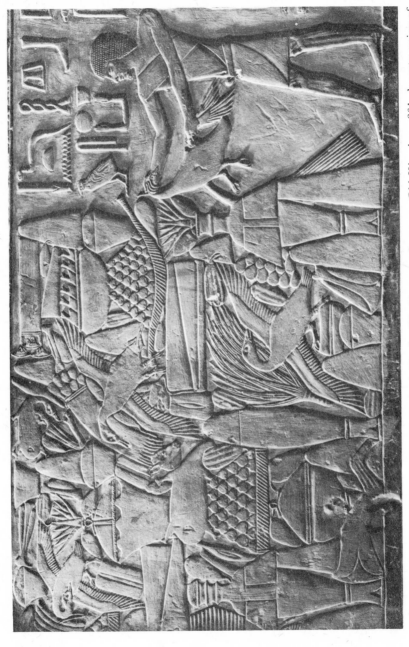

Fig. 6.19b. Fowl included among offerings of food. Tomb of Ptahhetep at Saqqara; Old Kingdom, fifth dynasty, reign of King Djed-Ka-Re, c. 2450 B.C. Photograph used with permission of the Ministry of Culture and the officials of the Centre for Documentation, Cairo, ARE (1969).

An official indication of the flourishing pigeon economy is the "pigeon house tax" (*dny ṣt mnt*) levied by Augustus (Octavian) (Lichtheim, 1957, 110). A byproduct of this industry was the dung deposited in the pigeon towers, which was considered highly valuable and of which a proportion was sometimes returned to the lessor as rent (Lindsay, 1966, p. 233). Today, pigeon dung is still the highest prized fertilizer in Egypt,[25] especially for vegetables and fruits of which it is said greatly to enhance the quality and yield.

It may be concluded that squab were commonly eaten in Egypt during the Greek and Roman Periods. A second century A.D. papyrus throws an amusing side-light onto everyday life

". . . the pigeons and small fowl which I am not used to eat, send to . . . the teacher of Heraidous . . . Whatever things I did not eat . . . send to the teacher of my daughter that he may be diligent with her . . ." (*S.P.*, 1932, 116)

Family Gruidae

Crane (Grus and Related Genera)

That crane and related species were kept for food is suggested by the large numbers depicted in illustration of poultry yards, where they were fed and tended by servants (Figs 6.18, 6.30 and 6.31). According to Moreau (1930, p. 68) the flocks had to be replenished with birds captured during the seasonal migration since they do not breed well in captivity.

Additional evidence is available from a text wherein Rameses III (nineteenth dynasty, *c.* 1198–1166 B.C.) offered a selection of "cranes" to the god Amon at Thebes (*A.R.*, IV, 242). Other texts also mention "crane," but all of these should be considered with caution since a detailed knowledge of ornithology cannot be expected from all Egyptologists, and the opposite is likewise true; it is not, therefore, certain whether the word depicted by (h)[26] was limited to cranes, or whether it equally designated other species such as herons, egrets, and the like.

The crane (*garnukh*) is eaten today by Bedouins living in the Western Desert in the vicinity of Borg el Arab where it is roasted and regarded as a great delicacy.

(h)

ḏȝt

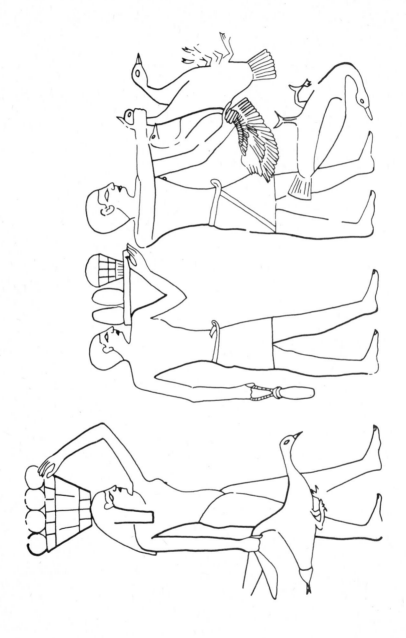

Fig. 6.20. Slaying fowl by wringing the neck. Tomb of Ukh-hotp (B2) at Meir; Middle Kingdom, twelfth dynasty, date uncertain. Redrawn from Blackman (1915b).

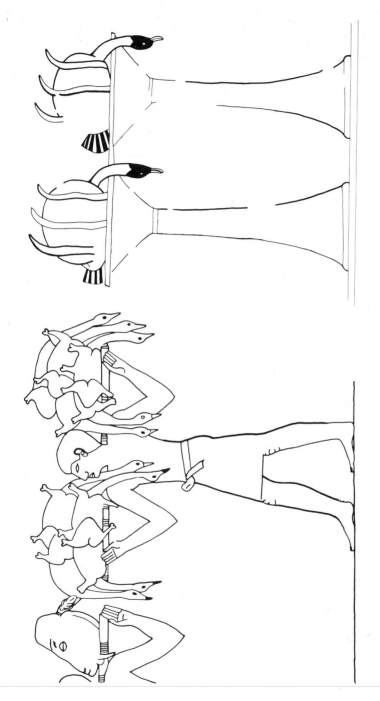

Fig. 6.21a. (Left) Food offering of plucked and dressed fowl. Tomb of Ukh-hotp at Meir; Middle Kingdom, twelfth dynasty, date uncertain. Redrawn from Blackman (1915b), plate 3.

Fig. 6.21b. (Right) A singed offering, Tomb of Menkheper (number 79) at Thebes (Upper Enclosure); New Kingdom, eighteenth dynasty, reign of King Thutmose III, *c.* 1475 B.C. Redrawn from photograph taken in 1969.

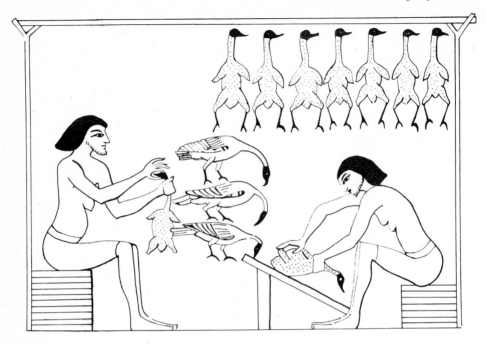

Fig. 6.22. Servants plucking fowl. From a tomb at Thebes; New Kingdom, date uncertain. Redrawn from Wilkinson (1878), Vol. 1, p. 364, Fig. 135.

Family Otididae

Bustard (Otis tetrax and Related Species)

One species of bustard is indigenous to Egypt; since this bird attains great size, it would have probably aroused considerable attention in antiquity. To our knowledge, however, there is no evidence to substantiate Wilkinson's suggestion (1878, Vol. 2, p. 103) that it was "prized for the table" during the Dynastic Period, for the mere presence of an animal or plant does not confirm its use as a dietary component. Considering the bustard as an item of food in Egypt prior to the Ptolemaic and Roman Periods remains, therefore, problematic, although it was apparently imported from Libya during the Greek Period (Athenaeus, IX, 44) and was appreciated by other Mediterranean people.

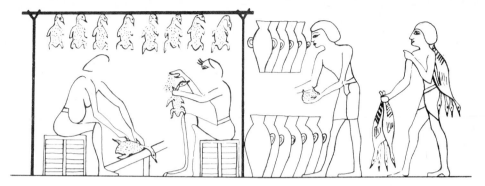

Fig. 6.23. Plucking and pickling fowl. From a tomb at Thebes; New Kingdom, date uncertain. Redrawn from Wilkinson (1878), Vol. 1, p. 290, Fig. 99.

Xenophon (*Anabasis*, 1, 5, 3) commented in part on the Persian method of capture

". . . the bustards on the other hand, can be caught if one is quick in starting up, for they fly only a short distance, like partridges and soon tire; and their flesh [is] delicious . . ."

At that time the common method of hunting the bustard was on horseback, as reported by Oppian (*Cynegetica*, 2, 432). Athenaeus (9, 390, D) described an unusual technique reportedly practiced in Egypt

". . . this creature is given to mimicry, particularly of anything which it sees a man doing. At any rate, it does the same things that it sees the hunters doing. So the hunters take a position in plain sight of the birds and smear their eyes with an unguent after preparing other unguents which cause eyes and eyelids to stick together; these they place at no great distance from themselves in small pans. The bustards, therefore, seeing the men smearing themselves, take the unguent from the pans and do the same thing, and are quickly caught . . .!"

Today, in Egypt, the Awlad Ali Bedouins on the northern coast capture and roast bustard which they relish. In adjacent countries the bustard is also highly appreciated as food, and in the Arabian peninsular it is hunted in the noble tradition of falconry, and is considered a delicacy fit to be served to sheikhs, princes and the most highly honoured guests.

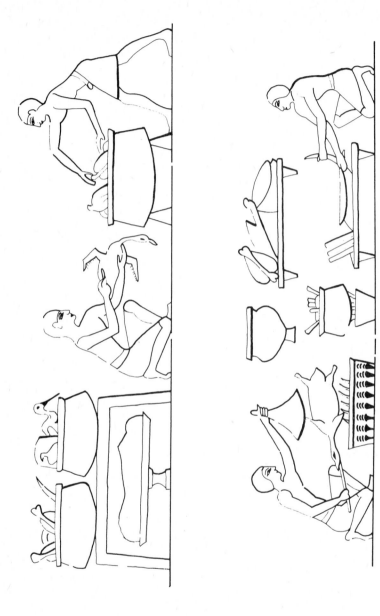

Fig. 6.24. Roasting and boiling. From an unknown tomb at Giza (?); Old Kingdom, date uncertain. Redrawn from Wilkinson (1878), Vol. 2, p. 35, Fig. 302.

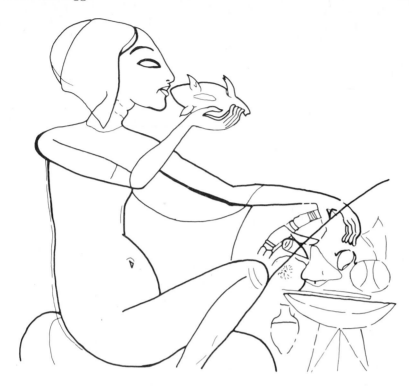

Fig. 6.25. Youth devouring a duck—trial sketch on limestone. Tell el Amarna; New Kingdom, eighteenth dynasty, reign of King Amenhotep IV (Akhenaten), *c.* 1360 B.C. Photographed and redrawn with permission of the Ministry of Culture and the officials of the Egyptian Museum, Cairo; ARE (1969).

Family Phasionidae

Chicken or "Domestic Fowl" (Gallus domesticus)

Historical information concerning the consumption of chicken (or chicken eggs) in Egypt prior to the Late Byzantine Period (sixth century) is ambiguous. Literary citations from this relatively late period are difficult to interpret owing to the uncertainties of translation (see *S.P.*, 1932, 48; Johnson and West, 1949, pp. 211 and 213).

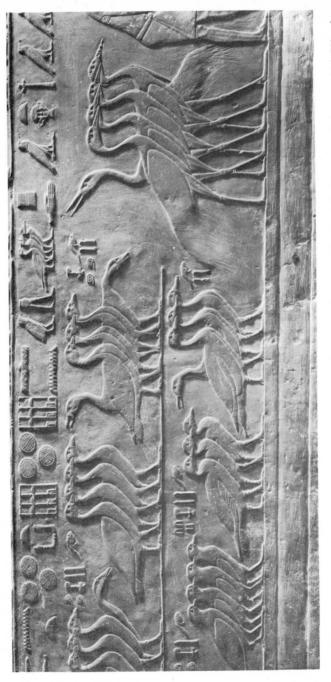

Fig. 6.26. A group of barnyard fowl including ducks, geese, pigeons, and a swan. Tomb of Ptahhetep at Saqqara; Old Kingdom, fifth dynasty, reign of King Djed-Ka-Re, *c.* 2450 B.C. Photograph used with permission of the Ministry of Culture and the officials of the Centre for Documentation. Cairo, ARE (1969).

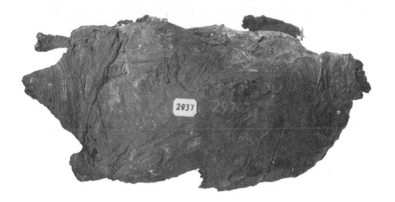

Fig. 6.27. A portion of the foods buried with King Thutmose IV; a dressed duck or goose wrapped in linen. Thebes (Valley of the Kings); New Kingdom, eighteenth dynasty, *c.* 1405 B.C. Photographed with permission of the Ministry of Agriculture and the officials of the Agricultural Museum, Dokki, ARE (1969).

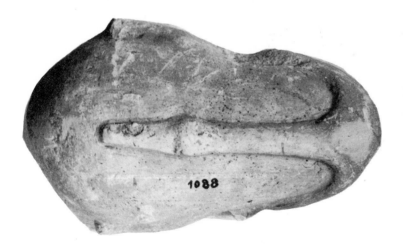

Fig. 6.28. Imitation food; a stone model of a goose. Old Kingdom; date and location uncertain. Photographed with permission of the Ministry of Agriculture and the officials of the Agricultural Museum, Dokki, ARE (1969).

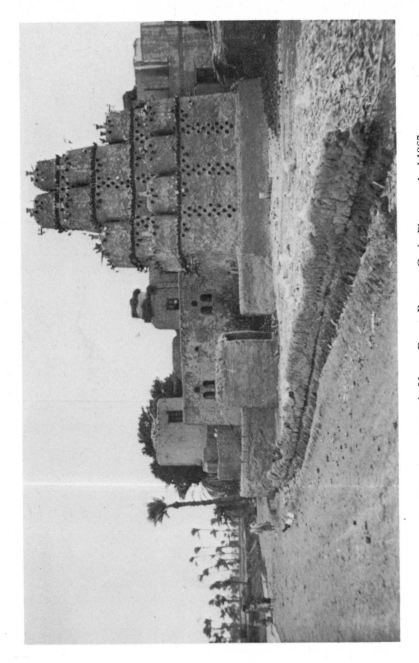

Fig. 6.29. Pigeon towers in Upper Egypt, Fayoum Oasis. Photographed 1967.

The earliest known remains of the "domestic fowl" in Egypt are the eggs and bones of a chicken dated to the eighteenth dynasty (Figs 6.32 and 6.33) kept in the Egyptian Agriculture Museum at Dokki. But these are not sufficient evidence in support of regular consumption of this bird. The dietary and economic importance of chicken during more modern times,[27] however, warrants a discussion of its history.

During his eighth campaign into Asia, King Thutmose III (eighteenth dynasty, *c.* 1504–1450 B.C.) received as tribute several birds that appeared so unusual that he ordered the event to be recorded

". . . four wild fowl of the country which ///////////// every day . . ." (*A.R.*, II, 483)

The lower portions of the partially erased word are still visible and were translated by von Bissing as "sing" (1896, 17–29), whereas Sethe (1906, 1916), reconstructed the phrase as "to give birth," paraphrased into English as "lay" (see Carter, 1923, p. 4).

From the New Kingdom comes the earliest pictorial evidence (Fig. 6.34) of the chicken in Ancient Egypt, a limestone fragment uncertainly dated between the years 1425 and 1123 B.C. It bears the distinctive profile of the red jungle fowl (Carter, 1923). The ornamentation on a rhyton vase from the Cretan (Keftiu) tribute in Rekhmare's tomb (Thebes number 100) is also said to show the head of a chicken (Müller, 1893, p. 348; Hornblower, 1935; Coltherd, 1966). Müller's sketch (Fig. 6.35) certainly resembles a rooster but, as early as 1943, this painting had been nearly destroyed (Fig. 6.36), and it could not be identified by the authors upon their examination of the tomb in 1969.

During the Late Period, chicken appear to have been better known. In the fourth century B.C. in the tomb of Petosiris at Tuna el Gobel, two paintings of fowl, easily identified as chicken, appear among the many offerings presented to the deceased (Figs 6.37 and 6.38), while further excavations at this site revealed other representations of the same bird (Gabra *et al.*, 1941).

During excavations at Memphis, Petrie *et al.* (1910, p. 45) discovered oil lamps decorated with camels and heads of roosters. But because of stratigraphic problems, these objects could only generally be dated to "before A.D. 70", and it is likely that they are not Dynastic in Period, but either Ptolemaic or Early Roman.

In addition, a fine collection of terracotta and bronze statues depicting roosters is on deposit in the Egyptian Agriculture Museum at Dokki.

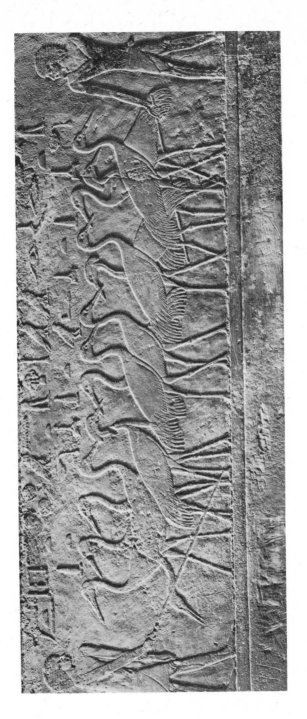

Fig. 6.30. Herdsmen tending a flock of cranes. Tomb of Ti at Saqqara; Old Kingdom, fifth dynasty, reign of Kings Nefer-ir-ka-Re and Ne-Woser-Re, *c.* 2500 B.C. Photograph used with permission of the Ministry of Culture and the officials of the Centre for Documentation, Cairo, ARE (1969).

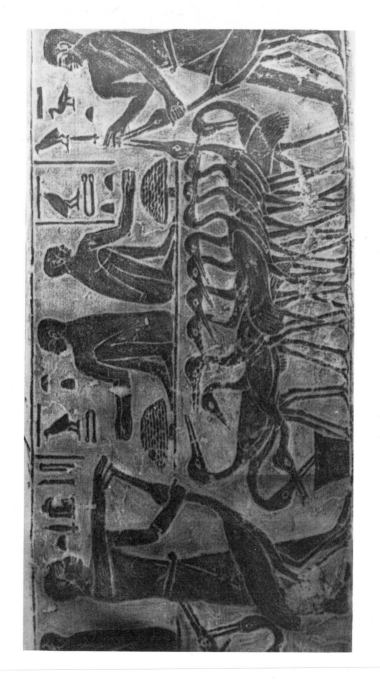

Fig. 6.31. The force-feeding of cranes. Tomb of Mereruka at Saqqara; Old Kingdom, sixth dynasty, reign of King Teti, *c.* 2390 B.C. Rubbing by Ward Patterson; used with permission (1969).

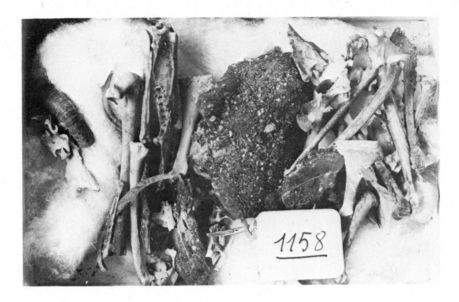

Fig. 6.32. Domestic fowl. Skeletal remains of a chicken (earliest known from Egypt). Thebes; New Kingdom, date uncertain. Photographed with permission of the Ministry of Agriculture and the officials of the Agricultural Museum, Dokki, ARE (1969).

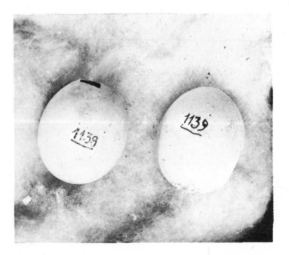

Fig. 6.33. Domestic Fowl. Eggs of a chicken (earliest known from Egypt). Thebes; New Kingdom; date uncertain. Photographed with permission of the Ministry of Agriculture and the Officials of the Agricultural Museum, Dokki, ARE (1969).

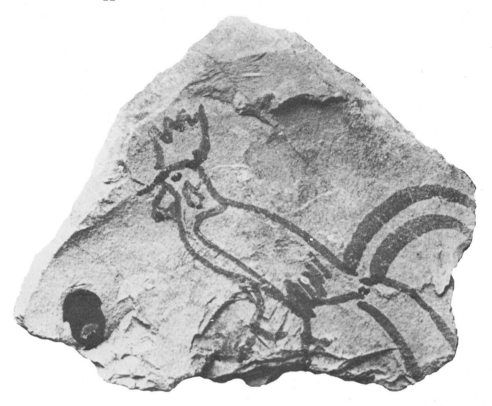

Fig. 6.34. Trial sketch of a rooster on limestone. Earliest known drawing of the domestic fowl in Egypt. Thebes (Valley of the Kings); New Kingdom, date uncertain (between 1425–1123 B.C.). From Carter (1923), plate 20, Fig. 1.

They were excavated at widely scattered sites in Egypt and are dated generally to the Roman Period (Figs 6.39 and 6.40).

On the basis of this scanty archaeological evidence, one cannot ascertain when the chicken was first introduced into Egypt. Moreau, (1927, p. 6) one of the major authorities on Egyptian birds, believed that it was unknown before the Ptolemaic Period. The evidence relative to the geographic dispersal of the chicken from its centre of domestication in southeast Asia was summarized by Simoons (1961, pp. 65–78). Concerning its arrival in Ancient Egypt, Carter (1923) and others, on the basis of etymological studies of ancient Sumerian words, believed it was imported from western Asia where they think it existed as early as

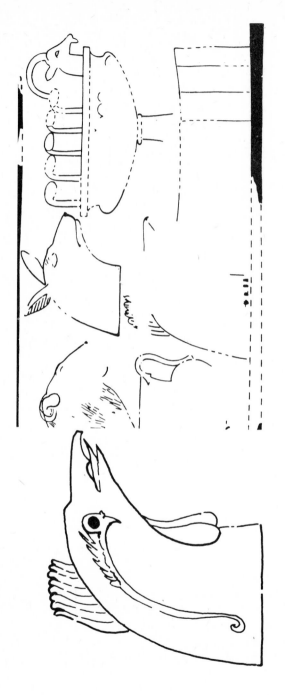

Fig. 6.35. (Left) Tribute vase from Crete. Tomb of Rekhmire (number 100) at Thebes (Upper Enclosure); New Kingdom, eighteenth dynasty, reign of King Thutmose III, *c.* 1475 B.C. Redrawn from Muller (1893), p. 348.

Fig. 6.36. (Right) Tribute vase from Crete. Tomb of Rekhmire (number 100) at Thebes (Upper Enclosure); New Kingdom, eighteenth dynasty, reign of King Thutmose III, *c.* 1475 B.C. Davies (1943), Vol. 2, plate 18. Photograph used and redrawn with permission of the Metropolitan Museum of Art, New York.

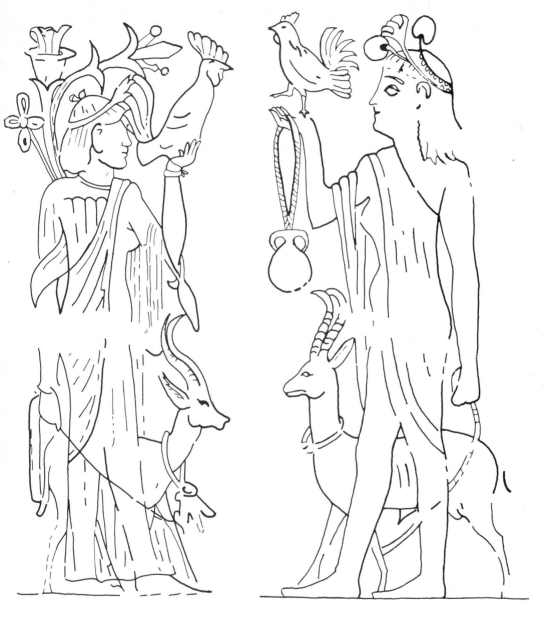

Fig. 6.37. (Left) Domestic fowl and gazelle among offerings of tribute. Tomb of Petosiris at Tuna el Gebel; Early Ptolemaic. Redrawn from Lefebvre (1924), part 3, plate 35.

Fig. 6.38. (Right) Domestic fowl and gazelle among offerings of tribute. Tomb of Petosiris at Tuna el Gebel; Early Ptolemaic. Redrawn from Lefebvre (1924), part 3, plate 46.

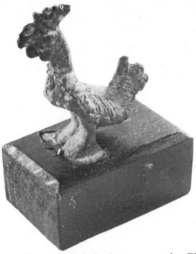

Fig. 6.39. Bronze rooster; Roman Period, date uncertain. Photographed with permission of the Ministry of Agriculture and the officials of the Agricultural Museum, Dokki, ARE (1969).

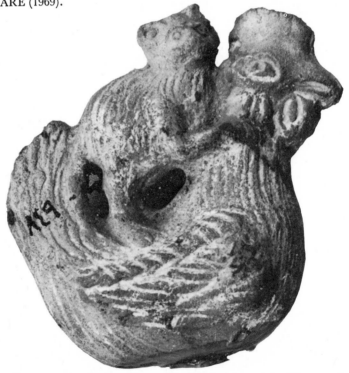

Fig. 6.40. Terra cotta hen and cat. Roman Period, date uncertain. Photographed with permission of the Ministry of Agriculture and the officials of the Agricultural Museum, Dokki, ARE (1969).

2500 B.C., i.e. nearly 1000 years before it was introduced into Egypt! But the finding of a rooster in eighteenth dynasty paintings of the Cretan tribute, although it could be argued that it represented an entirely foreign bird, suggests a possible diffusion into Egypt from the north, and further complicates the problem of introduction.

In antiquity, the main use of the hen in southeastern Asia and the eastern Mediterranean seems to have been sacrificial or divinatory rather than alimentary. This bird was held to be in affinity with the gods, since the cock signaled the coming of the rising sun (Simoons, 1961, pp. 71–72); hence its entrails were commonly inspected by priests for a wide variety of signs. Plutarch) *I. and O.*, 375, 61, E) wrote that the Egyptians of his day sacrificed chicken to the god Anubis

". . . they sacrifice to him on the one hand a white cock and on the other hand one of saffron colour, regarding the former things as simple and clear, and the others as combined and variable . . ."

It is known that Greek initiates into the rites of Maia[28] were required to abstain from eating chicken, as were initiates into the related celebrations in honour of the goddess Demeter held at Eleusis

". . . the initiated are ordered to abstain from domestic fowl, from fishes,[29] and beans, pomegranates, and apples, which fruits are as equally defiling to the touch, as a woman recently delivered, and a dead body . . ." (Porphyry, 4, 16)

There is no evidence, however, that the hen was ever used in Egypt as a divinatory tool, or that it was, at any time, subjected to a ban in Egypt.

Family Phasionidae

"Quail-like" Species

There is a wealth of information relative to "quail-like" birds in Ancient Egypt. It is most difficult, however, to identify the exact varieties described by the Ancients. Quail (*Coturnix* spp.), partridge (*Perdox* spp.), francolin (*Tetras* spp.), and pheasant (*Phasianus* spp.) all lie within this broad category and it is not certain how, or to what extent, they were differentiated by the Ancient Egyptians of different periods.

(i)

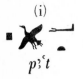

$p\underline{\imath}^{\varsigma}t$

According to Faulkner (1962, p. 87) the hieroglyph (i) was the term for quail; Thompson (1966, p. 215) suggests $p\underline{\imath}rt$ and bases this identification on linguistic similarities with the Coptic for quail. Such transformations of words are, however, common in Ancient Egyptian. It is certain that quail have been known from the earliest times in Ancient Egypt. Moreau (1930, p. 73) equated the Egyptian alphabetical sign *w* with the quail chick, a justifiable indication that the Ancient Egyptians knew the species (compare Coltherd, 1966, p. 218).

Emery (1962, pp. 6–7) described quail among the foods he found preserved in a second dynasty (*c.* 3000 B.C.) tomb at Saqqara. This discovery, coupled with the linguistic and phonetic evidence cited above, justifies the conclusion that quail was a relished food during the early years of the Old Kingdom.

During the Middle Kingdom, the archaeological record is apparently silent relative to quail; but, under the New Kingdom, this bird again occurs in a dietary context. Hayes (*S.P.*, II, p. 52) reports that dressed quail were identified from a royal burial dated to the reign of King Amenhotep I at Thebes (*c.* 1530 B.C.). But the first historical record that quail served as a substantial dietary element in Ancient Egypt is the statement made during the twenty-seventh dynasty by Herodotus (II, 77) who mentioned salted-quail as a dietary favourite of the Egyptians. Hipparchus, a little-known Greek traveller whose writings have been preserved in Athenaeus (9, 393, C) likewise wrote

". . . I liked not the life which the Egyptians lead, forever plucking quails and slimy magpies."

One may further suppose that quail were among the several varieties of small birds, unidentifiable as to species, that were pickled by the Ancient Egyptians of all periods, and so commonly depicted in tombs.

Quail, however, must have been only a seasonal item of diet. Two migrations occur yearly in Egypt, the northward in March–April and the southward in September–November. During their long overseas flight the quails returning to Egypt have few places to land except for an occasional island. Hence, they reach the shoreline of North Africa in an exhausted state and there are captured with relative ease by coastal residents from Sinai in the east, to Algeria and Morocco in the west. Sophisticated nets have long been devised to take advantage of this seasonal source of food. Diodorus (1, 60, 10) described a technique practiced by the residents of the poor village of Rhinocolura[30] situated along the coast of northern Sinai

". . . by cutting down reeds in the neighbourhood and splitting them, they made long nets which they set up along the beach for a distance of many stades[31] and hunted quails; for these are driven in large coveys from the open sea and in hunting them they caught a sufficient number to provide themselves with food . . ."

Such use of large nets is not identifiable in tomb artifacts of the Dynastic Period as a concerted effort directed at obtaining quail *per se*. The tomb of Mereruka at Saqqara contains a representation of a field net used to remove quail from a wheat field (Fig. 6.4) and similar scenes are known from the New Kingdom at Thebes (Vandier, 1969, Vol. 5, p. 319). In all such instances, however, the capture of quail is but part of a larger agricultural motif.

Modern quail nets used in Egypt are not very different in design from those described by Diodorus. Some are hundreds of yards long and elevated on poles higher than ten feet (Moreau, 1927, p. 9). Such techniques, in use for a minimum of two thousand years, have been highly successful. Gurney (1875 [?], p. 127) writes of one team who captured 80,000 quail in one day. More searching, however, are the reports by Moreau (1927, p. 13) and Meinertzhagen (1933, p. 71) that, between the years 1906–1913, over one million quail were exported yearly (not including those captured for domestic sale and consumption).

Organized collecting on such an enormous scale far overshadows the traditional techniques used by the Egyptians to capture quail, and the Egyptian government, cognizant of the threat to this valuable species, has attempted to limit the usage of such nets by forbidding placing them closer than 500 meters from the sea, and designating distinct passages for free-flight (Moreau, 1927, p. 10). On an individual scale, numerous writers have described the casting nets, snares, pitfall traps, spring-release traps, and other clever means by which sufficient quail can be collected by a trapper for himself and his family without his being accused of decimating a valued food resource (Lynes and Witherby, 1912, p. 185; King, 1925, p. 284; Dumreicher, 1931, p. 22; Al-Hussaini 1938, p. 546; Jarvis, 1938, pp. 260–261). Among the more unusual Egyptian methods, one that would be dismissed as fictitious were it not attested in the notebook of the famed ornithologist, Meinertzhagen (1954, p. 567–568), and indeed observable to this day, is that of using butterfly nets. In seaside locations during the months of quail migration, people gather at dawn in their favourite coffee shops along the beach; there they sit, drink tea, and catch the birds with their strange nets as they fly past. Such nets are also used to capture quail in parts of rural Greece (MacPherson, 1897, pp. 378–379).

There is a Biblical passage relative to quail that has excited a continuing controversy (Grivetti, 1971). During the Exodus and the march through Sinai, part of the diet of the Israelites consisted of quail

> ". . . and the people stood up all that day and all that night, and all the next day, and they gathered the quails . . . and while the flesh was yet between their teeth, ere it was chewed, the wrath of the Lord was kindled against the people and the Lord smote the people with a very great plague. And he called the name of that place Kibroth-Hattaavah,[32] because they buried the people that lusted . . ." (Numbers 11, 32–34; Philo, *Special Laws*, 4, 128–130; Josephus *Antiquities of the Jews*, 3, 13, 1)

Most early Christian works, mediaeval commentaries, and contemporary texts representing the fundamentalistic viewpoint have considered the Biblical quail incident as an act of God's avenging wrath or as an allegory, contrasting man's lust with God's never-ending patience. Sergent (1941, pp. 161–192) was the first to correlate this Biblical passage with the feeding habits of the quail. His work in Algeria brought him in contact with cases of food poisoning among peasants that occurred shortly after consumption of quail. He suggested a direct parallel with the Biblical report and believed that poisoning was due to toxic agents derived from the seeds of various alkaloid plants and concentrated within the musculature of the quail as a result of the dehydrating northward migration across the Sahara.

The same author (1948, pp. 249–252), in further discussions of this theme, documented incidents of quail poisoning from the southern coast of France. Later, Plichet (1952, p. 1189) and Hadjigeorge (1952, p. 1469) published brief accounts of quail poisoning, and extended the geographic distribution of the potential health problem eastward into Greece. Brehant (1966, pp. 1157–1158) compared the Biblical quail incident with an analogous occurrence where the Greek army under Xenophon was incapacitated by feasting on poisonous honey (*Anabasis* 4, 8, 15–21). Ouzounellis (1968, pp. 1863–1864), a Greek physician practising in the island of Lesbos (Mytilene), described cases of poisoning caused by quail which resulted in severe uremia and, occasionally, death. He further noted that the poisonings on Lesbos occurred during the southern migration of the quail and that the next major landfall for the birds is the northern coasts of Sinai—thus fitting the pattern described in the Biblical passage (Ouzounellis, 1970, pp. 1186–1187).

With present day information on the toxicity problem being at the most sketchy and incomplete, it is paradoxical that, in antiquity, the syndrome should have been described, possible causes identified, and antidotes and preventive measures prescribed. Aristotle (*On Plants*, 820b, 6–7) was among the first of the Ancients to consider this point

". . . some fruits are unfit for us to eat, but fit for others, like the henbane and hellebore, which are poisonous to men, but good food for quails . . ."

Didymus of Alexandria (*Geoponics*, 14, 24) likewise knew of this relationship and offered an antidote against the effect of the poison

". . . quails also feed on millet, wheat, darnel, and clean water: but as quails feeding on hellebore are pernicious to the persons who eat them, causing convusion and giddiness, you are to boil millet along with them: and if a person having eaten them be taken ill, let him drink a decoction of millet . . ." Lucretius echoed: ". . . moreover, to us hellebore is biting poison, but it makes goats and quails grow fat . . ." (*On the Nature of Things* 4, 639–640)

Pliny (10, 33) offered additional information on the toxic attributes of quail and mentioned that quail were avoided as food in Italy during his time (first century A.D.)

". . . the seeds of certain venomous plant are most highly esteemed by the quails as food; for which reason it is that they have been banished from our tables; in addition to which a great repugnance is manifested to eating their flesh, on account of the epilepsy, to which alone of all animals, with the exception of man, the quail is subject . . ."

Similar remarks can be found in the writings of other Greek and Roman authors (see Sextus Empiricus, *Outlines of Pyrrhonism*, 1, 57). Such commentaries indicate that between the fourth century B.C. and the third century A.D., quail were regarded skeptically as a safe food by the peoples of the northern shores of the eastern Mediterranean.

In the Middle Ages Arab and Jewish physicians also implied that quail were toxic. Avicenna (*The Canon*, lib. II, 2, 2, 5) noted that persons who eat quail are in danger of falling into convulsions and spasms. He added that this did not necessarily result from quail eating hellebore, but because the two have the same nature; whereas Maimonides stated

". . . many people who indulge greatly in eating quail meat develop cramps in the muscles because of the hellebore which is the nourishment of the quail . . ." (Rosner, 1970, p. 1544)

Van Veen (1966, pp. 174–175) summarized the information on quail toxicity and concurred with Sergent that the Biblical incident merely described the classical manifestations of food poisoning. Other writers, however, have taken different views. Jarvis (1938, p. 263) proposed that it was the fatty quality of quail flesh, coupled with the desert heat of Sinai, which caused acute gastric distress among the Israelites (compare Whymper, 1909, p. 107). Goodrich-Freer (1924, p. 223) reviewed the quail incident and believed the sickness was not somatic but psychological.

The thesis that the Israelites fed upon toxic quail was investigated further by one of the authors (L.G.) in the summer of 1969. He interviewed members of the Awlad Ali and Terebiyin Bedouin tribes who inhabit respectively the north-central Egyptian and Sinaitic coasts, where quail are most abundant. Additional interviews were conducted among others, Nubian and Sudanese residents of Egypt, urban and rural Moslems and Christians. None of those interviewed could recall any instance where persons within their respective family or tribe had become ill after eating quail. Nor does another of the authors of the present work remember having ever seen or heard of such a case despite his long medical practice both in towns and in the country (P.G.).

To our knowledge, the only modern evidence that suggests the existence of any problem relative to quail consumption in Egypt is the statement by Brown (1739, p. 313–314) that the flesh of some quail is black, hard, and ill-tasting, and that merchants at Alexandria were forced to raise the captured birds in coops in order to "remove the offensive bitterness."

Recently, Ouzounellis has expressed doubts that the source of the toxic agents can solely be attributed to the alkaloid plants on which the quail feed (personal communication 1971). Researchers at the University of Southern California currently are investigating the hypothesis that the offending toxic agents are metabolites which accumulate during the difficult trans-Mediterranean flight (Bessman, personal communication 1972). It would be interesting to correlate toxicity to the southward or northward direction of the migration, since it is known that meat from certain areas in the Soudan can cause a diarrhoea usually ascribed to cattle having eaten laxative herbs (senna?).

Family Struthionidae

Ostrich (Struthio camelus)

The potential value and uses of the ostrich are varied. A single bird could provide enough meat for several hunters.[33] If their nests were located, the eggs would serve as an additional source of food and the empty egg shells were useful to desert hunters as water containers.

The ostrich[34] was known and hunted by Pre-Dynastic Egyptians of both Upper and Lower Egypt and its bones have been found in strata correlated to the Sebilian horizon (Gaillard, 1934, p. 95; Sandford, 1934, p. 86). The numerous rock carvings and paintings dated to the Late Paleolithic/Mesolithic boundary suggest that early man was successful in capturing this game. In addition to the common rock carvings in Upper Egypt, ostriches frequently are depicted as a motif on pottery in this region.

In Lower Egypt rock carvings are not known, but beads made from the shell of ostrich eggs have been found in Fayoum sequences (Caton-Thompson and Gardner, 1934, p. 34); and Menghin and Amer (1932, p. 51) likewise found bits of ostrich egg shell at Maadi. Egg-shells, especially for use in bead-making, could be an article of commerce. and Debono (1948, p. 567) lists the ostrich among the fauna excavated at El Omari.

Representations of ostriches are rare in Old Kingdom art, but some slate palettes, like the "Hunter's palette" of the British Museum, do portray these birds. The Middle Kingdom tombs at Beni Hassan feature scenes in which ostriches are hunted with dogs, bows and arrows and trapped together with other desert species (Fig. 6.41). This relatively

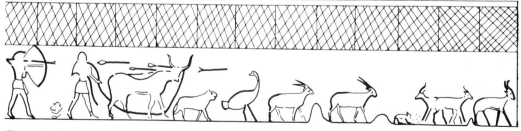

Fig. 6.41. Ostrich hunt. Tomb of Baqt III (number 15) at Beni Hassan; Middle Kingdom, eleventh dynasty, date uncertain. Redrawn from Newberry and Frazer (1893a), Vol. 1, plate 4.

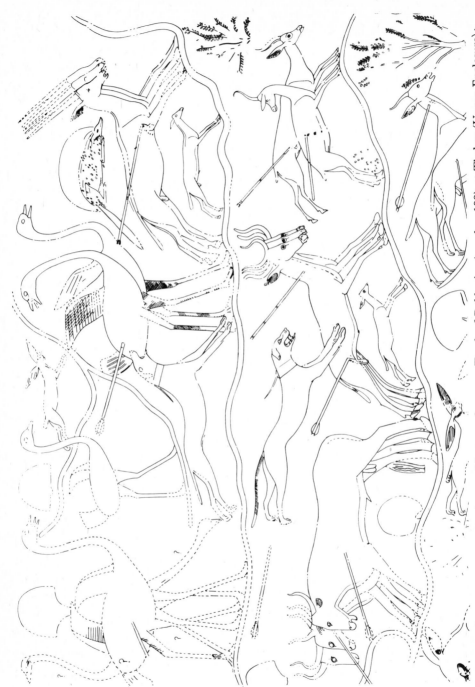

Fig. 6.42. Ostrich hunted with dogs and bows and arrows. Tomb of Rekhmire (number 100) at Thebes (Upper Enclosure); New Kingdom, eighteenth dynasty, reign of King Thutmose III, *c.* 1475 B.C. Davies (1943), Vol. 2, plate 43. Photograph used with permission of the Metropolitan Museum of Art, New York.

rare Middle Kingdom theme becomes frequent in New Kingdom paintings at Thebes where such hunts are commonly depicted and seem to have been a sport of the nobility (Fig. 6.42). Whereas in remote antiquity the primary purpose of hunting the ostrich was for food, with the rise and development of leisure and the evolution of fashion, design and ornamentation in Egyptian architecture and dress, the ostrich served not only as a potential source of food, but its plumes were highly valued for fans and head ornaments. Perhaps the inclusion of this bird among offerings (Fig. 6.43) is largely a reflection of its oddity. Possession of it might have served as a status symbol. Ostrich eggs obviously were desirable, for numerous New Kingdom tomb paintings illustrate them as components of tribute from Nubia and other southern regions (Fig. 6.44).

During the Byzantine Period ostriches were raised in special farms throughout Egypt (Johnson and West, 1949, pp. 42, 211). It may be presumed that they were then considered prestige birds much as in rich Egyptian households of the nineteenth and early twentieth centuries, and raised primarily for their plumes and secondarily for their eggs.

In modern times, evidence concerning the presence and consumption of the ostrich in Egypt is somewhat conflicting, although in the early years of this century an ostrich farm was kept near Heliopolis. Sonnini (1799, Vol. 2, p. 160) saw fresh ostrich eggs on sale in Egypt, stating that they were eaten, and that one would suffice for a man's meal (see also Gurney, 1875, p. 127). Brown (1739, p. 314) did not discuss eggs but stated that ostriches were found in the desert near Suez. Browne (1806, p. 16) saw ostrich tracks in the Western Desert along the way to Siwa oasis. In more recent times, Meinertzhagen (1930, Vol. 2, p. 650) stated that the ostrich was last seen in Egypt during the year 1916 and that, by 1930, it had been "extinct for at least 80 years." Etchecopar and Hüe (1967) likewise list the ostrich as extinct in Egypt. In 1935, however, an ostrich was killed in the Western Desert in the area connecting the oases of Kharga and Dakhla (Al-Hussaini, 1959, p. 3). In a personal communication, Dr Vivi Täckholm, botanist at Cairo University, stated that she saw ostriches on the plain between Gebel Alba and the Red Sea coast in January, 1962, but, prior to her, Hoogstraal *et al.* (1955–1956) had seen no ostrich in the Gebel Alba region. In February, 1967, while on a cooperative field trip with the Egyptian Ministry of Public Health to the same region of Gebel Alba, Osborn and his party reported sighting several small herds of ostrich, and collected study skins and eggs (Osborn, personal communication, 1967, 1969).

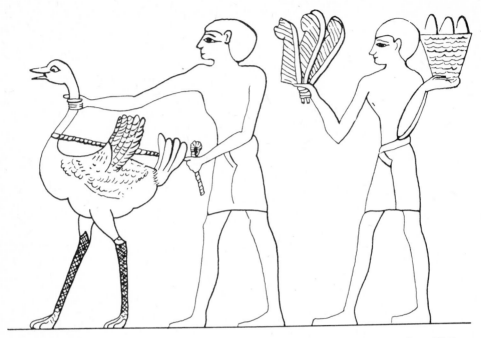

Fig. 6.43. Ostrich eggs and feathers; tribute from southern lands. From a tomb at Thebes; New Kingdom, date uncertain. Redrawn from Wilkinson (1878), Vol. 1, p. 282, Fig. 96.

In addition, Osborn and Helmi (personal communication, 1969) noted that the Rashaida tribesmen living in the vicinity of Gebel Alba probably ate ostrich meat, but they did not personally observe this custom. They reported the belief of the Ababda, a "Beja" tribe inhabiting the region near the southern Red Sea port of Mersa Alam, that fat extracted from ostrich bones is a valuable ointment for treating rheumatism.[35]

Uses of Fowl in Egyptian Medicine

Numerous medical prescriptions in Ancient Egypt included parts of birds—for example, "gall-of-a-*wjȝt*-bird" (*Eb.*, XXXII, 146) or "heart-of-a-*ms*-bird" (*Eb.*, XXII, 81). Even more frequently preparations

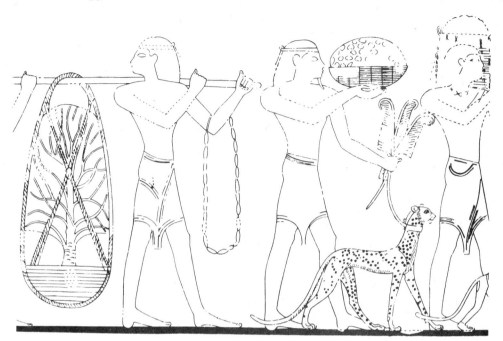

Fig. 6.44. Ostrich eggs and feathers; tribute from southern lands. Tomb of Rekhmire (number 100) at Thebes (Upper Enclosure); New Kingdom, eighteenth dynasty, reign of King Thutmose III, *c.* 1475 B.C. From Davies (1943), Vol. 2, plate 17. Photograph used with permission of the Metropolitan Museum of Art, New York.

included goose-fat or goose-grease (j)[36] and (k)[37], two often inter-changeable terms mentioned in several medical papyri (*Wb. Dr.*, 120). These latter ingredients usually were included in emollients, serving as bases for various external salves, but in some instances they were ingested

> "*To treat the belly and to treat the anus:* milk, goose-fat, powder of manna, colocynth, raisin; are strained and taken in one day" (*Eb.*, XXX, 132).
> "*To cause the stomach to receive bread:* sweet beer, *shpt*,[38] *dsrt*-beer,[38] powder of dates, powder of wheat, fruit of juniperus, frankincense, *smt*,[38] raisin, figs, goose-grease; are boiled, strained, and taken for four days (*Eb.*, LI, 285).
> "*To expel illness of the tongue:* bran (?), milk, grease-of-the-goose; rinse the mouth" (*Eb.*, LXXXV, 699).

Fat of birds other than the goose sometimes was used by physicians,

(j)

mrḥt

(k)

ʿd

but mainly in preparations for external application. Ostrich fat, for example, was an ingredient in a salve prescribed for disorders of the scalp (*Eb.*, LXV, 449); the fat of unidentified *gnw*-bird was applied to keep "flies-from-biting" (*Eb.*, XCVII, 845).

The whole carcass of a bird was incorporated in one external prescription to soften stiffness in all limbs

". . . hyoscyamus, beans, *sps*,[38] viscous fluid, grapes (?), crushed with the *ithwt*-bird and crushed with its feathers; [it] is bandaged therewith . . ." (*Eb.*, LXXXIV, 678)

Sacred or Forbidden Fowl

Some birds, held sacred, were forbidden as food. Those discussed in the following section were such, although they are perhaps the most commonly known birds of Egypt. Their inclusion in a history of food is important because of the light that their religious associations may throw on general food taboos. Three of these birds were real: the falcon/hawk identified with Horus, the Sun, and certain other gods; the ibis (*Threskiornis aethiopicus*), the bird of Thot; and the vulture (*Gyps* spp.), the personification of the goddess Nekhbet.

The fourth sacred bird, the *bnw* or phoenix, was a purely fictional creation that carried deeply mystical meanings.

Falcon-Hawk (Accipiter spp., Falco spp. and Related Genera)

This fierce but beautiful bird was greatly revered in Ancient Egypt and was primarily associated with the god Horus.[39] However, more than ten distinct deities with different relationships were named "Horus,"[40] and worshipped in different sites, the two most famous from the viewpoint of surviving mythology being Horus, son of the god Osiris and of the goddess Isis, the Harsiesis of Greek literature, and Horus the child, Harpocrates (1). But in the Egyptian pantheon this Horus-son-of-Isis was but a minor deity that received undue importance only in the very late Dynastic Period through a religious confusion with the earlier, stronger, and dominant Horus-son-of-Ra.

(1)

ḥr pʒ ḥrd

Horus-son-of-Ra, sometimes considered as the "Solar Horus," was visualized by Ancient Egyptians as a gigantic falcon/hawk whose right eye was the sun, and left eye the moon. During the Dynastic Period he was worshipped at Heliopolis. Religious dogma at Heliopolis did not remain constant throughout the Dynastic Period, and occasionally the importance and dominance of Ra shifted to that of Horus. The Heliopolitan theologians eventually combined this father/son concept into a third form, Ra-Harakhte, a combination of Ra with Harakhtes (m) a name that may be translated "Horus-of-the-Horizon" (compare Ames, 1965, p. 68).

(m)

Ḥr ꜣḫty

Another Horus of comparable eminence was the old primordial Horus, commonly known as "Horus-the-Elder" (n) and known to the Greeks as Haroeris. He was worshipped primarily at Latopolis, the modern Esna, although local centres of worship in the Delta existed in antiquity.

Horus-of-Edfu, yet another falcon/hawk god, was a local deity whose origins were related to and confused with those of the Heliopolitan "Solar-Horus." He was occasionally depicted as a bird, but more commonly he assumed the form of a winged sun-disc.

(n)

Ḥr wr

The falcon/hawk was also associated with Mont, and with Khonsu, the son of the reigning divinities at Thebes, Amon and Mut. At Kom Ombo, he was worshipped as Khons-Hor, and assumed the form of the head of a falcon/hawk.

The kings of Egypt also revered the old falcon god who had early become their ancestor and the dynastic god of Egypt. Two of the five "great names" (*rn wr*), that constituted the titulary (*nḥbt*) assumed by Pharaoh on the day of his accession, were compounded with the name of Horus. One was the "Horus name" or "*ka* name," written within a rectangular frame on which was perched the falcon Horus (Fig. 6.45). It asserted the king as the earthly embodiment of the old falcon-god Horus. The other was the "Golden Horus name" *Ḥr-nbw*[41] that has received various interpretations according to two different acceptions of the word *nb*, that may mean either "golden" or "The One of Ombos," i.e., Seth. The title has accordingly been variously translated "the falcon of gold" or "the victorious over Seth" (compare Ames, 1965, p. 68). In fact, from what is known of Ancient Egyptian mentality, it could have meant both.

So important was this god that great care was taken to embalm the dead hawks. Such mummies are prominent throughout Egypt but at Tuna el Gebel the embalming room is still stacked with these birds.

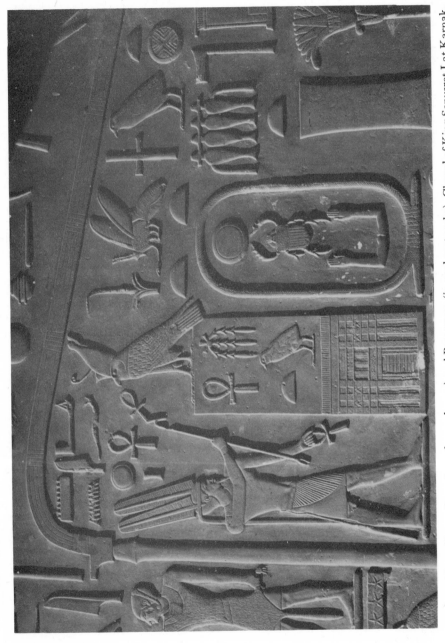

Fig. 6.45. Horus Name (in rectangular enclosure) and Prenomen (in oval cartouche). Chapel of King Senusret I at Karnak. Middle Kingdom, *c.* 1936 B.C. Photographed 1969.

Ibis (Threskiornis aethiopicus)

Visitors to modern Egypt frequently depart with the belief that they have seen thousands of sacred ibis nesting in the suburb of Giza, or flocking in the fields behind the farmers as they plow their rich Delta land.[42] These visitors have confused with the ibis the cattle egret (*Bulbulcus ibis*), known by the villagers as *abu gordan*.

The sacred ibis (Fig. 6.46) has been extinct in Egypt for many years. The last recorded sighting in Egypt was in 1876 near Damietta in the Delta (Meinertzhagen, 1930, Vol. 1, p. 438). So rare was the ibis in Egypt during the latter 1800s that Gurney (1875, p. 116) believed that it had always been rare, and that the large numbers of ibis needed for Egyptian religious purposes were imported from the southern lands. Today a species of black ibis (*Plegadis falcinellus*) is found in isolated regions of Egypt[43] away from human settlements.

The ibis (o)[44] was associated with the god Thot (Fig. 1.14), the master of knowledge and secret science.[45] So revered was this symbol of Thot that strict measures were taken to protect it

(o)

hby

> ". . . whoever kills an ibis or hawk, with intention or without, must die for it . . ." (*Her.*, II, 65)

According to the Greek travellers, one reason the ibis was so highly regarded concerned the "survival" of Egypt

> ". . . winged serpents[46] are said to fly at the beginning of Spring, from Arabia making for Egypt; but the ibis birds encounter the invaders in this pass[47] and kill them . . . the serpents are like water-snakes. Their wings are not feathered but most like the wings of a bat . . ." (*Her.*, II, 75–76)

This report is perpetuated in the writings of Pliny (10, 40, 75) and expanded by Aelian (2, 38)

> ". . . the black ibis does not permit the winged serpents from Arabia to cross into Egypt, but fights to protect the land it loves, while the other kind [white variety] encounters the serpents that come down the Nile[48] when in flood and destroys them. Otherwise there would have been nothing to prevent the Egyptians from being killed by their coming . . ."

Strabo (17, 2, 4) called the ibis the "tamest of birds," but did not consider them clean

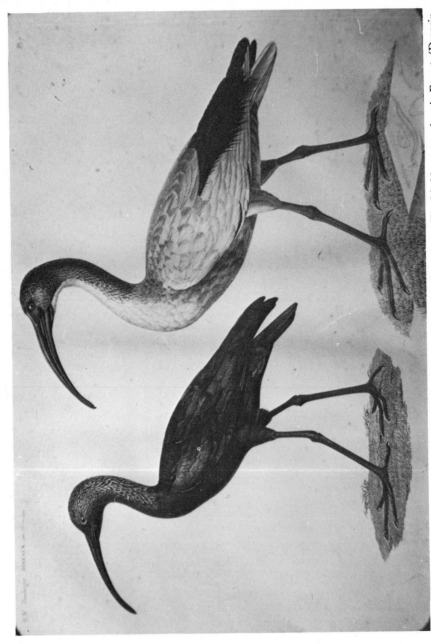

Fig. 6.46. The sacred ibis as drawn *c.* 1799 by scientists accompanying Bonaparte. The bird is now extinct in Egypt. (Description de l'Egypte. Histoire Naturelle, plate 7). Darby Collection.

". . . every cross-road in Alexandria is full of them; and though they are useful in one way, they are not useful in another. The bird is useful because it singles out every animal and the refuse in the meat-shops and bakeries, but not useful because it eats everything, is unclean, and can only with difficulty be kept away from things that are clean and do not admit of any defilement . . ."

The unclean aspects of the ibis were discussed by Aelian (10, 29)

". . . it thrusts its beak down into every place caring nothing for any filth and treading upon it in the hope of tracking down something even there . . ."

Yet other passages in the writings of the Greek and Roman travellers describe the ibis as a discriminating fowl

". . . for she does not drink water if it is unwholesome or tainted, nor will she approach it . . ." (Plutarch, *I. and O.*, 381, 75, D)

Aelian (7, 45), in contrast to his earlier quoted position cited above, seemed to agree on this point

". . . for they [the priests] know full well that this bird would never drink water that was dirty or that had been tainted with any drugs; for they believe that the bird possesses a certain prophetic faculty . . ."

This dual attitude may perhaps be compared with an earlier belief that the ibis taught mankind the medicinal use of the enema. This belief is not a part of Ancient Egyptian tradition, and, apparently, the Ancient Greek and Roman writers perpetuated (or invented?) a fictitious tale that later was to become engrained in Egyptian lore. They believed that the ibis went every morning to the Nile, filled its mouth with water and, using its long curved beak, injected the water into its rectum. Plutarch (*I. and O.*, 381, 75, C) is equally guilty in perpetuating the fabrication

". . . the Egyptians assert that a knowledge of clysters and intestinal purges is derived from no discovery of man's but they commonly affirm that it was the ibis that taught them this remedy . . ."

The association of the ibis with the god Thot easily explains the relationship between the Ancient Egyptian sage/architect, Imhotep, and the millions of mummified ibis found at Saqqara in a vast subterranean gallery of winding passages and different depths that Emery and el-Khouli believe to be built around his burial site (Emery, 1966, 1967, 1970).

Imhotep, chief architect of King Zoser (third dynasty, *c.* 2770 B.C.), was, among his other achievements, responsible for the design and construction of the "step pyramid" of his king (Fig. 1.16), and of the surrounding first monumental structures in the world built of stone. During the Ptolemaic Period the Greeks identified him with their physician/sage/god, Asklepios, and pilgrims and patients from all the known world trekked to Saqqara, the necropolis of Memphis, to pay homage to this god and to seek healing at the site of his burial. There they piously deposited ibis as tokens of devotion and gratitude. One is intrigued, however, by the overwhelming numbers of these birds, in contrast to the statements of Herodotus (II, 65) and Diodorus (1, 83, 6, 8–9) that death was the punishment of even the accidental killing of an ibis. The explanation of the source of what must have been a flourishing market in ibis religious-tokens is not clear, unless the birds had died natural deaths and were embalmed by priests for special offering at this site.

Vulture (Gyps spp.)

(p)

nrt

(q)

w3dt

The vulture *nrt*—see (p)[49] was the graphic personification of the goddess Nekhbet (Fig. 1.7), the protective deity of Upper Egypt. In the north, her counterpart was the cobra goddess of Buto (*Dp*), Uadjit (q). Together, these "two ladies" benevolently protected Egypt. Since the earliest dynasties, combined into one of the five royal names (the *nbty* name,[50] i.e., the "two ladies") they symbolized rule over both Upper and Lower Egypt.

Like the falcon/hawk, the vulture was combined with several distinct deities. Apis, sacred bull at Memphis, was sometimes depicted with the protective wings of the vulture along its back. Both the goddesses Mut and Isis were sometimes depicted wearing vulture wings, that might be outstretched to protect the royal personage.

Freud (1947, pp. 33–49) utilized the homonomy of "mother" and "vulture" in Ancient Egyptian (both *mut*) to explain a childhood dream of Leonardo da Vinci where the image of a vulture recurred. He pointed to the resemblance between *mut* and German *mutter* (also mater, mother, etc.) and he traced the identification of the vulture with motherhood to an old belief that vultures were all females and were impregnated, when flying, by the wind. This was an argument from nature used by the early Christian fathers against those who denied the Virgin birth.

There is a passage from *The Pyramid Texts* that sounds a curiously resonating note

> ". . . He [The King] has come to these his two mothers, the two vultures, . . . they of the . . . pendulous breasts . . . They draw their breasts to his mouth and never do they wean him." (Erman, 1927, p. 9)

bnw-Bird or Phoenix

Many birds played leading roles in various mythologies, e.g. the Stymphalian (Greek), Roq (Arabic), Garuda (India), and Simur (Persia). Avian folklore and mythology have been widely discussed by Ingersoll (1923) and Armstrong (1958). But few mythological birds in the cultural history of either the Old or New World have captured the imagination, and interest of man as powerfully as did the *bnw*-bird (r) or Phoenix of Egyptian/Greek literature (Fig. 6.47). The name *bnw*[51] comes from the same etymological root as the verb *wbn*[52] (s) that means "to rise" (the sun); hence, the Egyptian theologians, who believed in the identity of homonymous sounds and words, had ample opportunity to play on these words. The Phoenix was sacred at Heliopolis, and in art is figured resting atop the *bnbnt*,[53] the pyramidion or pyramidal summit of the obelisks that symbolized the primordial mound of earth which rose from the sea, on which the Egyptian believed the sun first shone and engendered life (Wiedemann, 1878; Daumas, 1965). Hence, the Phoenix was said to exist before all else.

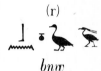

(r)

bnw

(s)

wbn

A correlative belief held that the essence of life (*hike*) was brought by the Phoenix from a distant "Island-of-Fire," lying somewhere beyond the recognized boundaries of the earth, where the gods were born and revived, and whence they were sent to the world. The Phoenix was its chief messenger and the prime communicating link binding earth with this distant "island." The victorious soul on a coffin text compared itself to the Hike-filled bird

> ". . . I come from the Isle of Fire having filled my body with Hike like that bird who [came and] filled the world with that which it has not known . . ." (de Buck, 1935, p. 945)

Coupled with these beliefs was the underlying Egyptian concept of time and regularity. Life was composed of recurrent cycles, day-night-day, life-death-rebirth, flood-planting-harvest-flood, etc.; hence the cyclic

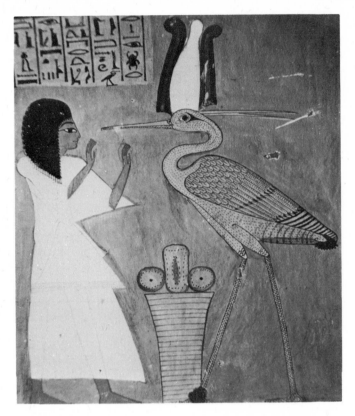

Fig. 6.47. The Phoenix or *bnw*-bird. Tomb number 359 (owner unknown) at Thebes (Deir El Medina); New Kingdom Ramessid Period, date uncertain. Photographed 1969.

visit of the Phoenix to Heliopolis was but another instance of the order and regularity without which chaos would have persisted. The Phoenix or *bnw*-bird, therefore, occupied a key position in Egyptian beliefs and was not a minor deity as so often portrayed in the Greek and Roman writings (compare Clark, 1949, 1950 and 1959).

Herodotus (II, 73) was among the first visitors to describe the Phoenix, but acknowledged that he had not viewed the bird

". . . indeed, it is a great rarity even in Egypt, only coming there once in five hundred years, when the old phoenix dies . . ."

Despite such reports Herodotus doubted the veracity of the Egyptian priests

". . . they tell a story of what this bird does which does not seem to be credible . . ." (II, 73)

In point of fact, Herodotus entirely misunderstood the mystical meaning of the phoenix. Many writers in antiquity discussed the *bnw*-bird, among them Pliny (10, 2, 3–5), Ovid (*Metamorphoses*, 15, 391–407), Tacitus (*The Annals*, 6, 28), and Achilles Tatius (3, 25, 1–7). Rather than summarize the numerous variations according to each author, the traditional story of the Phoenix as gleaned from these sources is paraphrased below

> The Phoenix lived in either Arabia, Assyria or Ethiopia. As death approached, the Phoenix prepared a ball of myrrh and spices (in some versions the ball was prepared after his death by the new Phoenix). The Phoenix died and from his body was born the new, a son who tended his father's remains and placed them inside the ball of wonderful spices. The young Phoenix then flew up the Nile Valley carrying the encased body of his father, the goal being Heliopolis and the temple of the sun. After reaching his destination, he presented the body of his father to the priests for interment; then, in order to authenticate his birthright, he submitted to inspection from the Heliopolitan priests. After being declared as the "true" Phoenix he returned to his native land. The cycle was repeated every 500 years, although some accounts give 1461, 7006, or even 12,954 years between visits.

Eggs

An egg today better than a chicken tomorrow
(Popular saying)

". . . eggs possess a fortifying and nutritious element but produce flatulence. They are fortifying because they have a generating value; they are nutritious because they are, so to say, the milk of the hatching bird, they produce flatulence because though small in bulk they diffuse considerably . . ."
(Hippocrates, *Regimen II*, 50)

Artificial hatching of fowl from eggs was a well established technique employed by the ancient Egyptians during the Late Dynastic Period. Aristotle (*History of Animals* 6, 2) described the method

". . . in some cases, as in Egypt, they [eggs] are hatched spontaneously in the ground, by being buried in dung heaps . . ."

Numerous Greeks and Romans were amazed at this method

". . . for they do not use the birds for hatching the eggs, but in effecting this themselves artificially by their own wit and skill in an outstanding manner . . ." (Diodorus 1, 74, 4–5)

Pliny (10, 75, 153) likewise observed this unusual procedure

". . . in some cases nature hatches of her own accord even without the hen sitting, as on the dung-hills of Egypt . . ."

Reports of artificial hatching of eggs continued into the Arabic Period. Abd al Latif al Baghdadi (1965, pp. 79–89), a physician and traveller of the thirteenth century A.D., gave a most complete description and concluded

". . . nothing is more rare than to find in Egypt chickens hatched naturally by incubation of the hen; one frequently sees among the Egyptians people to whom this natural process is unknown . . ."

During the nineteenth century hatching ovens were commonly used in rural Egypt. Browne (1806, pp. 83–84) believed that the "artificial" technique originated in the idea that, during certain seasons, eggs hatched by hens were uncommonly sterile. St John (1834, Vol. 2, pp. 328–329) described hatching ovens with a capacity of 100,000 eggs (20 chambers each containing 5,000 eggs) and contemplated the impact of such production if adopted in England! Despite this long history of hatching eggs in Egypt by artificial means, we are unable to arrive at an accurate evaluation of the practice and its extent in Egypt today. Modern hatcheries, of course, exist in the vicinity of the major cities and supply urban needs. Our experience with village markets throughout Egypt shows eggs as a primary non-seasonal product, but they are not common items in the diet of the very poor.

With such a history of fowl production one could assume that eggs were commonly eaten through Egyptian history. Most archaeologists, historians, and ornithologists would concur that eggs stolen from the nests of marsh and river fowl have been part of the diet of man in Egypt during all periods, but it is impossible to document this belief. The presence of egg-shells at archaeological sites is no proof that their contents were eaten, they might as well have been made into beads. The same may be said of many tomb paintings and reliefs from the Dynastic Period that depict eggs among funerary offerings, for it can be argued that they were merely to assure a supply of eggs for hatching fowl rather than to serve as a food in after life.

The earliest reference to consumption of eggs in Egypt that we have identified is attributed to Hermeias of Methymne, a little-known author of the third century B.C.

". . . if a Naucratite gives a wedding banquet, it is forbidden, following the prescription of the marriage law, to serve eggs and honey-cakes . . ." (Athenaeus, 4, 150, A)

It is not clear whether this avoidance was a Greek custom, or was originally Egyptian and later adopted by the Greeks living in the Delta near Naucratis.

Medicinal Use of Eggs

The Ancient Egyptians were not completely ignorant of the edibility of eggs, however, and they commonly incorporated them in medical prescriptions, although most of these were meant for external application (*Eb.*, XXXII, 146). "Egg yolk", however, was one of the ingredients of a prescription used to control diarrhoea, according to Ebbell (XIV, 45). In the view of von Deines and Grapow (*Wb. Dr.*, pp. 295, 433) the yolk is not mentioned; only "egg," and an unidentifiable part of it. In other parts of the papyri, a substance called "flour of egg," presumably powdered egg-shell, is recommended. In general, the ostrich egg, possibly because of its size and consistency, is the only variety consistently encountered throughout Egyptian history.

During the Late Roman Period (A.D. 327) governmental restrictions were imposed on Egyptian egg dealers

". . . I acknowledge that I am to carry on the retailing of eggs in the market-place publicly, for the supply in retail of the said city [Oxyrhynchus] every day without intermission, and that it shall not be lawful for me in the future to sell secretly or in my house . . ." (*S.P.*, 1934, 331)

Secret dealings were most probably forbidden because of governmental concern over loss of revenue.

Modern Attitudes towards Fowl and Eggs

Eggs, possibly because they potentially contain the essence of life, were and still are the subject of many curious beliefs. Ever since the beginning of the Christian era, the ostrich egg has figured prominently in Coptic churches, usually hanging from the central chandelier, to urge patient-goers to meditation. Priests explain this symbolism by a current lore

". . . as the ostrich does not keep its eye off its eggs during the whole period of incubation, so does Christ carefully watch over and protect his Church . . ."

In Southern Sudan, the Nuer adult males do not eat eggs, believed to be fit only for women and children. In remote Greek villages egg and chicken taboos are still effective. Simoons (1961, p. 72) suggests that these reflect vestiges of the Eleusian and Maian mysteries.

Modern Egyptian lore regarding eggs and fowl covers sickness, childbirth, and marriage, and is not untainted with magic. There is thus a common belief, now being slowly dissipated, that eggs are bad for *bard*, a word which literally means "a cold" but which covers a variety of non-specific complaints such as upper respiratory infections, "rheumatic" pains, and gastro-intestinal disorders.

Another modern popular belief, not specific to Egypt, is based on the obsolete medical opinion that eggs, because of their sulphur content, increase the risk of sulphaemoglobinaemia from "sulfa" drugs, and should be avoided while under that therapy.

Regarding chicken, it is believed that chicken or pigeons eaten before and during delivery, supply the strength needed during and after child-birth. Chicken is thus given during the first week of the puerperium, a sacrosanct custom so well established that it is followed even in govern-ment hospitals, and that a popular expression says of a greedy person "He would eat the chicken of a delivered woman." Other foods that are held as equally important are butter, vegetable soup, rabbit, or milk and sugar. One woman interviewed remarked that eggs speed delivery and ease pain.

Poultry plays an important role in scattered rural marriage customs, although these are not general throughout the country. A woman from Shebin El Qanater reported that a chicken is fed for a months killed, then eaten by both the bride and groom before their marriage. In parts of Egypt a meal of boiled chicken is prepared by the parents of the bride, placed in a skillet, and put under the marriage bed for the bride and groom to share during their first breakfast together. These current customs do not seem to stem from antiquity.

Pigeons are believed to promote virility; hence, they are fed to the prospective bridegroom for several days prior to the marriage celebration. Chicken soup may be substituted in some instances. Among the Kenuzi in Nubia, pigeons roasted in *semna* (molten or clarified butter) are eaten for forty days by the bridegroom, after which he must prove his strength . . . bread made from sorghum is toasted to a very hard consistency, and he must crush the roll in one hand and let the crumbs fall into a bowl of soup. If he accomplishes this fact, it is believed that his marriage will be strong and lasting. Otherwise, he is further fed to gain sufficient strength.

Many other superstitious beliefs that smack of magic linger, although they are opposed by modern physicians. In the vicinity of Luxor and elsewhere in Egypt it is believed that chicken blood can break the spell of female sterility. A chicken is slain, and the sterile woman then steps seven times over the blood; custom asserts that she will thereafter be able to conceive.

There is also a traditional avoidance of certain birds because their "call" is imagined to imitate an appeal to God. Thus, the dove (yamam), eaten with delight by many, is avoided by others because its call imitate, the words ". . . *Ya Rahman, ya Rahman* . . ." (Oh, all merciful, oh, all merciful), this being one of the Divine names. Other birds included in this category are the hoopoe (*hodhod*) that cries ". . . *Ya Raouf, ya Raouf* . . ." (Oh, all pitiful, oh, all pitiful); and the stone curlew (karawan) the call of which resembles: ". . . *Al Moulk lak, lak, lak, ya Sahib al Moulk* . . ." (The universe is yours, yours, yours, oh Master of the Universe.) These beliefs date to very old lore and appear in such old works as Al Demiry's and Qazwiny's Books on Animals (1956).

Other reasons for avoidance of specific varieties of fowl concern the help and aid the birds render man. The cattle egret (*abu gordan*) for example, is not eaten because it is considered the "farmer's friend." It follows behind man as he plows his fields and devours worms that, otherwise, might damage valuable crops. Not only is it forbidden by law to hunt it but it is considered extremely bad luck to kill one.

These present-day attitudes illustrate the difficulty of interpreting from archeologic finds and/or portrayals in tombs, alone, the manner in which a particular species might have been regarded by the Ancients. Contemporary accounts may be helpful, but often do not exist.

Notes: Chapter 6

1. *F.*, 3
2. *F.*, 278, *ḳbḥw*
3. *F.*, 157, *h ꜣ w*
4. *F.*, 117, *myst*
5. *F.*, 274, *šdw*
6. *F.*, 70, *wšnw*
7. *F.*, 199, *ḫt ꜣ w*
8. Fowling by "throw net" is not uncommon in Egypt in the vicinity of Port Said in the northeastern Delta. Browne (1806, p. 407) was among the first to describe such casting nets. Gurney (1875, pp. 94–95) accompanied one such "fowling" excursion and remarked that the Egyptians were accurate in casting their nets up to 25 feet.
9. *šḫty* (*F.*, 240).
10. The Egyptian variety of fowling stick would not return to the thrower. It was called *ꜥmꜥmt* (*F.*, 42).
11. *h ꜣ rw* was the Egyptian word for decoy ducks, or bait in general (*F.*, 163).
12. Pliny wrote "There is also a method of treating the livers of sows as of geese, a discovery of Marcus Apicius, they are stuffed with dried fig, and when full killed directly after having been given a drink of mead" (*N.H.*, VIII, LXXII, 209).
13. *F.*, 70.
14. We know of no other method of cooking represented in Ancient Egypt. Unusual methods practiced nowadays are cooking fowl wrapped in a banana leaf or in the belly of a lamb (see note 27); or, as do the Bedjas of southeastern Egypt, to bake them in clay. Before eating, the outer "earthenware" crust is broken. The latter method, a refined mode of cooking that preserves all the juice of the fowl is practiced in France and Italy and is called by Italians "pollo alla creta."
15. *F.*, 206; *G.*, 587.
16. Also means bird, in general (*F.*, 3; *G.*, 550, however, translates this term as goose).
17. *F.*, 228; *G.*, 590.
18. *F.*, 146; *G.*, 577.
19. *F.*, 235; *G.* 591.
20. *F.*, 288; also *gbb*, *G.*, 597.

21. *F.*, 306; *G.*, 601.
22. *F.*, 108; *G.*, 568.
23. *F.*, 49.
24. From Campania, a district in southwestern Italy.
25. According to Adams (1870, p. 26) doves were raised in Egypt *only* for their dung.
26. *F.*, 318.
27. Avicenna (Ibn Sina) the learned Arab physician wrote ". . . the flesh of chicken is moist and relaxing to the bowels, whereas that of partridge is dry and constipating. Roast fowls are better if they have been prepared in the belly of a kid or lamb because that preserves their moisture. Chicken-broth tempers the humours strongly; more so than fowl-broth, though the latter is more nutritious . . ." (Gruner, 1930, 796).
28. An earth goddess originally worshipped in Phrygia in Asia Minor.
29. See pp. 383, 395.
30. The name of this village means "clipped nose." Mutilation by severing the nose was a method by which criminals were distinguished from honest citizens. It is not clear whether Rhinocolura was a penal colony, or a village founded by mutilated exiles living together to avoid public ridicule.
31. A unit of linear measurement, variously given as 600, 607, or 630 feet.
32. Hebrew for "graves of lust."
33. Osborn, informed us that freshly cooked ostrich meat is not particularly pleasing (personal communication, 1967, 1969). This would be, however, a matter of personal taste.
34. *niw*: *F.*, 125; *G.*, 572.
35. Ostrich eggs, when obtainable, are eaten by the Kenuzi in Nubia to alleviate rheumatism.
36. *Wb. Dr.*, 120. This word stands also for oil (*F.*, 112). See Chapter 19.
37. *Wb. Dr.*, 120. This term, however, is also used for fat or grease in general (*F.*, 51). See Chapter 19.
38. Unknown products.
39. *F.*, 173; *G.*, 582.
40. Ames (1965, p. 68–71) has cleared much of the confusion surrounding the identification and separation of the various Egyptian gods named "Horus."
41. *G.*, 72–73; *F.*, 174.
42. This tame relationship was noted by Aelian (2, 1) ". . . and they fall in with the Egyptians as they are sowing their fields, and in the ploughlands they find, so to speak, a generous table, and though uninvited partake of the Egyptians' hospitality . . ."
43. We have seen them at Qara Oasis in March, 1966.
44. *F.*, 158; *G.*, 579: *hby*.
45. The god Thot is also represented as a baboon. The Ancients observed the

social chattering of baboons at dawn and concluded therefrom a close affinity with the sun.

46. Might these have been locusts?

47. The narrow pass discussed by Herodotus was placed near a town called Buto ". . . I saw innumerable bones and backbones of serpents; many heaps of backbones there were, great, and small, and smaller still . . ." (II, 75).

    This could not have been the "northern" Buto in the Delta, but must have represented the "southern" Buto, i.e., Edfu, where Wadi El Miyah (Valley of Waters) connects the Nile Valley with the Red Sea. Interpretation of the "serpent backbones" is unclear. Might they be weathered nummulitic fossils which closely resemble intervertebral cartilage discs? Or could they have been the actual vertebrae of fish trampled, buried, and left in the plains north and east of Edfu, later disturbed and uncovered by winds (see p. 387)?

48. The association of the ibis with domination over snakes was also reported by Aelian (1, 38) who states that ibis feathers frightened serpents. One is also intrigued with his description of "serpents that come down the Nile." Is this perhaps the "messenger fish" (p. 391)? If so, might this "fish" have been an eel?

49. *F.*, 134; *G.*, 469.
50. *F.*, 129; *G.*, 469.
51. *G.*, 470.
52. *F.*, 162; *G.*, 560.
53. *F.*, 82; *G.*, 564.

Chapter 7   *Fish*

Introduction

". . . put forth thy hand boldly, O flourishing fisherman; behold, fish are caught, the Silurus fishes appear with the Hippopotamus; it is the doing of Horus . . ." (Tomb of Tehuti-Nekht, El Bersheh; Middle Kingdom, twelfth dynasty. Griffith *et al.* [1894], p. 20.)

". . . we remember the fish, which we did eat in Egypt freely . . ." (Numbers, 11, 5)

Judging from the many excavated remains of fish, fishing implements, pisciform palettes and from the idioms, metaphors or expressions in the daily language, which indicate familiarity with fish, or from the number of signs of fish in hieroglyphic writing, fish, an important source of protein and minerals, filled an important role in the Ancient Egyptian's diet, especially before he learned the arts of agriculture and husbandry. The Nile, said Diodorus (I, 36),

". . . contains every variety of fish and in numbers beyond belief; for it supplies the natives not only with abundant subsistence from the fish freshly caught but it also yields an unfailing multitude for salting."

The volume of fish production may be judged from the ancient texts. Taxes to the State were paid by fishermen as early as the eighteenth dynasty (*A.R.*, IV, 243 and 394) and Lake Moeris alone brought into the treasury a silver talent per day for the six months during which water flowed from the lake into the river, and twenty minae for each day of the flow of water into the lake (*Her.*, II, 149). This enormous revenue was allotted as "pin-money" to queens (Diodorus, I, 52) to buy the perfumes, ointments, jewels and other objects connected with their toilet. According to Rawlinson (see also *Her.*, II, 149, n. 9) a talent was equivalent to £193 or £243, according to various estimates, and 20 minae to £64.60 or £81.80, this would amount to an annual revenue, at the lowest calculation, of £47,000. These estimates were made in 1880, and would be considerably higher nowadays. But Rawlinson remarks that a talent could not have been raised daily from that one fishery, and that it would more probably include revenue from all fisheries in Egypt.

History and Development of Fishing in Ancient Egypt

Sources of food for early inhabitants of Egypt were discussed in the first century B.C. by Diodorus Siculus

". . . a second way by which the Egyptians subsisted was, they say, by the eating of fish, of which the river provided a great abundance, especially at the time when it receded after its flood and dried up . . ." (1, 43, 3)

Aelian, sometimes considered an unreliable source because of his flights into ecstatic expression,[1] was objectively descriptive when he confirmed the method described by Diodorus Siculus

". . . later the river retreats and returns to within its naturally proper limits, while the fish, bereft of their sire and abandoned by the floodwater, are left behind, nurtured in the thick slime to provide a meal for the farmers. This then, though the expression is somewhat violent, is the Egyptian fish-harvest . . ." (10, 43)

Collecting fish in this manner, certainly the simplest of all methods, has been current in Egypt throughout history, and even into recent decades, before the construction of the Aswan dam made the flood an event of the past. An Old Kingdom song told it in poetic form

". . . the shepherd is in the water among the fish. He speaketh with the shad (?) and greeteth the (?)-fish . . ." (Erman, 1966, p. 131)

Other fishing techniques developed in Egypt have had long developmental histories (Bates, 1917). Such factors as the development of leisure time, spread of religion, discovery of copper and increased food requirements, have influenced them. For example, fishing by trap or net is more economical in terms of time and catch than line-fishing. Spear-fishing may have been in later periods primarily a sport; but, in early Egypt, it was a practical and important method of obtaining food. Thus, specific fishing techniques are linked with a variety of technologic, economic and social parameters, some of which are outlined in Table 1, but as early as the twelfth dynasty they were all well developed. The

Table 1

Technological, economic and social aspects of fishing

Techniques by which fish are obtained	Quantity of catch	Degree of patience	Level of technical development	Relative level of skill	Presumed Theoretical Division of Labour	
					Lower classes and servants	Upper classes[b]
Catching of fish by hand: (fish stranded in pools left by the Nile flood)	Abundant	None	None	None	Youth and adults (food)	Youth (play)
Spearing of fish	Limited	High	Bone and metal	High	Youth and adults (food)	Youth and adults (sport)
Hooks; "drop-line"	Limited[a]	Low	Bone and metal	Medium	Youth and adults (food)	Youth (play)
Hooks; "fishing-rod"	Limited	High	Bone and metal	High	Youth (play) Adult servants (food)	Youth and adults (sport)
Traps; permanent	Abundant	None	Low	Low	Youth and adults (food)	(not practiced)
Traps; individual	Limited	Low	Basketry	Medium	Youth and adults	(not practiced)
Corded nets	Abundant	Low	Weaving	High	Youth and adults	(not practiced)

[a] A qualified evaluation; fishermen using multiple lines with many hooks can bring abundant catches.
[b] The Upper Classes probably obtained their fish mainly from servants or from local markets.

Eloquent Peasant (Lefebvre, 1949, p. 61) comparing the ruthlessness of the Governor of his province to a fisherman, said

" . . . O Great Steward, My Lord, the *Khoudou*[2] fisherman slaughters the *iy*[2]—fish; the fisherman with the trident spears the *aouseb*[2] fish; the *Djabhou*[2] fisherman against the *paqer*[2] fish, the net fisherman, he devastates the river. Well, You, are the like of them! . . ."

Traps

Construction of simple fish traps requires little technical skill. Several Late Paleolithic drawings (Fig. 7.1), discovered at a sheltered cliff site

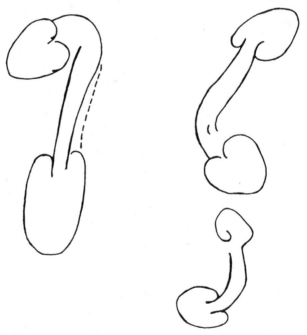

Fig. 7.1. Fish traps (?). Late Paleolithic; Upper Egypt. Redrawn from Winkler (1938), Vol. 1, plate 32, Figs 1 and 2.

situated along the Ancient migratory route connecting the Nile Valley with the western desert oasis of Khargah, have tentatively been identified as "fish-traps" (Winkler, 1938, I, p. 32), but as fish are not actually depicted inside, or associated with the "traps," even though they are illustrated at the same site, these drawings may represent another type of game trap, or may be unrelated to either hunting or fishing.

Ruffer (1919, p. 32) believed that spear-fishing, as practiced during the Pre-Dynastic and Dynastic Periods, was less the pitting of hunter's skill against fish, than the simple channelling of fish into shallow waters by means of "stake" traps where they could be more easily speared or captured by hand. Construction of such traps was dependent upon a gradually sloping lake-bed as at Lake Moeris in the Fayoum, and a supply of stout, aquatic reeds. Present archaeological information cannot determine, however, whether the Fayoum "A" settlers used traps of this sort, even though fish-spears have been found at this site (pp. 354, 355).

To our knowledge, no examples of such fish barricades or traps have been depicted in Egyptian funeral art. During the Graeco-Roman Period, however, this method is mentioned by foreign observers as one of the primary means whereby the Egyptians obtained fish

". . . now the Cestreus,[3] he says, runs up the river in spring when it is carrying its spawn, but for the purpose of spawning comes down in schools before the setting of the Pleiad,[4] at which time they are captured, being caught in schools by the fenced enclosures . . ." (Strabo, 17, 2, 5)

This description recalls the elaborate spiral system of traps employed today by Egyptian fishermen along the southern shore of Lake Mariut. These are set in shallow water with the reeds arranged in a curved wall that forms an ever tightening spiral. The fishermen take to their boats and by thrashing the water, drive the fish toward the mouth of the spiral trap where they are channelled into the centre of the enclosure and netted with ease. Such traps are also found in areas of the Arabian/Persian Gulf (Serjeant, 1968).

Although these barricade traps are not represented in Egyptian tombs, portrayal of small basket traps is not uncommon in Old Kingdom tombs at Saqqara and Deir el Gebrawi. These traps were sometimes supported by floats and placed just below the surface of the water. In the tomb of Mereruka at Saqqara artists have portrayed hosts of tiny fish swimming towards them (Fig. 7.2).

Seines

Although it is not certain whether the Neolithic settlers at Fayoum "A" used fish traps or barricades, there is evidence that they probably were

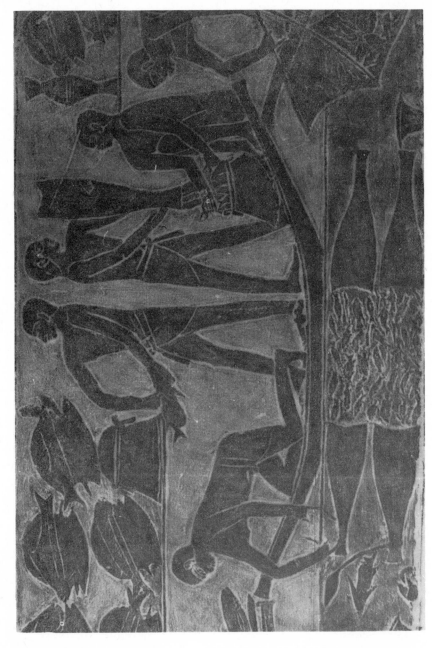

Fig. 7.2. Tomb of Mereruka at Saqqara; Old Kingdom sixth dynasty, reign of King Teti, *c.* 2390 B.C. Rubbing by Ward Patterson; used with permission (1969).

familiar with large fishing nets. Grooved limestone balls that presumably functioned as "sinkers" have been found in great numbers at this locality (Caton-Thompson, and Gardner, 1934, pp. 67 and 89).

Large seines (Figs 7.3, 7.4, and 7.5) that required the efforts and energy of a team of fishermen are a common feature of Old Kingdom tombs. These nets were primarily deployed from the shore with the assistance of fishermen in other boats. The upper edges of the nets, as depicted by the ancient artists, reveal a series of triangular objects identified as "floats", and the lower edges are lined with either rectangular or ovate "sinkers". Sometimes slings were attached to the nets and slipped over the shoulders of the fishermen to facilitate the drawing in of the catch. Illustrations of this technique are found at Saqqara, Giza, Meir, Deir el Gabrawi, El Bersha, Thebes and elsewhere. Their wide distribution indicates their common use, and implies a ready acceptance of Nile fish as food. But, though they are profusely represented in drawings and models of the Middle Kingdom, they are less common in the New Kingdom tombs where they give way to scenes of harpooning.

Hand Nets

Several varieties of open-mouth "V" nets are known from scattered sites of the Old and Middle Kingdoms (Figs 7.6, 7.7). They varied in individual construction, but the basic form consisted of two sticks lashed together at the bottom and strengthened laterally with a brace. A net was attached to this pre-formed "V" which could be opened or closed by manipulation of a longitudinal cord. Boulenger (1907, pp. 39–40) drew attention to two modern varieties of Egyptian nets, known as the *Shilb* and *Lawafa*, that appear to be identical with the ones used during the Old and Middle Kingdoms. We have observed these in use by fishermen in Cairo and Fayoum.

It is not clear from examination of the paintings whether the "V" net was dragged through the water as boatmen poled along, whether it was used to collect fish which had been channelled into a fenced barricade, or whether it was used in both these ways. If a modern parallel may be drawn, the latter, combined technique seems more probable. Today Egyptian village boys near Saqqara construct barricades in shallow canals; they then re-enter the canal a hundred meters up-channel and drive the fish towards the barricade, where other boys net the fish with the "V" nets.

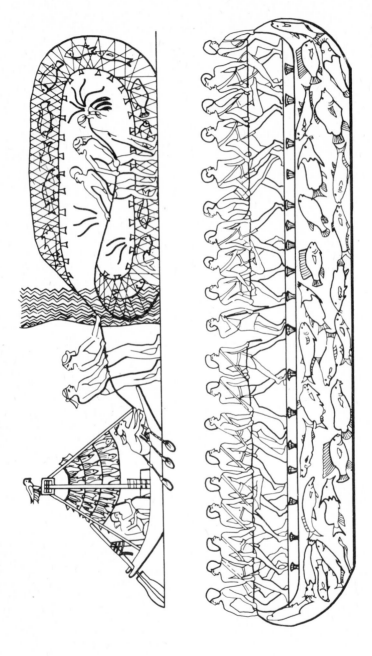

Fig. 7.3. (Upper) Hauling in a large sein. Tomb of Horemheb (number 78) at Thebes (Upper Enclosure); New Kingdom, eighteenth dynasty, reign of King Thutmose III, *c.* 1475 B.C. Redrawn from Wilkinson (1878), Vol. 2, p. 102, Fig. 361.

Fig. 7.4. (Lower) Hauling in a large sein. Tomb of Mereruka at Saqqara; Old Kingdom, sixth dynasty, reign of King Teti, *c.* 2390 B.C. Redrawn, with permission, from Gaillard (1923), p. 6, Fig. 4.

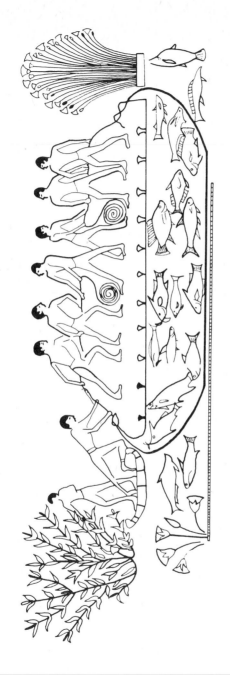

Fig. 7.5. Hauling in a large seine. Tomb (number 5) at El Bersheh; Middle Kingdom, date uncertain. Redrawn from Griffith, *et al.* (1894), plate 16.

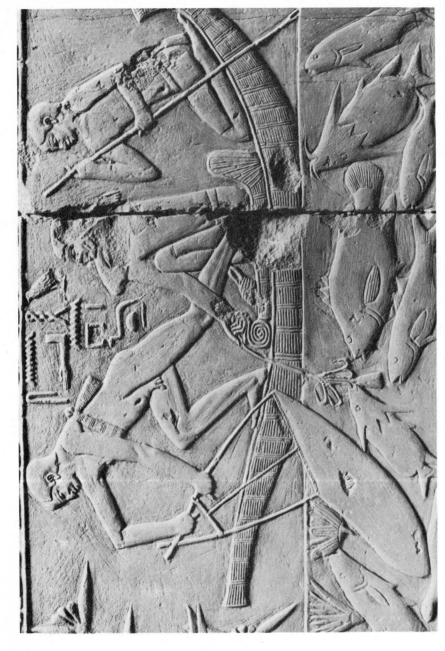

Fig. 7.6. Hand fish net. Tomb of Ka-Gem-Ni at Saqqara; Old Kingdom, sixth dynasty, reign of King Teti, *c.* 2390 B.C. Photographed 1969.

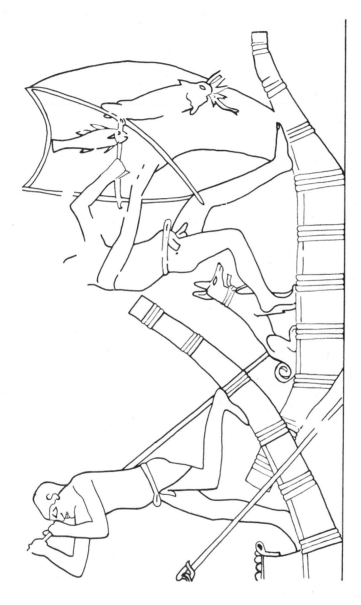

Fig. 7.7. Open-mouth "V" net. Tomb of Ukh-hotp at Meir; Middle Kingdom, twelfth dynasty, date uncertain. Redrawn from Blackman (1915a), plate 4.

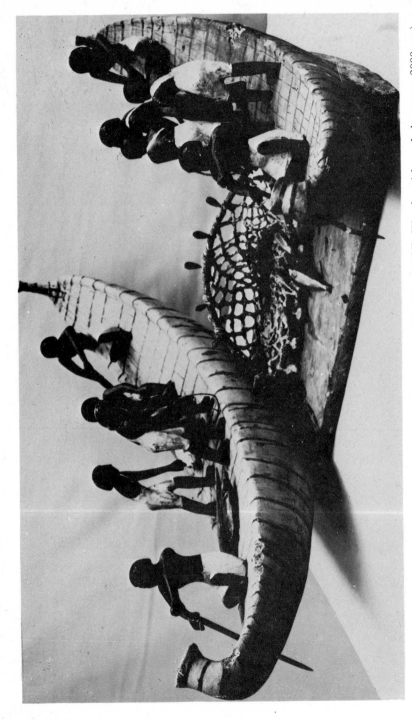

Fig. 7.8. Small-scale model from the tomb of Meket-Re, an important noble of the Middle Kingdom (eleventh dynasty, *c.* 2000 B.C.). Thebes. Cairo Museum. Two fishing boats dragging a trawl net stretched between them. The net is re-inforced by a heavy rope around the edge of the opening and along the centre of the bottom. Sinkers and floats keep the net in position. The men hauling the net wear a white band over the left shoulder to protect the shoulder when hauling the net. Fish can be identified as bolti, bynni, mormyrus and perch.

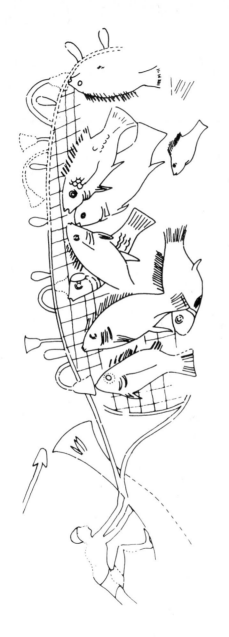

Fig. 7.9. Tomb of Sebeknekht at El Kab. A fisherman, called "the very clever fisherman", Anqetsa, drawing an elliptical net full of fish within reach of his master's spear. Redrawn from Tylor and Clarke (1896), plate IV.

A variation of this technique (Fig. 7.8) is illustrated in a small scale model from the tomb of Meket-Re (eleventh dynasty). Two fishing boats drag a trawl net stretched between them. The net is reinforced by a heavy rope around the edges of the opening and along the centre of the bottom. Sinkers and floats keep the net in position (Winlock, 1955).

The only illustration we know of the circular or elliptical cast net, that is so common in modern Egypt, is from the tomb of Sebeknekht (Tylor and Clarke, 1896) where the "very clever fisherman Anqetsa" is shown drawing the net full of great fish within reach of his master's spear (Fig. 7.9). Radcliffe (1926, p. 317) quoting Julius Pollux of Naucratis, a writer of the second century A.D., states that the Ancient Egyptian vocabulary included words for "nets that are cast" and a passage from Herodotus (II, 95) is certainly indicative of a large hand net, rather than a huge seine or a "V" hand net

> ". . . every man of them has a net, with which he catches fish by day, and for the night he sets it round the bed where he rests, then creeps under it and so sleeps. If he sleeps wrapped in a garment or cloth, the gnats bite through it; but through the net they do not even try at all to bite . . ."[5]

Bates (1917) commenting on the scarcity of illustrations of this kind of net, believes it due not to unfamiliarity with its use, but to the fact that, quite apart from the greater productivity of the seine, the crew which worked it could more easily be shown hauling on the ropes than could the single fisherman engaged in flinging his cast net.

Hooks: Drop-line and Rod-fishing

> ". . . He [Antony] was fishing once, and had bad luck, and was vexed at it because Cleopatra was there to see. He therefore ordered his fishermen to dive down and secretly fasten to his hook some fish that had been previously caught, and pulled up two or three . . ." (Plutarch, *Lives*; *Antony*, 29, 3–4)

Fishing by hook and line is a very ancient practice in Egypt. Hooks of various types have been found in Pre-Dynastic settlements in both Upper and Lower Egypt. Though absent in excavated Fayoum "A" sequences (Caton-Thompson and Gardner, 1934), a barbless variety made from horn, discovered at Merimda Beni Salama indicates its early use in Lower Egypt (Junker, 1929, pp. 71–72; *MAE*, pp. 110–111). In addition, fish hooks of shell and horn have been excavated at El Omari (Debono,

1948, p. 567) and hooks made of copper have been found at Maadi (Menghin and Amer, 1936, p. 48).

Initial excavations at El Badari in Upper Egypt did not at first reveal fish hooks, although the finding of large vertebrae of *Lates niloticus* (Nile perch; Fig. 7.23) indicated that the inhabitants ate this species (Brunton and Caton-Thompson, 1928, pp. 41 and 94). Subsequent excavations at this site, however, did unearth fish hooks (*MAE*, p. 111).

Daumas (1964, p. 83) analysed numerous Old Kingdom tomb illustrations that depicted "drop-line" fishing and concluded that these represented a survival in art of Pre-Dynastic techniques used by early man before the expansion and development of a broad-based fishing technology. According to him, the inclusion in tomb art of such methods was a heritage of religion and did not depict the principal method of obtaining fish. Daumas noted further that all illustrations of line-fishing from the Old Kingdom show the hook unbaited (Fig. 7.10). He considered this not a true representation of the technique of Egyptian line-fishing, but rather an artistic convention that showed only the essential part of the object.

The baits used by the Ancient Egyptians are not identifiable with certainty. One literary source, however, indicates that the Egyptian fishermen would not use as bait the flesh of the same kind of fish they sought

". . . I have not caught fish [with bait made of] the bodies of the same kind of fish . . ." (*Papyrus of Nu; Book of the Dead*, Budge, 1960, p. 575)

There is speculation concerning the relation of ancient methods of fishing to modern Egyptian methods. Geoffroy St Hilaire (1829) observed Egyptian fishermen using dates (*Phoenix dactylifera*) as bait. Gaillard (1923) reported the same practice by fishermen in Upper Egypt at Asyut and Qena. Such observations, however, offer little basis for projecting into the Dynastic Period the use of dates as bait.

Boulenger (1907, pp. 26–27) reported on other Nile fishermen who used "mud-baits," balls of mud mixed with either millet (*Sorghum vulgare*) or barley (*Hordeum* spp.), affixed to the hooks, and Gaillard (1923) likened these "balls" to the objects seen attached to fishing lines in Old Kingdom tomb pictures (Fig. 7.11).

Among other bait used by modern fishermen, Geoffroy St Hilaire (1829, pp. 285–286) reported bait from bread, and Boulenger (1907, p. 27) recorded the use of worms from Aswan to the Delta.

One may argue that the absence of baited hooks in tomb art may not

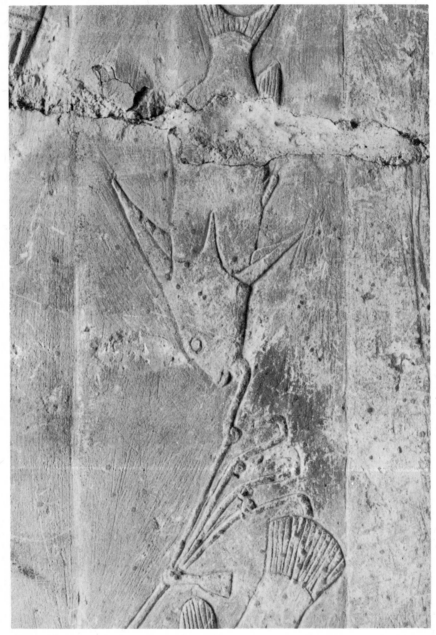

Fig. 7.10. Drop-line fishing with unbaited hooks. Tomb of Idut at Saqqara; Old Kingdom, fifth dynasty, reign of King Unas, *c.* 2423 B.C. Photographed 1969.

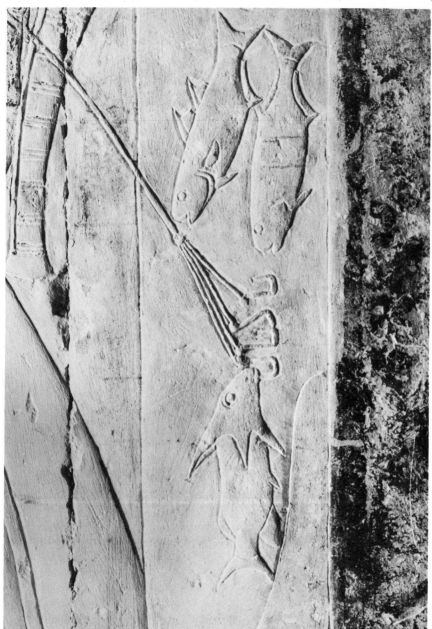

Fig. 7.11. Drop-line fishing with unbaited hooks fitted with "sinker/spinner". Tomb of Idut at Saqqara; Old Kingdom, fifth dynasty, reign of King Unas, *c.* 2423 B.C. Photographed 1969.

have been a mere artistic convention. The modern Egyptian fisherman is skilled at "snagging" fish. Boulenger describes a technique whereby long fishing lines on which are attached hundred of hooks are played out behind the boat. A skillfully timed tug on these lines may bring a catch of soft-bodied varieties that feed on the bottom (1907, p. 26).

The Fishing Rod

Some rare tomb paintings depict the use of fishing rods. Drawing upon modern parallels, one might anticipate that this method was employed during periods of leisure enjoyed by the upper classes; but in the preserved paintings, both the nobility and servants are shown using the pole. For example, a picture at Beni Hassan dating to the Middle Kingdom shows a servant fishing in this manner (Fig. 7.12). Others, all badly damaged, are known from New Kingdom tombs at Thebes. Our examination of Theban tombs in the summer of 1969 included a specific search for the famous "fishing noble" depicted by Wilkinson (Fig. 7.13) and by Vandier (Fig. 7.14), but we were unrewarded; apparently the picture has been destroyed. Furthermore, we were unable to locate any of several other published tomb paintings illustrating the "fishing pole" technique.

As artistic motifs, fishing by hook, net and trap become increasingly rare at the conclusion of the Old Kingdom; at the same time there is a proportional increase in scenes of harpooning. The significance of this shift is not clear; it might reflect an increased interest in the sporting aspect of fishing, or be purely a function of artistic design. It cannot be interpreted in terms of acceptance or avoidance of fish.

Further evidence concerning ancient fishing methods exists in the Egyptian Agricultural Museum at Dokki where there is displayed a fine collection of tackle, including hooks, nets and fish net floats (Figs 7.15, 7.16, 7.17, 7.18). These, however, are Post-Dynastic.

Spear- (harpoon) Fishing

Fish spears made from bone or fish spines have been found in the Fayoum "A" sequences (Caton-Thompson and Gardner, 1934, pp. 22 and 34). As discussed above, spear-fishing as an artistic motif is less frequently encountered in tombs dated to the Old Kingdom (Fig. 6.12), where seines, hand nets and drop-lines predominate. During the Middle and New Kingdoms, however, these latter techniques probably lost favour as decorative designs, and spear-fishing was more widely exhibited (Fig. 7.19), each scene being artistically balanced against a stereotyped representation of fowling. It is not clear whether spear-fishing was depicted because of its sporting aspects, to recall a pleasant outing, because of its religious connotations (spearing the enemies of Osiris and Horus), or because of its decorative value. In any case, the technique could not result in abundant catches (Table 1). One interesting detail of these scenes is the "water mountain" rising in front of the sportsman. One explanation is that this was to obviate painting the nobleman in an undignified bent posture.

Identification of Freshwater Fish Consumed by Ancient Egyptians

Knowledge of the freshwater fish consumed by Ancient Egyptians rests, on the one hand upon the correct identification of unearthed finds and of tomb drawings and, on the other, on interpretations of the Ancient Egyptian, Greek and Roman names of species. The most fruitful of these efforts were those that were based on the analysis of Old Kingdom bas-reliefs, because of the outstanding artistry of their execution and the meticulous attention to detail they exhibit.

But a valid interpretation of the Egyptian, Greek and Latin names for fish in terms of modern scientific and Arabic colloquial usage is thwarted by the substantial changes in nomenclature, especially during the past century. The descriptions of Geoffroy St Hilaire (1829), a member of Bonaparte's Expedition to Egypt in 1798, bear only a rudimentary resemblance to the modern taxonomy proposed by Boulenger (1907), Gaillard (1923) and others. The difficulty is compounded by the fact that colloquial names of fish in any language vary within the same country, or between different groups of fishermen speaking the same language. When such problems of identification were encountered, we have followed the suggestions of Montet (1913), Gaillard (1923), d'Arcy Thompson (1928), Cerny (1937–1938), and Keimer (1948).

A further difficulty arises from the possibility of changes in the aquatic fauna in the last 5000 years, resulting either in the disappearance of old varieties or in the appearance of new ones. This is possibly the case with

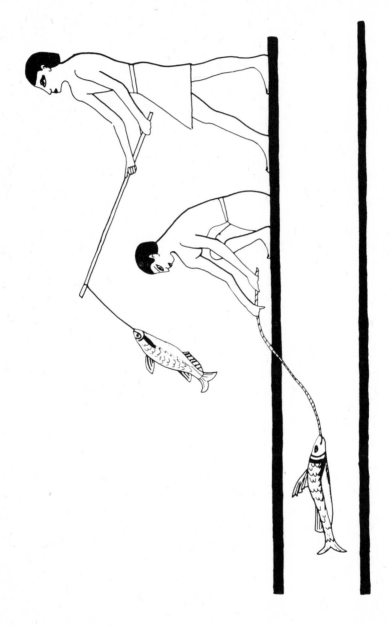

Fig. 7.12. Servants using a drop-line and "rod". Tomb of Khnum-hotep (number 3) at Beni Hassan; Middle Kingdom, eleventh dynasty, date uncertain. Redrawn from Wilkinson (1878), Vol. 2, p. 116, Fig. 371.

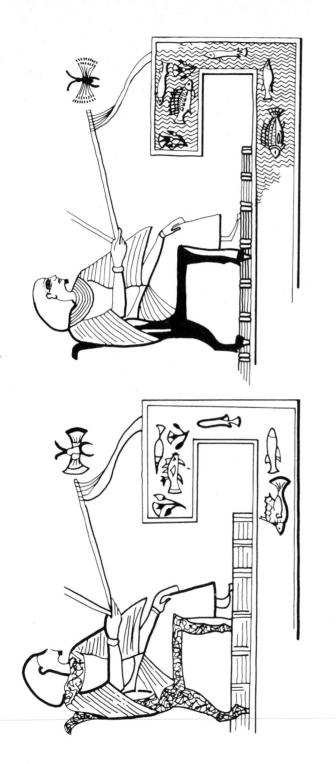

Fig. 7.13. (Left) "An Egyptian Gentleman Fishing". Tomb of Nebunenef (number 157) at Thebes (Drah abu el Naga; southern tombs); New Kingdom, nineteenth dynasty, reign of King Rameses II, *c.* 1250 B.C. Redrawn from Vandier. (1969), Vol. 5, part 1, p. 609, Fig. 248.

Fig. 7.14. (Right) "An Egyptian Gentleman Fishing". Tomb of Nebunenef (number 157) at Thebes (Drah abu el Naga; southern tombs); New Kingdom, nineteenth dynasty, reign of King Rameses II, *c.* 1240 B.C. Redrawn from Wilkinson (1878), Vol. 2, p. 115, Fig. 370.

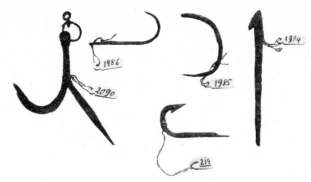

Fig. 7.15. Fish hooks. Roman Period; date uncertain. Photographed with permission of the Ministry of Agriculture and officials of the Agricultural Museum, Dokki, ARE (1969).

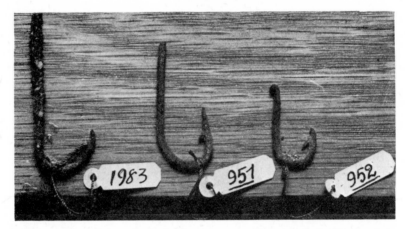

Fig. 7.16. Fish hooks. Roman Period; date uncertain. Photographed with permission of the Ministry of Agriculture and the officials of the Agricultural Museum, Dokki, ARE (1969).

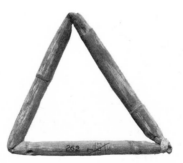

Fig. 7.17. Fish float (compare with Fig. 7.5). Fayoum Oasis (Kom Ouchim); Roman Period, date uncertain. Photographed with permission of the Ministry of Agriculture and the officials of the Agricultural Museum, Dokki, ARE (1969).

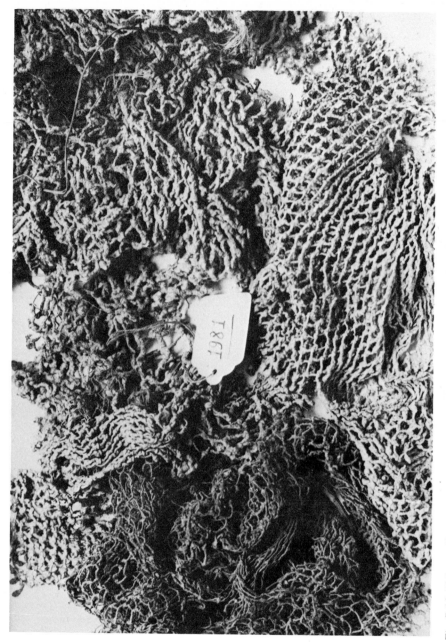

Fig. 7.18. Fish net. Fayoum oasis; Roman Period; third century A.D. Photographed with permission of the Ministry of Agriculture and the officials of the Agricultural Museum, Dokki, ARE (1969).

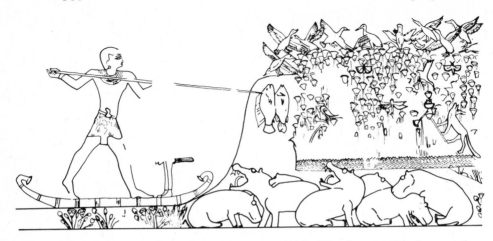

Fig. 7.19. Spear fishing. Tomb of Senbi at Meir; Middle Kingdom, twelfth dynasty, date uncertain. Redrawn from Blackman (1914), plate 2. Note: (a) the "water mountain" arising in front of the spearer; (b) papyrus and lotus in the water.

some Hydrocyons, Alestes and Polyptera, found today in Egypt but that, according to Gaillard, are untraceable either in hieroglyphs or in illustrations. He is contested, however, by Keimer (1948), who pointed to a drawing in Ankhtifi's tomb at Moalla (Upper Egypt) that, he felt sure, represents Hydrocyon, to a specimen in the Agricultural Museum at Dokki that is probably Alestes, and to a drawing in the *Book of the Dead* that could be a Polypterus.

In spite of these difficulties, Gaillard in a detailed study of 118 fish silhouettes from the tombs of Ti and Mereruka, a cast in the Lyons University, and a schist plaque from Hierakonpolis, could identify 24 species. These are: *Mugil cephalus, M. capito, Tilapia nilotica, Clarias anguillaris, Cl. lazera, Synodontis schall, Anguilla vulgaris, Mormyrus kannume, Morm. caschive, Morm. niloticus, Tetrodon fahaka, Citharinus citharus, Cith. latus, Malopterurus electricus, Gnathonemus cyprinoides, Synodontis batensoda, Petrocephalus bane, Petr. bovei, Lates niloticus, Barbus bynni Labeo niloticus, Schilbe mystus, Hyperopisus bebe,* and *Heterobranchus longifilis.*

He commented that small fish were not represented, probably because the artist did not think it worth while drawing them. Only one silhouette he could not identify, although it had been carved by one of the best artists of the Old Kingdom, and he suggested that it belonged to a now extinct species.

One cannot categorically state, however, that all fish depicted in tombs were eaten, for whereas fishermen discard unprofitable species from their hauls, artists may indiscriminately portray all the catch or, alternatively, select those that appeal to them or with which they are familiar. Recognizing this selectivity of artists Gaillard adopted, as a basis of assessment, present-day attitudes of Egyptian fishermen. Another criterion could be the frequency of utilization in Ancient Egyptian medicine. The Ebers papyrus mentions nine kinds of fish of which Montet (1913) identified four. Medical information must be viewed, however, with several reservations, the familiarity of physicians and patients with fish might be different; homeopathic concepts might lead to treatment of a dry skin disease with consumption of dry fish, or a "vile" disease with consumption of a "vile tasting" fish; or mythological legends may have been at the base of their therapeutic use.

We have tabulated these against Gaillard's and our experience among fishermen and urban dwellers (Table 2). We may tentatively conclude from this comparison that the frequency of illustration is in part related to popularity as food. This is the case with *Claria anguillaris*, *Mugil cephalus*, and *Tilapia nilotica*. On the other hand, a discrepancy is observed with *Lates niloticus* and *Synodontis schall*, possibly a result of cultural shifts unknown to us, for it would be presumptuous to assume that our present taste is more "correct" than that of the Ancients (see Figs 7.20 to 7.29).

When one comes to actual remains of fish, one encounters another difficulty, that of selective preservation or recognition. It is often stated, for example, that both *Lates niloticus* and *Synodontus* were widely eaten. Is this because of the peculiar skeletal elements that allow easy identification of these fish, or of better preservation of the large vertebrae of *Lates* and the cranial spines of *synodontus* with their greater structural density?

Until more definitive evidence is available, for example, preserved meals including fish, or papyri describing more fully the banquet fares of different periods, it is hazardous to be dogmatic as to the varieties most commonly used as food by the Ancient Egyptians of all periods.

Freshwater Fish Preferences of the Greeks and Romans in Egypt

Greek travellers and subsequent Roman observers discussed the merit of various Nile fish. Strabo (17, 2, 4) prepared a list of fish that were available but did not identify those varieties eaten:

Table 2

Identification and frequency in tomb art of selected Nile fish[a]

Scientific Latin name	Old Kingdom frequency: Saqqara tomb art	New Kingdom frequency: Ebers Medical Papyrus	Modern attitudes in Egypt
Barbus bynni[b]	14th	—	Esteemed
Clarias anguillaris	3rd	1st	Esteemed
Lates niloticus	13th	4th	Esteemed
Mugil cephalus	1st	3rd	Esteemed
Petrocephalus bane	12th	—	Esteemed
Schilbe mystus	16th	—	Esteemed
Tilapia nilotica	2nd	3rd	Esteemed
Citharinus citharus	8th	—	Little Esteemed
Synodontis schall	4th	2nd	Little Esteemed

[a] Gleaned from Ebbell (1937), Gaillard (1923), Montet (1913a), Wreszinski (1913).
[b] Illustrations of the species appear in Figs 7.20 through 7.29.

". . . as for fish in the Nile, they are indeed many in number and different in kind, with a special indigenous character, but the best known are the Oxyrhynchus, and the Lepidotus, Latus, Alabes, Coracinus, Choerus and Phagrorius, also called Phagrus, and besides, the Silurus, Citharus, Thrissa, Cestreus, Lychnus, Physa and Bos . . ."

Athenaeus (7, 312, A–B), on the authority of the Athenian comic poet, Archippus, likewise listed the common fish of the Nile

". . . the fishes of the Nile, if I can still recall them after many years absence from the country are: Narke, Choerus, Simos, Phagrus, Oxyrhynchus, Allabes,[6] Silurus, Synodontis, Eleotris, Enchelis, Thrissa, Abramis, Tephle, Lepidotus, Physa, Cestreus. But there are many others besides . . ."

May one tacitly assume that such lists define species taken for food? Or should we require contextual gastronomic evidence, as is provided, for example, by Athenaeus (7, 311, F–7, 312, A) in his description of a Nile fish famous for its flavour, and known by several names

". . . the Nile also produces many kinds of fish, all of them very good, especially the Crow-fish . . ."

and

". . . the river Crow-fish from the Nile, which some call crescent but which among the Alexandrians is known by the specific name of half-salt is rather fatty, quite well-flavoured, meaty, filling, easily digested and assimilated, and in every way superior to the mullet . . ." (3, 121, B–C)

He further discusses the Crow-fish, that he also calls "Coracinus," and describes its colour, method of preparation, and medicinal properties

". . . [it] is the special product of the Nile. The black is inferior to the white, the boiled to the baked. For the latter is good both for stomach and bowels . . ." (8,356, A).

So renowned was this fish that Martial of Bilbilis immortalized it in an epigram

". . . you of all fish are scrambled for, Coracinus, in the markets of Nile; to Alexandria's gourmets no fish has renown surpassing yours . . ." (13, 85)

Where such comments appear, there is no question about consumption.

The flavour of some Egyptian freshwater fish was, however, disagreeable to foreign palates, if we believe Athenaeus

". . . it appears that no one, sir, has mentioned in this list [of desirable edible fish] the Mendesian fish[7] of you Alexandrians; fish which even a mad dog would not taste . . ." (3, 118, F)

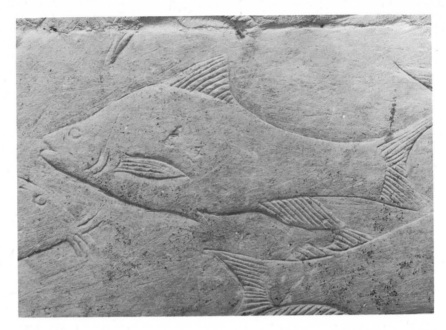

Fig. 7.20. Representative Nile fish. *Barbus bynni.* Tomb of Mereruka at Saqqara; Old Kingdom, sixth dynasty, reign of King Teti, *c.* 2390 B.C. Photographed 1969.

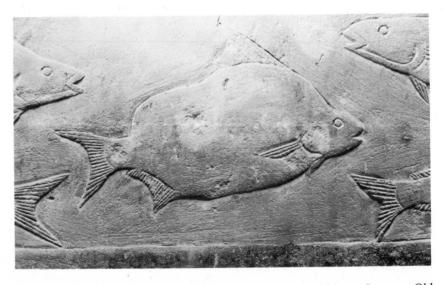

Fig. 7.21. Representative Nile fish. *Citharinus citharus.* Tomb of Idut at Saqqara; Old Kingdom, fifth dynasty, reign of King Unas, *c.* 2423 B.C. Photographed 1969.

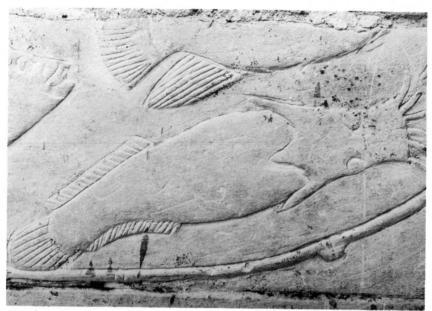

Fig. 7.22. Representative Nile fish. *Clarias anguillaris.* Tomb of Mereruka at Saqqara; Old Kingdom, sixth dynasty, reign of King Teti, *c.* 2390 B.C. photographed 1969.

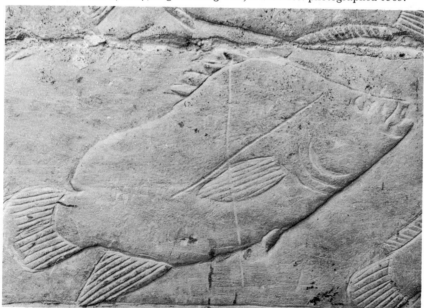

Fig. 7.23. Representative Nile fish. *Lates niloticus.* Tomb of Mereruka at Saqqara; Old Kingdom, sixth dynasty, reign of King Teti, *c.* 2390 B.C. Photographed 1969.

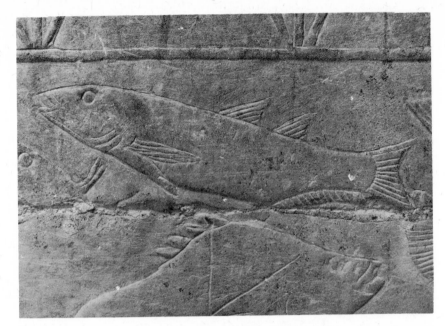

Fig. 7.24. Representative Nile fish *Mugil cephalus*. Tomb of Mereruka at Saqqara; Old Kingdom, sixth dynasty, reign of King Teti, *c.* 2390 B.C. Photographed 1969.

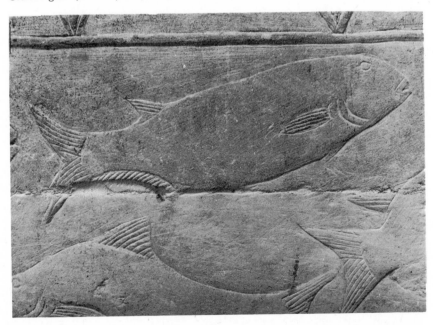

Fig. 7.25. Representative Nile fish. *Petrocephalus bane.* Tomb of Mereruka at Saqqara; Old Kingdom, sixth dynasty, reign of King Teti, *c.* 2390 B.C. Photographed 1969.

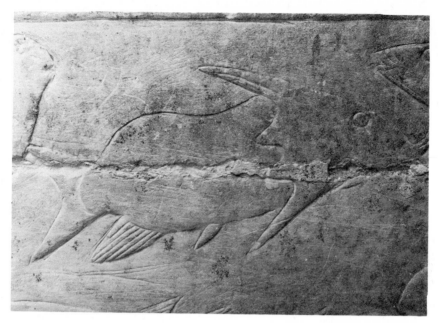

Fig. 7.26. Representative Nile fish. *Synodontis schall.* Tomb of Mereruka at Saqqara; Old Kingdom, sixth dynasty, reign of King Teti, *c.* 2390 B.C. Photographed 1969.

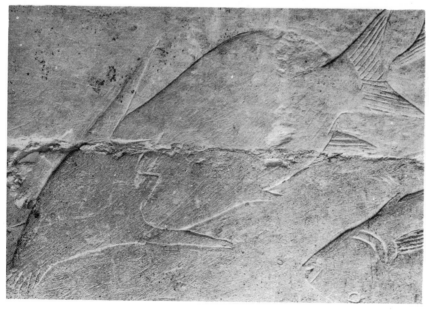

Fig. 7.27. Representative Nile fish. *Synodontis schall*; inverted position. Tomb of Mereruka at Saqqara; Old Kingdom, sixth dynasty, reign of King Teti, *c.* 2390 B.C. Photographed 1969.

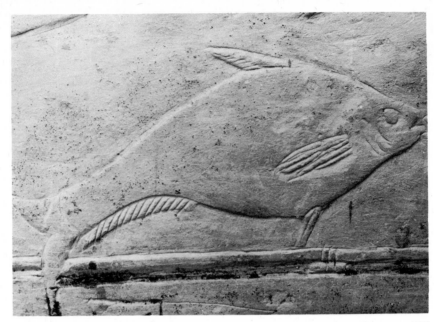

Fig. 7.28. Representative Nile fish. *Schilbe mystus.* Tomb of Mereruka at Saqqara; Old Kingdom, sixth dynasty, reign of King Teti, *c.* 2390 B.C. Photographed 1969.

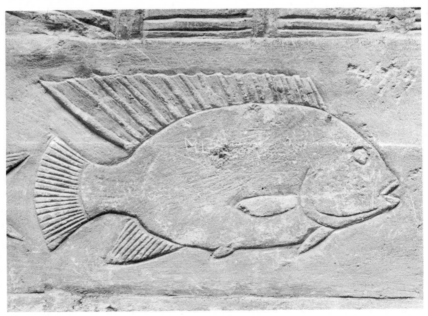

Fig. 7.29. Representative Nile fish. *Tilapia nilotica.* Tomb of Idut at Saqqara; Old Kingdom, fifth dynasty, reign of King Unas, *c.* 2423 B.C. Photographed 1969.

Preparation and Preservation of Fish

Tomb art from all Dynastic Periods documents the preparation of fish and its preservation. Once caught, fish were hauled aboard, and vicious ones clubbed (Fig. 7.30). Further preparation was sometimes carried out on the boat (Fig. 7.31); but, more commonly, this was accomplished on shore (Fig. 7.32). In some scenes fish is seen being broiled, held on a long stick passed through its mouth and tail, while a cook fans the fire with a fan. Nearby, other cooks make round fish balls of chopped or shredded fish, like the cakes reportedly made by the Ichthyophagi (Bates, 1917, p. 265).

The majority of fish, however, probably were salted, pickled or sun-dried to preserve for later use. Baskets of fish are commonly shown being carried, presumably to preparation or salting areas.[8] The New Kingdom reliefs of Tell el Amarna illustrate the storage of fish thus prepared (Fig. 7.33). It is not evident whether large species or specimens were salted, but that they were considered desirable is indicated by numerous representations of "trophy-size" catches (Figs 7.34, 7.35, 7.36).

The slabbing and drying of fish, and its subsequent hanging on the rigging of large fishing boats (Fig. 7.3) is also often depicted in extremely fine detail, even down to the vertebral column and rib arrangement. Confirmation of the illustrated procedure of slabbing of fish exists in the discovery of a preserved fillet of salted fish at Deir el Medina and dated to the Ramessid Period (Fig. 7.37).

This information is complemented by Greek and Roman descriptions. Herodotus cites a group of Egyptians who lived entirely on fish

". . . [the fish] are gutted as soon as caught, and then hung up in the sun; when dry, they are used as food . . ." (II, 92)

The salting areas are also described by several ancient authors

". . . there are twenty-two different kinds of fish in the lake [Lake Moeris], they say, and they are caught in such abundance that the people engaged in salting them, though exceedingly many, can scarcely keep up with their task . . ." (Diodorus, 1, 52, 5–6)

Fish was pickled for both domestic consumption and export. A document dated to the late twentieth dynasty, entitled *The Tale of Wenamon*, tells of the commercial adventures of Wenamon, sent by King Rameses

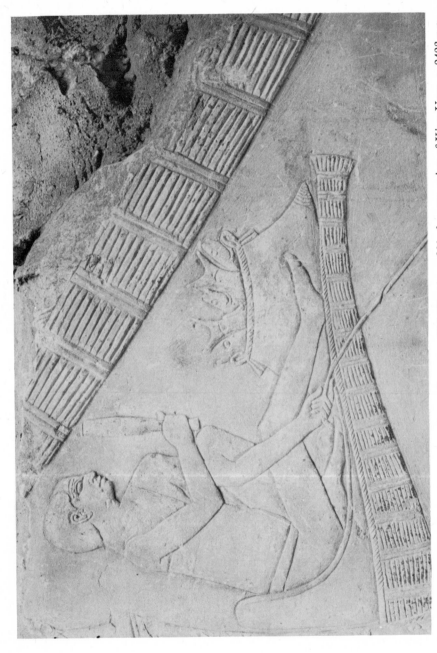

Fig. 7.30. Clubbing the catch. Tomb of Idut at Saqqara; Old Kingdom, fifth dynasty, reign of King Unas, *c.* 2423 B.C. Photographed 1969.

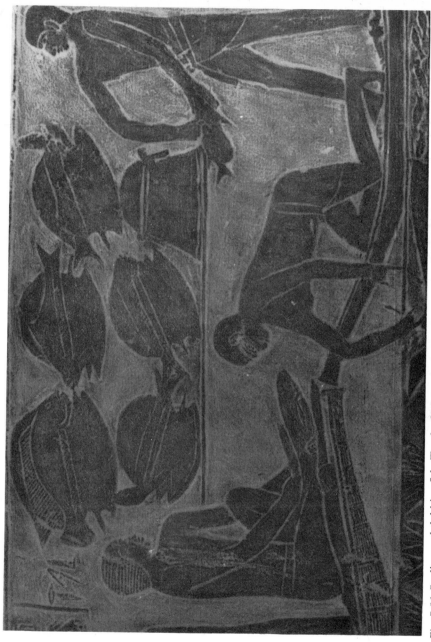

Fig. 7.31. Scaling and slabbing fish. Tomb of Mereruka at Saqqara; Old Kingdom, sixth dynasty, reign of King Teti, *c.* 2390 B.C. Rubbing by Ward Patterson; used with permission (1969).

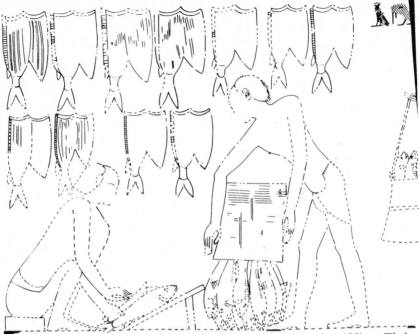

Fig. 7.32. Scaling and slabbing fish. Tomb of Rekhmire (number 100) at Thebes (Upper Enclosure); New Kingdom, eighteenth dynasty, reign of King Thutmose III, *c.* 1475 B.C. Davies (1943), Vol. 2, plate 46. Drawing used with permission of the Metropolitan Museum of Art, New York.

XII as emissary to the Prince of Byblos. Thirty baskets of salted Egyptian fish were to serve as partial payment for cedar wood needed by the Egyptians for ship construction (*A.R.*, IV, 582).

The great demand for salted fish most probably was unchanged in Egypt during the Post-Dynastic Period. The delight with which salted fish was eaten is recorded by several authors, like Lucian of Samosata

". . . in the name if Isis, remember to bring us those delicate pickled fish from Egypt . . ."[9] (*The Ship or the Wishes*, 15)

In modern Egypt the most appreciated salted fish is prepared from mullet (*Mugil* spp.), and called *fassikh* or, in Upper Egypt, *melouha*. Different kinds are produced in several centres, but the best come from Damietta and Nabaro. It is a traditional item on all tables at the Spring festival of Sham en-Nessim.

One particular delicacy relished today both in Egypt and throughout the Near East is the ovary of fish, usually mullet. This may be eaten fresh

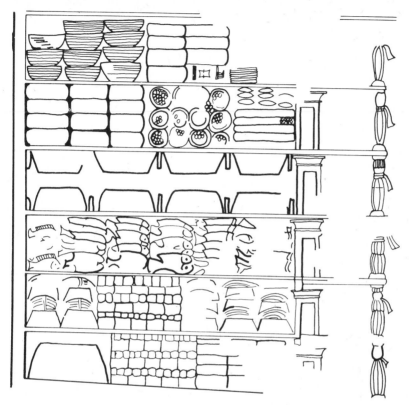

Fig. 7.33. Fish as desired food. Provisions at a royal storehouse. Tomb of Mery-Ra at Tell el Amarna; New Kingdom, eighteenth dynasty, reign of King Amenhotep IV (Akhenaten), *c.* 1360 B.C. Redrawn from Davies (1903), plate 31.

but, more commonly, it is washed, salted, pressed in layers between wooden boards, and dried. The dried fish roe, locally called *batarekh* (from Coptic *pi-tarikh*?), was mentioned by early travellers in Egypt from the sixteenth century. It was prepared then, as it is today, mainly in Lake Manzaleh. It is exported thence to all parts of Egypt, to Turkey, and elsewhere, where it fetches fairly high prices.

Keimer (1938–1939), commenting on the frequency of illustrations of mullet (mugil) in Egyptian tombs, pointed to some scenes that clearly show the extraction of roe from these fish, and he gave several examples of these from the tombs of Ptahhetep and others in Saqqarah and Giza (Fig. 7.38). In these scenes, a seated fisherman opens up with a knife a mullet placed on a low sloping block; near the fish and often all over the

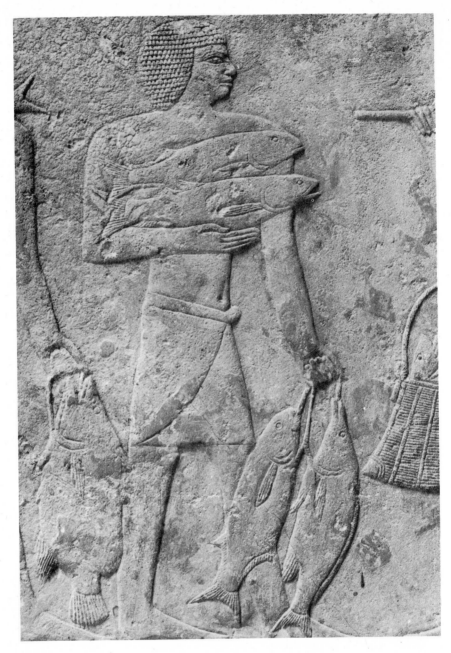

Fig. 7.34. Fish as desired food. Tomb of Ka-Gem-Ni at Saqqara; Old Kingdom, sixth dynasty, reign of King Teti, *c.* 2390 B.C. Photographed 1969.

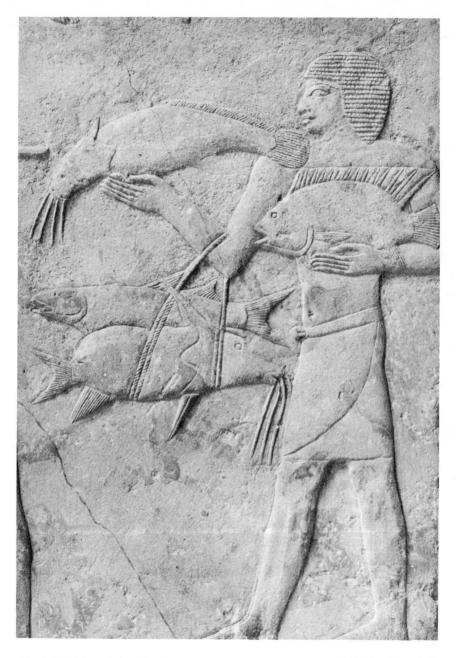

Fig. 7.35. Fish as desired food. Tomb of Ka-Gem-Ni at Saqqara; Old Kingdom, sixth dynasty, reign of King Teti, *c.* 2390 B.C. Photographed 1969.

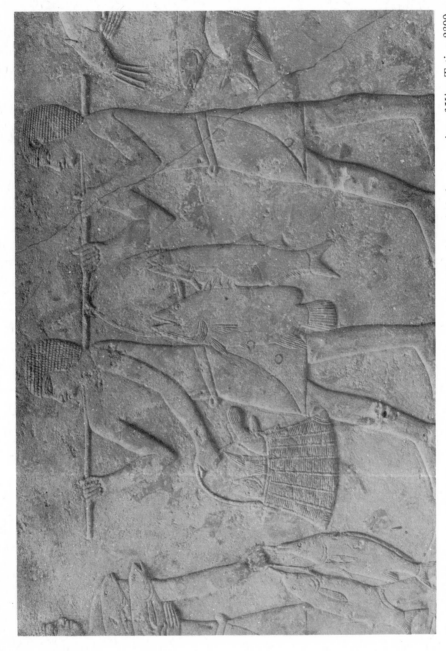

Fig. 7.36. Fish as desired food. Tomb of Ka-Gem-Ni at Saqqara; Old Kingdom, sixth dynasty, reign of King Teti, *c.* 2390 B.C. Photographed 1969.

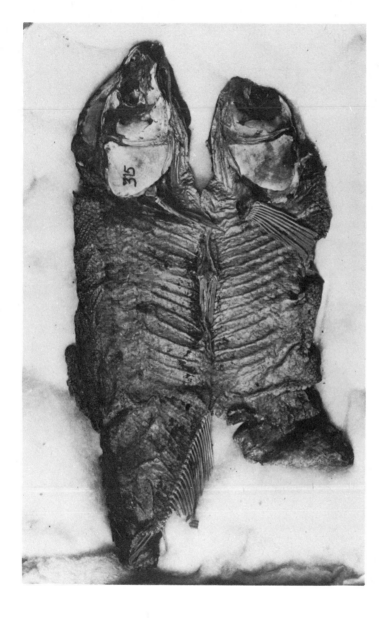

Fig. 7.37 Fish as desired food. A preserved slabbed fish. Thebes (Deir El Medina); New Kingdom, Ramessid Period, date uncertain. Photographed with permission of the Ministry of Agriculture and the officials of the Agricultural Museum, Dokki, ARE (1969).

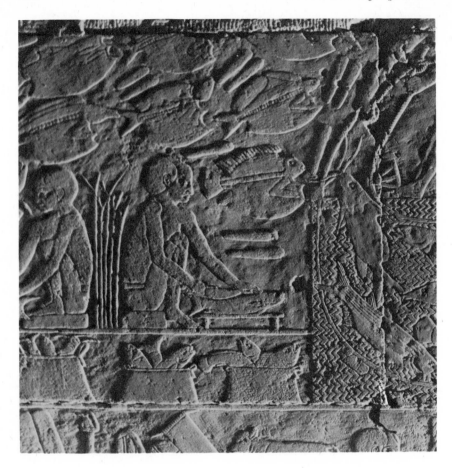

Fig. 7.38. Fishermen slitting fish open. Long ovoid bodies between the slit fish probably represent roe. Ti's tomb. Saqqara. Ancient Kingdom. Courtesy of Centre of Documentation, Cairo.

scene, long ovoid bodies represent the extracted roe, which is sometimes depicted placed in a vessel or hanging on a rope tied to a horizontal pole.

Although actual salting and pressing are not illustrated, the regular oblong shape of the roe, as drawn in these pictures, provides evidence, according to this author, that they were so treated. The same interpretation was given by Bates (1917, p. 265). The actual name of fish roe is, however, uncertain. The Berlin Wörterbuch tentatively suggests ᶜmm, a word that Faulkner (1962, p. 43) translated "brain", and Dawson rendered by fish otolith or insect larvae in the skin (*Wb. Dr.*, 95, 96). On the other hand, Ebbell translated *iꜣrt*, sperm of a synodontis fish (*Eb.*, CV, 861), without this interpretation being attested elsewhere. The only relevant find is one of very young fry seemingly just hatched from roe, that was interred, wrapped in linen, in special burials (Lortet and Hugounenq, 1902, p. 16).

Fish and Medicine in Ancient Egypt

Prescriptions in the Ebers Medical Papyrus include nine varieties of fish in preparations for external application. One recommends the application of fish (ꜣ *bdw*) gall in a compound for an ophthalmologic disorder

". . . To expel white spots that have arisen in the Eye: gall of *bdw* fish, stibium,[10] water, are ground fine and put into the eyes . . ." (*Eb.*, LXII, 405)

This use of the fish, ꜣ *bdw*, was probably an instance of religious association: this fish reputedly guided the boat of the sun god "Ra" on its journey through the underworld; hence it could relieve blindness. It is curious to find a parallel to the use of the ꜣ *bdw*-fish to relieve "white spots" in the story of Tobit[11] who captured a giant fish from the Tigris River and took from it the gall, heart, and liver as directed by the Angel Raphael

". . . as for the gall, anoint with it a man who has white film in his eyes, and he will be cured . . ." (Tobit, 6, 8)

Upon the recommendation of the angel, Tobit applied this substance to the blind eyes of his father

". . . and when his eyes began to smart he rubbed them and the white films scaled off from the corners of his eyes. Then he saw . . ." (Tobit, 11, 12–14)

Even if Tobit's story be apocryphal, it dates at least to the third or fourth centuries B.C., a period when Ancient Egyptian traditions were still alive (Davies, 1965, p. 44)

Another prescription of the Ebers papyrus (*Eb.*, LVIII, 360) prescribes gall of tortoise to expel white spots in the eyes; and it is, likewise, curious to find Arab physicians like Ibn el Baitar (quoted by Loret 1892a), and Avicenna (*The Canon*, lib. V, 2, 2) ,recommending the same medication.

Other prescriptions of, which some are listed below, illustrate the use of fish for external application

"To remove a thorn: burnt skull of a Silurus-fish with oil is applied to its opening until it comes out . . ." (*Eb.*, LXXXVIII, 730)

"To Expel Affliction in the Head: the interior of $\underline{d}$*ꜣ rt*,[12] *ḥ*s of tamarix, natron, *sfꜣft*,[13] burnt bone of the Lates-fish, burnt bone of the Synodontis-fish, honey, ladanum, the head is anointed therewith for four days . . ." (*Eb.*, XLVII, 248)

"To relieve Effluency: *int*[14] -fish, *tmt*[15] -fish, *ḏꜣrt*, wax, dung of a crocodile, honey, are ground fine, mixed together, and is bandaged therewith . . ." (*Eb.*, LXXI, 542)

Acceptance and Avoidance of Fish in the Diet

Like fish, naked and vain
(popular saying)

The study of the intricate problem of acceptance *vs* avoidance consists in sorting out contradictory statements and evidence, in clarifying ambivalent attitudes and trying to fit them into a valid framework.

Bates (1917, p. 268), underlining the contrast between the absence in the Old Kingdom of fish in offering lists of the viands provided for the deceased, and the profuseness of fishing scenes and of excavated fishing tackle and fish remains, observed that the Egyptian monuments distinguish clearly between the facial types of the peasantry and the nobility, that the Delta must have been the main centre of fishing as an industry, and that the fishermen in that region perpetuated one of the oldest anthropological types in the country. The absence of fish in offering lists indicated that the upper classes in that period entertained a prejudice against that food, possibly because they represented a small but dominant class of cattle owners averse to the idea of a fish diet.

From a study of the relative chronology of fishing implements, he further concluded that the consumption of fish among the peasantry was unbroken from the earliest period; that the beginning of the Middle Kingdom was marked by a decline of that aversion to fish displayed by the Old Kingdom nobility. This was accompanied by a return of fish-shaped vases, and by the invention of new kinds of fishing implements. What took place, he thinks, was a partial recrudescence of elements in the population which, from the beginning of the Dynastic Period to the economic breakdown of the Old Kingdom, had been in a state of subjection and repression.

The dual regard to fish is best illustrated by the finding, side by side, of prehistoric culinary remains of a fish, and of a fish cemetery, probably of Pharaonic, i.e. later times, where each fish was carefully interred in a small individual grave, the whole resembling the emblem of the local nome (Debono, 1948; Drioton, 1952).

An example of self-contradiction occurs in Nu's papyrus where the deceased had to pronounce the following uttering

". . . I am the great and mighty Fish which is in the city of Qem-ur, I am the lord to whom bowing and prostrations are made in the city of Sekhem . . ." (Budge, 1949, p. 279)

although, later, it prescribed a rite to be performed by

". . . a man who is clean and ceremonially pure, one who hath eaten neither meat nor fish and who hath not recently had intercourse with women"

a prescription that, incidentally, indicates that, in that particular instance, meat was as defiling as fish (Budge, 1949, p. 420). The following examples illustrate acceptance

". . . his Majesty increased that which was furnished to the army in ointments, ox-flesh, fish, and plentiful vegetables without limit . . ." (*A.R.*, III, 207)

". . . when a child is born first they let him suck his mother's milk a while; but after they feed him with fishes taken in the lake and roasted in the hot sun . . ." (Heliodorus of Emesa, 1587, p. 4.)

". . . He [god] made for them [mankind] plants and cattle, fowls and fishes, in order to nourish them . . ." (*The Ancient Egyptians. Instruction of Merikere*, Erman, 1966, p. 83)

One version of *The Hymn to Amon*, dated to the reign of King Amenhotep II (*c.* 1450 B.C.) contains a passage which likewise indicates religious appreciation of fish

". . . He who made that whereupon live the fish in the river . . ." (Erman, 1966, p. 286).

A second religious text, *The Hymn to Aton*, dating to the reign of King Amenhotep IV (Akhenaten) (*c.* 1370 B.C.) which represents a philosophy opposed to Amon worship, also illustrates high regard for fish

". . . the fishes in the river leap up before thy face [the god Aton]. Thy rays are in the sea . . ."[17] (Erman, 1966, p. 298)

Egyptian deities other than Amon and Aton were honoured with offerings of fish during both the Middle Kingdom (Fig. 7.39) and the early dynasties of the New Kingdom. Amenhotep III had carved upon his funerary temple at Thebes[18]

". . . Lord of fish and fowl . . ." (*A.R.*, II, 833)

—a certain implication that fish were not detested during his reign. Furthermore, on the basis of eighteenth dynasty paintings at Thebes, one may conclude that no religious stigma against fish existed (Fig. 7.40).

During the nineteenth and twentieth dynasties, which witnessed a partial return to Seth worship under Seti I and the succeeding Ramesids, texts continued to indicate tolerance to fish and even the existence of an official cadre of fishing officials.

One of the first citations that directly state that fish was eaten is an inscription at Gebel Silsileh, attributed to Seti I, that we partly quoted on p. 381. This inscription lists the rations distributed to the king's messengers and standard bearers sent to transport a religious monument

". . . good bread, ox flesh, wine, sweet oil, olive (?) oil, fat (?), honey, figs, fish, and vegetables every day." (*A.R.*, III, 208)

Seti's son, Rameses II, had inscribed oh his father's temple at Abydos a text in his honour

(a)

wḥ ʿw

". . . I put fishermen [(a)] . . . on the waters, on every pool, in order to furnish for thee taxes by the shipload . . ."[19] (*A.R.*, III, 276)

The same Rameses II included fish in his offerings to Ptah in Memphis

". . . there is joy and laudation at seeing thee for plenty of fish and fowl are under thy feet . . ." (*A.R.*, III, 404)

Rameses III waived tax payments by fishermen in the service of the Theban god Khnum (*A.R.*, IV, 148), and the king, himself, offered numbers of fish to Amon-Ra

". . . 400 jars [of the canal] filled with fish, 2,200 white-fish, 15,500 *sn*-fish, 15,500 fish cut up, 441,000 fish whole . . ." (*A.R.*, IV, 243)

We next find King Rameses IV (*c*. 1166 B.C.) sending 200 officers in the "division of the court fishermen" to Wadi Hammamat in order to quarry building stone and to obtain blocks for statuary (*A.R.*, IV, 466).

Finally, in a love poem of the New Kingdom, a maiden tells her beloved

". . . My brother, it is pleasant to go to the [pond] to bathe me in thy presence, that I may let thee see my beauty in my tunic of finest royal linen, when it is wet . . . I go down with thee into the water, and come forth again to thee with a red fish, which lieth(?) beautiful on my fingers . . . Come and look at me . . ." (Erman, 1927, p. 243)

How could a taboo strike such a fish! These texts are in support of the previously collated evidence from finds of prepared fish (Fig. 7.37), and from the inclusion of fish in offerings (Figs 7.39, 7.40).

Other texts, however, express an avoidance or distate of fish, such as the statement of Porphyry

". . . they [the priests] abstained from all fish that was caught in Egypt . . ." (Porphyry 4, 7)

or the desperate cry of the "One who was tired of life"

". . . Lo! my name is abhorred, Lo! more than the odour of fishermen, more than the shores of the swamps, when they have fished . . ." (Erman, 1966, p. 86)

which recalls a local saying

"Like a fessikh [salted fish] pond, plenty and squalor."

Interpretation of these contradictions may be attempted within one or more frameworks: the Osiris-Seth conflict; the deification of fish not associated with the Osirian epic; class differences; and imposition of dietary restrictions by foreign conquerors.

Sacred Fish Associated with the Osiris Myth

The Osiris myth (Chapter 1, pp. 14–20) illustrates the reason for the exclusion of fish from the diet of the priests who served Osiris and the

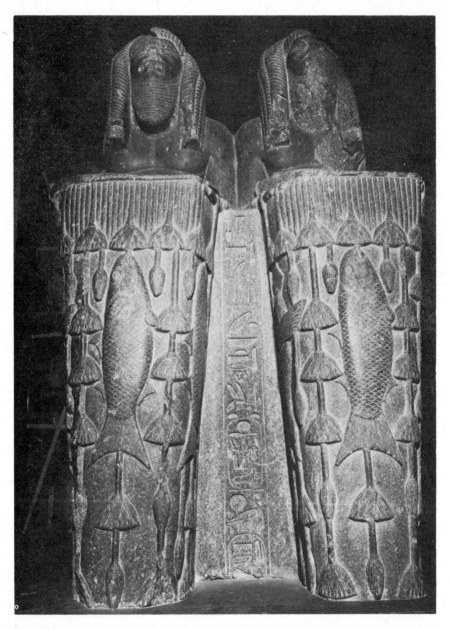

Fig. 7.39. Presentation of fish and other Nile products to the gods. Tanis. Middle-Kingdom, date uncertain (the name of King Psusennes of the New Kingdom appears on the statue). Photographed with permission of the Ministry of Culture and the officials of the Egyptian Museum, Cairo, ARE (1969).

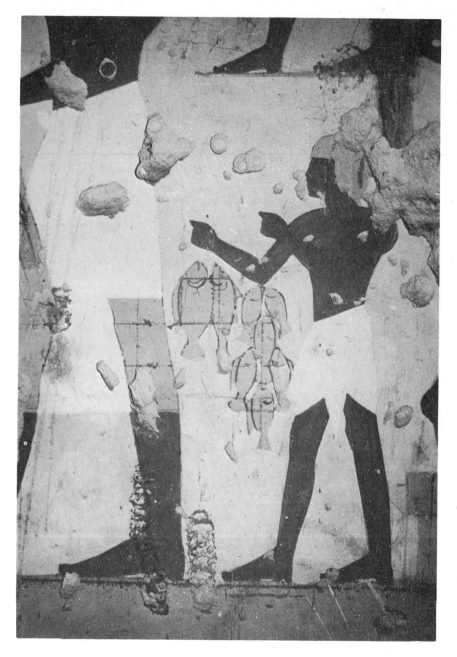

Fig. 7.40. Tomb of Suemnut (number 92) at Thebes (Upper Enclosure); New Kingdom
eighteenth dynasty, reign of King Amenhotep II, *c.* 1440 B.C. Photographed 1969.

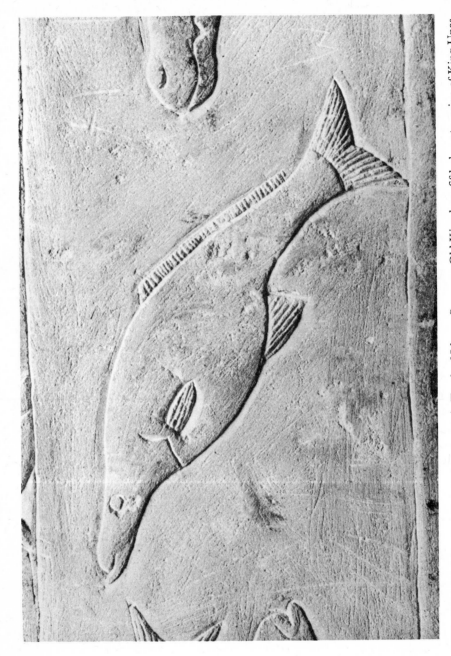

Fig. 7.41. The Oxyrhynchus (*Mormyrus* spp.). Tomb of Idut at Saqqara; Old Kingdom, fifth dynasty; reign of King Unas, *c.* 2423 B.C. Photographed 1969.

related gods, since it told that the Oxyrhynchus, Lepidotus and Phagrus had fed upon the phallus of Osiris and

". . . it was from these very fishes that the Egyptians were most scrupulous in abstaining . . ." (Plutarch, *I. and O.*, 358, 18, B)

Conversely, worship of these fishes by the followers of Seth is also explained; and likewise, the extension by a contagious process, of abstinence to all varieties of fish on the part of the clergy.

The intensity of feelings aroused by the Osiris-Horus conflict may be judged from the behaviour of worshippers at a ceremony annually performed at Edfu, the site of the decisive victory of Horus over Seth, to commemorate the ending of Isis's widowhood. There, carrying symbols of the three fishes, they threw fish on the ground and hacked and hewed them with knives saying

". . . Cut ye wounds on your bodies, kill ye one another; Ra triumphs over his enemies; Horus of Edfu triumphs over all evil ones." (see Kees, 1961, p. 92)

Of the three offending fish, only the Oxyrhynchus can be identified with certainty. Several authors have proposed identifications of the Lepidotus and Phagrus, but these remain questionable.

The Oxyrhynchus

Gaillard (1923, pp. 24–30) equated the oxyrhynchus with any species of the genus *Mormyrus*, and with the Ancient Egyptian hieroglyph (b). This identification is easy since the ancient texts clearly describe the downward-curved beak of this fish (Fig. 7.41), and the Egyptian Arabic name for the *Mormyrus* (*abu bowez*), means "the beaked."

(b)

ḫꜣt

Despite the fact that it is one of the most commonly depicted fish in Old Kingdom tombs, there is little specific information on the Oxyrhynchus prior to the later dynasties and most of our knowledge is gained from Greek and Roman sources.

The Oxyrhynchus was worshipped at the Egyptian village of Bahnasa, known during the Post-Dynastic Period as the hieroglyph (c) (Oxyrhynchus). It was adored by the followers of Seth, and numerous bronze statuettes of the fish, dated to the Late Dynastic and following Ptolemaic and Roman Periods were found throughout Egypt (Fig. 7.42).

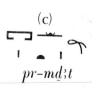

(c)

pr-mdꜣt

One might imagine that it was avoided by followers of both Horus and Seth; the former because of abhorrence; the latter, reverence.

Avoidance of the Oxyrhynchus because of reverence for this fish was noted by other Greek and Roman writers. Aelian (10, 46) recorded a custom attributed to fishermen in the vicinity of Oxyrhynchus/Cynopolis

". . . and whenever fish are netted, they search the nets in case this famous fish has fallen in without their noticing it. And they would rather catch nothing at all than have the largest catch which included this fish . . ."

Aelian would also have us believe that the regional fishermen avoided fishing by hook and used only nets

". . . should the inhabitants catch a fish on a hook, they will never eat it for fear that the aforesaid fish [Oxyrhynchus] may have chance to impale itself on the hook . . ." (10, 46)

This report might be treated as an imaginative literary excursion were it not for corroborative evidence from Egyptian sources dated to the first century A.D. Fishermen living near Oxyrhynchus were required to sign a religious pledge

". . . we swear that we never have been or will be privy to fishing or dragging a net or casting a net to catch the images of the divine *Oxyrhynchi* and *Lepidoti* . . ." (S.P., 1934, 329)

Although fishermen at Fayoum and Oxyrhynchus so obliged, this might well have been a mere formality, disregarded when the first large haul was pulled, unobserved, aboard.

Plutarch (*I. and O.*, 380, 72, B–C) told an entertaining and revealing tale of the religious feelings that could be aroused . . .

"in my day the people of Oxyrhynchus caught a dog and sacrificed it and ate it up as if it had been sacrificial meat, because the people of Cynopolis [Greek for 'dog's city'] were eating the fish known as the Oxyrhynchus. As a result of this they became involved in a war and inflicted much harm upon each other . . ."

Such retaliation by the citizens of Oxyrhynchus, of course, does not suggest that they habitually ate dogs, jackals or wolves; it was merely a religious ripost.

Despite these literary reports, Egyptian tombs of all periods frequently portray the Oxyrhynchus among fish being netted for food (Fig. 7.3) interpretable as indicating that the tomb owner did not consider the fish as either abominable or sacred. The speculation that the Egyptian tombs which portrayed the Oxyrhynchus belonged to followers of Seth, or that they were only of local significance, may be discarded purely on the basis of the widespread geographic and chronologic depiction of the Oxyrhynchus. All of these tombs could not belong to worshippers of Seth. Furthermore, if one uses the criteria set in Table 2, Chapter 1, to indicate with any probability which varieties of foods were favoured, the reliefs in these tombs strongly indicate that the Oxyrhynchus was an accepted food.

Might, therefore, the placement of the Oxyrhynchus in direct opposition to Osiris be a relatively late innovation? Or are we to believe that oxyrhynchus was widely consumed throughout much of Egypt despite basic religious attitudes? Or, since representation in tombs does not by itself absolutely imply consumption, could this inconsistency be a mere construction in the minds of modern researchers?

The Lepidotus

The name of this fish, "scale fish," suggests as its distinguishing characteristic the possession of large and unusually distinctive scales, a qualification found best, among Nile fishes, in *Barbus bynni* (Gaillard, 1923, p. 47). This fish was found among the mummies brought from Thebes by Passalacqua, enveloped in wrappings and placed in boxes made in its shape (Geoffroy St Hilaire, 1829, Vol. 24, p. 288). Boulenger (1907) reproduced two statuettes of this fish. The interior of a wooden one, described by Lortet and Gaillard (1909, p. 305, Fig. 219) contained scales of the fish enwrapped in cloth stained by resinous natron. A statue of Lepidotus is also on exhibit at the Dokki Museum (Fig. 7.43). Its name, as well as the discovery of mummified specimens and its scales, support the identification of it with the sacred Lepidotus, already suggested by Sonnini (1799) and Geoffroy St. Hilaire.

Judging from the shape of the fish used as determinative for the fish called *bwt*, this may have been the Ancient Egyptian name of *B. bynni*; but the same determinative was used also for other species, like the *Schilbe* (Montet, 1913, Figs 5 and 6).

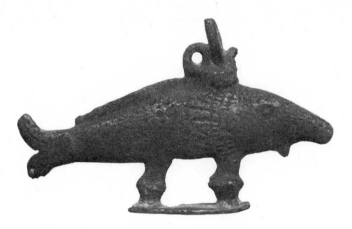

Fig. 7.42. Bronze statuette of Oxyrhynchus (*Mormyrus* spp.). Provenance unknown; Late Period *c.* 700 B.C. Photographed with permission of the Ministry of Agriculture and the officials of the Agricultural Museum, Dokki, ARE (1969).

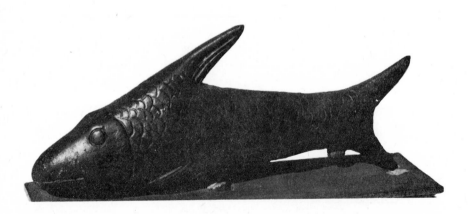

Fig. 7.43. Lepidotus (?) (*cf. Barbus Bynni*). Provenance unknown; Graeco-Roman Period, date uncertain. Photographed with permission of the Ministry of Agriculture and the officials of the Agricultural Museum, Dokki, ARE (1969).

The Phagrus

Identification of the phagrus remains, likewise, uncertain. Strabo (17, 1, 40) cites an unidentified city and nome of Phagrioropolis, mentioned by earlier authors, that he situated near the Bitter Lakes. The tale relative to the ibis (see p. 323) hinted to Rawlinson (1885, Vol. II, p. 104, n. 8) that it might have been an eel, but this view is now abandoned. Deiber (1904) identified Phagrus with a fish he calls *annu* but that should probably read *int*, now tentatively regarded as *Tilapia* (see later). Geoffroy St Hilaire, arguing from its name phagrus, "the voracious," and from two characteristics mentioned by Clement of Alexandria, its remarkable voracity, and its heralding of the flood (which is the reason why the Syenites did not eat it) identified it with the long-teethed *raschal* (*Hydrocyon forskalii*). The latter has gained from its predatory habits the colloquial name "kalb el-bahr," Nile dog, and like the Phagrus, it appears with the first wave of the flood. Gaillard, however, could not recognize *Hydrocyon* among the species illustrated in the tombs he examined, and suggested that it was a late-comer in Egypt; but Keimer (1948), who agreed to the identification, described what seems to be a unique illustration of this fish.

Greek and Roman texts imply a dual attitude towards Phagrus. Whereas it was said by Aelian (10, 19) to be revered because it signalled the flood, Plutarch (*I. and O.*, 358, 18, B) wrote that it was detested because it had fed upon the phallus of Osiris. This again illustrates that attitudes towards a foodstuff are not simple and reducible to single generalization.

The Maeotes

Another species of fish, the *Maeotes*, was worshipped near Syene (Aswan) where the Phagrus was venerated

> ". . . the people of Syene worship the Phagrus; the inhabitants of Elephantine, another fish, the Maeotes . . ." (Clement of Alexandria, *Exhortations* 2, 34)

Deiber (1904) identified it with the *nar* (a siluride) that swallowed the phallus of Bitiou in the "Tale of the Two Brothers" of the Orbiney papyrus (Lefebvre, 1949) and Wilkinson (1878, Vol. III, Ch. XIV) places it in the same species. But Aelian (10, 19) stated that the phagrus worshipped at Syene was the same fish that was called *Maeotes* by the people of Elephantine. Bates (1917) contended that, as Syene and Elephantine are within gunshot of each other, and that Plutarch (*I. and O.*, 353, 7) says of the phagrus what Aelian relates of the *Maeotes*, namely, that it was held sacred because its appearance indicated the impending rise of the Nile, there is little question that the two names were applied to one fish. Logic favours these arguments.

Sacred Fish not Associated with the Osiris Myth

In addition to the above varieties of fish several others were venerated elsewhere, like the much discussed fishes of Mendes, and possibly the Latus, the *ꜣ bdw*[20] and the *int*.[21]

The Latus

The Latus (*ꜥha*) (Engelbach, 1924), schilbe or Nile perch, said by the Greeks and Romans to be a fish of good quality (Strabo 17, 2, 4), has been identified by Gaillard (1923, pp. 81–84) with *Lates niloticus* (Fig. 7.23). This fish was worshipped principally at Esna in Upper Egypt; indeed, the Greek name for this site was Latopolis or "City of the Latus." Thousands of mummified Latus have been found there, and so revered was the fish that even its roe was wrapped in linen and interred in special burials (Lortet and Hugounenq, 1902, p. 16). Other examples of mummified Latus have been found in Lower Egypt as, for example, at the site of Abu Gourob (Loat, 1904, pp. 4–6). The primary focus of its worship and adoration, however, was certainly Esna. But reverence at one place did not exclude consumption at another.

The *ꜣ bdw* and int Fishes

The *ꜣ bdw* was so revered, that Anubis, the god of embalming, was occasionally depicted preparing its body. The large size of the picture of a fish called *abet* in a Theban tomb, led Foucart (1917) to identify it with either *Lates niloticus* or *Tilapia nilotica*, although its forked tail was different from these fishes' tails (Gaillard, 1923, p. 88). On the other hand, both Gaillard, and Faulkner (1962, p. 23), believe that *Tilapia nilotica* was the *int* fish. Whatever the identity of these two fish, their consumption was limited by religious considerations.

Avoidance Imposed by Foreign Domination

During the First Intermediate Period, a time of general anarchy, Libyan tribesmen harassed the northern Delta settlements and occupied limited portions of the land. An Egyptian document dated to this era, or to the early years of the Middle Kingdom, describes the general despair in Egypt resulting from these attacks

> ". . . moreover, those good things are ruined, the fishponds, where were the slittings, which shone with fish and wild fowl. All good things are passed away, the land is laid low through misery, by reason of yon food of the bedouins who traverse the land . . ." (*Prophecy of Neferrohu*, Erman, 1966, p. 113)

Other literature from this period of anarchy, however, indicates that Egyptian fishermen were regarded as lowly and inferior

> ". . . it goeth more ill with him than any other calling . . ." (*Instruction of Duaf*, Erman, 1966, p. 70)

Also from this period is the *Dispute of a Man With His Soul*, a text that deprecated fish and fishermen in a poetic manner. This document further related that human corpses were sometimes thrown into the Nile where they were fed upon by fish

> ". . . the flood hath taken its end [of them] and likewise the head of the sun, and the fish of the river-bank, hold converse with them . . ." (Erman, 1966, pp. 88–89)

This text offers striking parallels with the Nubian "grandfather legend" discussed later.

Nearly 1500 years after these Libyan incursions, the Ethiopians, led by Pi-'Ankhi, invaded Egypt. The culture and background of these southerners is not well known, but contemporary documents reveal that they considered the consumption of fish abominable

". . . these kings and princes of the Northland [Egyptians] who came to behold the beauty of his majesty [Pi-ʿAnkhi], their legs were as legs of women. They entered not into the King's house because they were unclean[22] and eaters of fish; which is an abomination for the palace. Lo, King Numlot, he entered into the King's house because he was pure and he ate not fish . . ." (*A.R.*, IV, 882)

Approximately 300 years after Pi-ʿAnkhi conquered the "abominable fish-eaters", Herodotus visited Egypt. He was among the first Greek visitors to report an ingrained fish-avoidance among the Egyptian priests

". . . sacred food is cooked for them, to each man is brought every day flesh of beeves and geese in great abundance, and wine of grapes too is given to them. They may not eat fish . . ." (II, 37)

It is, however, unclear whether the fish avoidance to which the Greeks and, later, the Romans referred, stemmed from the Osirian tradition, or from dietary usage introduced by Pi-ʿAnkhi during the twenty-fifth dynasty. The attitudes towards fish during the later dynasties reflected diversity of origins; and these may have resulted in prohibitions that lingered into the first period of Persian occupation, when Herodotus visited Egypt.

Fish, Medicine and Diet during the Ptolemaic and Roman Periods

Plutarch, in discussing the Egyptian priests' abstinence from fish, found it to be in harmony with the words of Homer who, in his poetry, represents neither the Phaeacians, who lived amid a refined luxury, nor the Ithacans, who dwelt on an island, as making any use of fish. Nor even did the companions of Odysseus during their long voyage and in the midst of the sea eat fish until they had come to the extremity of want (1, 80, 353). The deduction was made by Dio Chrisostomus that

"Homer does not give such details without a purpose and that he is evidently declaring his own opinion as to what kind of nourishment is best." (*Second Discourse on Kingship*, 47–48)

Although Babbitt, who edited Plutarch, comments that the deduction that fishing was despised in Homeric times is not warranted, Radcliffe (1926, p. 201), interested in the origins of such a dislike for fish on the part of a people whose country has one of the longest coastlines, was of the opinion that the avoidance arose from Greek mythology that connected each brook, lake, river and spring, to a specific nymph. Hence, to eat the fish that lived therein would be a sacrilege—an attitude that was transferred to marine species.

On the other hand, the origin and distribution of this early eastern Mediterranean fish avoidance was also investigated by Issel (1971), who concluded that the practice arose from an association with sacred fish.

The non-consumption of fish portrayed in Homeric writings, however, did not persist. Hippocrates discussed the dietary varieties from the medical point of view

". . . all those fish that feed in muddy and marshy places, as mullet, cestreus, eels and the like are heavier because they feed upon muddy water and other things which grow therein—pickled fish are drying and attenuating; oily ones are gently laxative. The driest of pickled fish are those of the sea, the next those of the rivers, while the moistest are those of the lakes. Of pickled fish considered by themselves, those are driest which are made from the driest fish . . ." (Hippocrates, *Regimen* II, 48).

Several papyri dated to the Ptolemaic Period give also possible information on fish as therapy. One document, *c.* 259 B.C., tells of Cydippus, an Egyptian Greek invalid who wrote to his friend, Zenon, asking him to purchase "salted fish" at a local market; a possible implication that custom or medical advice considered such food beneficial for his condition (*S.P.*, 1932, 170).

The famed medical writer, Celsus, highly recommended fish and discussed the relative superiority and status of specific varieties

". . . the fish in use belonging to the middle class; the strongest are, however, those from which salted preparations can be made, such as the mackerel [*Lacertus*]; next come those which, although more tender, are nevertheless firm, such as the gilthead [*Aurata*], gurnard [*Corvus*], sea bream [*Sparus*], eyefish [*Oculata*], then the flat fish (*Plani*), and after these all rock fish . . ." (*On Medicine*, 2, 18, 7)

Celsus, likewise, classed edible fish according to habitat, and believed that their use in human nutrition was partly related to their ecologic niche

". . . fish living among rocks are less nutritious than those in sand, and these again are less than those in mud. Hence it is that the same classes of fish from a pond or lake or river are heavier, and those which live in deep water are lighter food than those which live in shallows . . ." (*On Medicine* 2, 18, 9)

Thus both Greek and Roman medical thought reflected the interplay between ecology and descriptive opposite qualities, such as "heavy-light" or "dry-wet", and how these related to characteristics of specific diseases.

The medicinal use of salted fish continued into the Arabic Period. Until lately, salted fish (*fessikh*) was a household remedy for typhoid along the northern seacoast of Egypt, and we recall a legend told to us at Siwa, where salted fish is favoured by women during pregnancy. This tradition, was first recorded by Belgrave (1923), and it was retold to us at the oasis, as summarized below.

> Long ago, salted fish was unknown at Siwa. One day, a pregnant woman, seized by an unreasonable craving for this food, screamed in anguish, but no one knew how to assist her.
>
> Far to the north, along the sea, a miraculous bird heard her entreaties. It gathered a fish in its mouth and flew to Siwa, where it landed at the window of the stricken woman and dropped the gift into her lap. Shortly later, the woman bore a son and named it Soliman. As Soliman matured, his religious piety and reputation for honesty and justice were unbounded and, after his death, he was venerated as a saint.
>
> To this day the women of Siwa eat quantities of salted fish during their pregnancies in the hope that their sons will be as just and honorable as was Soliman.[16]

Assessment and Evaluation of the Patterns

The information that seemingly indicates a dietary restriction of fish during some periods of Egyptian history is thus counterbalanced by evidence supporting that fish was an acceptable food. It seems obvious that avoidance patterns, when they occurred, were primarily localized, and that they were mainly a reflection of attitudes exhibited by the clergy and nobility, either because they belonged to a different, cattle-raising culture, or because they were more interested in, and better financially able to conform to religious restrictions that the poorer could not afford to keep.

Fish were always an easily obtainable source of food for the poor: "No chicken, eat fish" says a common proverb. Even during periods of alternating Seth and Osiris domination, or when disruptive clashes occurred between the followers of Amon and Aton, fish were seemingly acceptable to them, regardless of their religious following.

Localization is further suggested when one considers the revered position of *Lates niloticus* and *Tilapia nilotica* (if we accept their identity with the ꜣ *bdw* and the *int*) which did not prevent these species from being widely consumed throughout the land. It appears, therefore, that the instances of strict fish avoidance, as reported by Greek and Roman observers, were of late origin. They may possibly be interpreted as residues of impositions instituted by Pi- ꜥAnkhi, although, against this view, is the fact that the Ethiopian venture lasted a little less than seventy years, and was marked by continuous fights, first between the Egyptians and Nubians, later between the invaders and the Assyrians. In the end the invasion was ruthlessly put to an end.

Fish in Ethiopia

The possible extension into Egypt of the Ethiopian fish avoidance attitude by King Pi- ꜥAnkhi poses several interesting questions. Were the people of northern Ethiopia, of the kingdom of Napata or Kush, averse to fish, or are we mistaken as to their traditions? These people who lived adjacent to the Nile were certainly familiar with fish and must be considered differently from the Libyan "bedouins" to whom fish was alien (p. 393). If, however, the Napatan monarchs and their subjects avoided fish, as indicated by the Pi- ꜥAnkhi stele, Greek and Roman literature set the framework for an interesting evaluation of a cultural and dietary difference between northern Ethiopians (Napata) and the lands of Meroe further to the south.

The Egyptian King Psammetik, who deposed the Ethiopian rulers in 663 B.C. and founded the twenty-sixth dynasty, reportedly kept fish-eating slaves because he wished to discover the sources of the Nile (Clearchus of Athens, on authority of Athenaeus 8, 345, E).

Herodotus, likewise, related that Cambyses, conqueror of Egypt in 525 B.C., needed fish-eating guides to lead him southward into Ethiopia

". . . Cambyses was resolved to send the spies, he sent straightway to fetch from the city of Elephantine those of the fish-eaters who understood the Ethiopian language . . ." (III, 19)

How is one to reconcile these reports with those which relate that the Ethiopians of King Pi- ʿAnkhi, ruler of the northern kingdom of Napata, considered fish abominable?

Might Pi- ʿAnkhi's kingdom at Gebel Barkal, near the present Sudanese city of Dongola, have been situated between two "fish-eating" countries, Egypt to the north and a fish-eating Southern Ethiopia? Otherwise, why would both Psammetik and Cambyses need fish-eating slaves or guides to speak the language beyond the Napatan capital?

Another question is who were the "fish-eaters" who spied for Cambyses (*Her.*, III, 23) and where did they live? Were these "interpreters" the same as the Ichthyophagi mentioned by Strabo (16, 4, 13) as a people who baked fish in the sun

> ". . . when they have thoroughly baked them, they pile up the bones, tread the flesh with their feet and make it into cakes; and again they bake these cakes and use them for food—they live in caves, or in pens roofed over with beams and cross-beams, consisting of bones of whales and small fish . . ."?

The familiarity of these ichthyophagi with whales or other large sea animals would situate them, however, far from the Nile, and near to the Red Sea.

Marine Species of Fish in Egyptian Antiquity

There is little evidence that marine fish were eaten during the Dynastic Period in any quantity. Scenes from the temple of Queen Hatshepsut at Deir el Bahari (Fig. 1.17) depict a sea journey to the southern land of Punt. Vessels sent by the queen are shown in waters teeming with salt water fish, molluscs, and crustacea. Danelius and Steinitz (1967) attempted to pinpoint the geographic position of Punt on the basis of species identification from the reliefs of Deir-el-Bahari. Their success was limited, for the varieties so depicted represent both Indian Ocean and Red Sea forms.

But, although Egyptian artists of the eighteenth dynasty were thus cognizant of marine fish, there is no indication that they ate it. On the contrary, Plutarch (*I. and O.*, 363, 32) stated that priests eschewed it because of the association of the sea with Typhon (Seth). Our only information on seafood in Egyptian antiquity stems from descriptions of banquets held in Alexandria. Machon of Corinth (third century B.C.), told of a feast offered by Ptolemy I (Soter I) shortly after his return from Athens

". . . a fat casserole was brought in containing three sliced gobies at which all the guests were amazed. Archephon[23] was enjoying greatly his fill of parrot-fishes together with the red mullets and the forked hake; he was a fellow gorged with sprats, minnows, and Phaleric anchovies . . ."[24] (Athenaeus 6, 244, B–C)

Most Ancient Egyptians could not have had the opportunity of eating fresh seafood, since distribution to inland markets would have been prevented by difficulties of preservation,[25] and we have no evidence indicating that marine forms were salted or preserved as opposed to fish in general (see p. 369). But things were different on the seacoast. The Roman gourmet, Apicius, noted that grilled fish was part of the Alexandrian diet, and offered an inviting recipe for "grilled fish in the Alexandrian manner

". . . pepper, lovage, fresh coriander, onion, stoned damsons, *passum*, liquamen,[26] vinegar, and oil, pounded, mixed, cooked, then spread over the fish as it cooked . . ." (10, 1, 6–8)

He does not, unfortunately, indicate the varieties thus prepared. But the consumption of fresh seafood in Alexandria should not be interpreted as indicating familiarity with it elsewhere.

Nowadays, Egyptians betake themselves to the small village of Abukir, twelve miles east of Alexandria, where seafood is the best in Egypt. Few realize that the Egyptians, Greeks, and Romans went to this site for the same "gourmand" purpose. The ruins of Canopus lie not far from Abukir, and the marine varieties caught there were renowned among the Ancients; indeed, there are recipes for Canopic Ribbon-Fish (*Tainiai*), prepared with cheese and oil (Mithaecus,[27] on the authority of Athenaeus 7, 325, F–7, 326, A). The dominant influence of geographic locations upon local food habits and attitudes is strikingly evident throughout the ages at this site!

Fish Avoidance Patterns During the Arabic and Modern Periods

". . . permitted to you is the game of the sea and the food of it, as a provision for you and for the journeyers . . ." (Holy Koran, 5, 97)

Attitudes towards fish in modern Egypt represent customs existent prior to the Arab conquest, blended with those introduced by Eastern invaders.

The Arab army, led by Amr Ibn El-Ass may be considered to have been composed of two dietary groups: those who were familiar with fish (men whose homes or camps were adjacent to rivers, lakes, or seas) and those pastoralists who habitually abstained from eating fish because they had not previously seen or tasted it. Chief among the barriers to dietary acceptance is unfamiliarity with the food. Nomads who had never tasted fish rejected this unfamiliar food when offered it the first time, preferring their customary diet of milk, cheese, yoghurt, meats and dates.

Early Arabic medical tradition regarded the consumption of fish dangerous if eaten in combination with certain other foods. Avicenna recorded this opinion without committing himself

> ". . . Experienced people from India and others said that milk must not be taken with fish, for they cause chronic disease like leprosy (*The Canon*, lib. 1, fen 3, 2, 8)

It may be noted that the association of fish and milk with scabrous diseases almost exactly parallels ancient beliefs in regard to swine and consumption of pork.

There is a tendency to look upon the fish/milk avoidance as originating from the traumatic contact between two rival cultural groups; the cereal, vegetable and fish-eating settled farmer-fishermen, and the nomadic herdsmen whose diet is principally composed of meat and dairy products. This view is particularly tempting in regard to Egypt where the avoidance nowadays extends not just to fish and milk, but to fish mixed with cheese, cream, yoghurt or any dairy product.

On the other hand, "traumatic contact" does not adequately explain why in modern Egypt, fish mixed with eggs is likewise avoided, being believed by urbanites and peasants alike to cause severe stomach distress and "cold" (see p. 332).

It would be incorrect to argue that fish/milk avoidance stemmed solely from events in Egypt, for the width of its distribution across North and West Africa, into Europe, Southwest Asia, and even into America, is but one indication of the antiquity and complexity of this tradition.

The precise period at which it arose is, however, unclear. The Arabic language offers one clue that may extend it to a period when trade relations with East Africa and India were well established. An idiom commonly used in colloquial Egyptian Arabic, *samak, laban, wɛ tamrhindi* translated as "fish, milk and tamarind" is used to express the absurdity of any given situation. It is difficult to determine when tamarind (*Tamarindus indica*), a bland fruit used as a refreshing drink or a mild laxative, was introduced from India into Egypt or East Africa. The fact that the idiom is so ingrained in the Egyptian vernacular strongly indicates an early origin, but we know of no Latin, Coptic or Greek parallel that would carry it back to before the Arab era.

We may further conclude from the fact that Athenaeus did not criticize the fish and cheese recipe of Mithaecus, that he quoted (p. 399) that the Graeco-Egyptian nobility in his time (third century A.D.) did not look down upon this combination.

Nowadays, no variety of fish is forbidden in Egypt, but different kinds enjoy varying favour among different classes. The electric eel (*Malopterurus electricus*), known in Egyptian Arabic as *ra ʿad*, is usually avoided, although we were informed by a man born at Beni Mazar in Upper Egypt that fishermen in his village will sometimes eat it. Freshwater fish would not be touched by dwellers on seashore locations. The catfish (*Clarias* spp.), (Fig. 7.22), known to the Egyptians as *garmut* or *qarmut* is classed as a food of low quality by some; by others, it is held among the best of all edible Nile fish. Interestingly, one finds that the catfish occupies a similar dual position in the United States. Avoidance of *Clarias*, however, is primarily found among Egyptians of Nubian extraction, because of a legend concerning their traditional ancestor

> "Grandfather" was a most noble and pious man revered by all. One day, while walking near the Nile he accidentally slipped into the water and was drowned. When his body came ashore, the catfish (garmut) was found clinging to a huge gaping hole which it had eaten in the corpse! Henceforth the catfish was considered taboo and avoided by all subsequent generations.

This legend may be a remnant of the Old Osirian myth; or it may reflect a parallel with the "Dispute of a Man with his Soul," quoted on p. 393. On the other hand, a zoologist we consulted dismissed it as an "afterthought" that arose from the observation of food poisoning commonly associated with the catfish in Egypt. He stated that *Clarias* needs to be cooked within a very short time after it is caught; otherwise, its flesh spoils rapidly.

As stated in Chapter 4 (p. 171), it is widely held that association of pork ingestion with disease led to its avoidance. Mullet, *Mugil cephalus* (Fig. 7.24), is likewise, a source of the parasitic disease heterophyiasis, but it has never suffered from any ban. The discrepancy between the two sets of evidence certainly offers no support for the hypothesis that pork avoidance arose from ancient observations relative to consumption and disease.

A general study on fish avoidance among societies in Africa recently has been concluded by Kloos (1971). The geographic distribution of this custom reflects the non-fish diet of African pastoralists, yet it does not sufficiently explain why fish, likewise, are avoided by some agricultural peoples. Kloos prefers a multiple origin for the dietary prohibition, one stemming from pastoral, religious, and totemistic attitudes and beliefs.

In concluding, we recall an instance in which the innocent ignorance of the fish/milk avoidance pattern in Egypt nearly led to a serious misunderstanding between American and Egyptian co-workers. The story illustrates the importance of food attitudes in cross-cultural understanding:

> On a medical field trip to a remote desert area American and Egyptian scientists had worked long, hard hours. The American in charge of the expedition wished to compliment his co-workers for their efforts and announced that he would prepare the evening meal, prefacing his remarks with the statement that the meal would be typical of American "fare." The Egyptians were pleased at the suggestion and turned to talking among themselves, paying no attention to the dinner preparation. After lengthy fanfare the meal was served; but it was received by the Egyptians with stony silence and no one raised a fork or spoke a word. The huge pot of simmering spiced *creamed tuna* was left untouched!

> The American felt insulted and believed the Egyptians had showed him a great discourtesy when, in fact, he had tried his very best to please. The silence was eventually broken by a query—do Americans actually eat such food? The Egyptians could not believe anyone could possibly prepare such a mixture and serve it for dinner! A new meal was prepared and feelings smoothed over. A strangely tense situation had changed into one of laughter.

Would that all of our prejudices could be so lightly resolved!

Notes: Chapter 7

1. Aelian described music as a method of gathering fish ". . . those who live by the lake of Marea catch the sprats there by singing with the utmost

shrillness accompanying their song with the clash of castanets. And the fishes, like women dancing, leap to the tune and fall into the nets spread for their capture. And through their dancing and frolics the Egyptians obtain an abundant catch . . ." (6, 32). Aelian probably mistook a fish drive destined to scare the fish into stake nets. But this seemingly literary fantasy had a modern parallel in Egypt during the flood. Where sweet water meets salt water at the Nile estuaries, mullet and other fish leap out of water to escape the predatory fish and often land into barges.

2. Unidentified varieties of fish.
3. According to Hippocrates (*Regimen* II, 48) the Cestreus fish was edible but of "heavy" disposition because it fed upon muddy water.
4. This constellation of seven stars rises in May and sets with the approach of the harvest season in October. In Greek mythology the stars were originally seven maidens who were pursued by Orion until they were changed into stars and set into the heavens by Zeus; another version stated that they committed suicide over the despair they felt towards their father, Atlas, who was forced to support the heavens upon his shoulders (see Graves, 1955, Vol. 1, 41, E).
5. Much is made of a similar tradition relative to the American cowboys' rope, or lariat, which, placed in a loop around his bedroll, is believed to repel snakes and keep him safe at night. The connecting bond between the two widely divergent customs may stem from the smell of old fishnets and that of a well-used lariat!
6. A spelling variation of the Alabes described by Strabo.
7. The identification of the Mendes fish is discussed by Engelbach (1924).
8. According to Ruffer (1919, p. 341) centres for pickling fish were established in the Delta adjacent to the Pelusaic, Canopic and Mendesian branches of the Nile.
9. A humorous vignette is provided by Archippus of Athens ". . . an Egyptian, Hermaeus, is the most rascally pedlar of fish. Why? He forcibly peels off the skin of file-sharks (?) and dog-fish (?) and offers them for sale, and he disembowels sea-bass (?), so they tell me . . ." (Athenaeus, 6, 227, A).
10. According to Ebbell. This translation has not been accepted by all Egyptologists, e.g. Faulkner (1962, p. 118) translates the term as "black paint".
11. Holy Bible, Catholic edition. The London Catholic Truth Society, Tobit, 6, 1, 11–21.
12. *Caroub? Colocynth?*
13. Slime?
14. See p. 368 *Tilapia nilotica* (Fig. 7.29).
15. Unidentified fish; according to Grapow, a small fish (*Wb. Dr.*, 558).
16. We observed great quantities of imported salt-fish on sale at local stores in Siwa. In other oases, before modern routes connected them with the Nile

valley, fish was unknown. An Oasian, being shown one, is known to have believed it a demoniac monster.

17. The phrase "thy rays are in the sea" would seemingly demonstrate a tolerant attitude toward marine species. From the Late Dynastic Period and well into the Ptolemaic era there is literary evidence that the Egyptian priests avoided salt (considered to be the "spume" of Seth), and the avoidance likewise extended to fishermen and sailors that associated themselves with the sea.

18. His temple now is completely in ruins; the only surviving portions are negligible foundation stones and broken statue bases. In front of the temple facing the rising sun stood two colossi erroneously known as the Colossi of Memnon (in memory of the "Ethiopian" king who fought in the Trojan War). These statues are presently more famous than the temple of which they originally were a portion.

19. Inclusion of the inscription at Abydos is an indication that fish were accepted by the priests of both Osiris and Seth. A parallel position, relative to the finding of porcelain pigs at Abydos, is discussed in Chapter 4, p. 180.

20. *F.*, 3. An unknown variety of fish commonly discussed in Egyptological literature under various spellings: *abtu* (Budge, 1960, p. 116), *abdu* (Joachim, 1890, p. 96, 104).

21. An unknown variety of fish sometimes discussed in Egyptological literature as *ant* (Budge, 1960, p. 166), *'int* is the standard reading (*F.*, 23).

22. Unclean, *m'm'* with the determinative of a phallus, sometimes rendered "uncircumcized" (*A.R.*, IV, 882, n.d.).

23. A court parasite who feasted on the generosity of King Ptolemy I.

24. Such anchovies were netted either along the eastern rocks of the great harbour of Alexandria or taken off the port of Phaleron south of the modern seaport of Piraeus in Greece. Both sites were named after Phalerus, son of Alcon in Greek mythology.

25. Though Cairo is only 90 miles from the Red Sea and 120 miles from the Mediterranean, wise shoppers avoid buying fish except in the very early morning; and only rarely in summer. More extensive use of refrigerated transport and fish displays is alleviating this limitation.

26. A basic sauce used for flavouring. The whole formula sounds very much like "poisson à la grecque" a favourite recipe today in Greek restaurants at Alexandria.

27. Nothing is known of his life.

Chapter 8

Reptiles, Shellfish, Molluscs and Arthropods

Reptiles

The artistic endeavours of the Pre-Dynastic Egyptians indicate their acquaintance with reptiles such as the crocodile, lizard and snake, but they provide no evidence of their use as food. The Greek chronicles, however, relate that the crocodile was eaten on specific occasions, perhaps in ritualistic retaliation for its attack on unwary humans; and one learns from the medical papyri that various "humours" and parts of some reptiles were used medicinally. One suspects that their role in the Egyptian diet was only a minor one, but it is of interest to examine what evidence exists.

Crocodile

". . . I am troubled for her children that are broken in the egg, that behold the face of the crocodile before they were yet alive . . ." (*Dispute With His Soul of One Who is Tired of Life*, Erman, 1966, p. 88)

". . . the people of Elephantine are so far from considering these animals as sacred that they even eat their flesh . . ." (*Her.*, II, 69)

South of the Egyptian city of Qena, on the eastern shore of the Nile, lies the tiny village of Qous, known in antiquity by the Egyptian name *Ks*. During the Greek and Roman periods this same village was called Apollonopolis Parva; the Arabs have retained the Egyptian name, whereas the Greeks and Romans substituted one of their own.

At *Ks*, the local deity was Horus-the-Elder,[1] a member of the Osirian cycle. Across the Nile lay the village of Ombos[2] where the crocodile, a Sethian animal, was worshipped.

Aelian (10, 21) underlined the inimical attitudes of these two up-
holders of rival allegiances

". . . in Egypt there are some, like the people of Ombos, who venerate
crocodiles, and when, as often happens, their children are carried off by
them, the people are overjoyed,[3] while the mothers of the unfortunates are
glad to go about in pride in having, I suppose, borne food and a meal for
the god . . ."

This contrasted with their neighbours' customs

". . . the people of Apollonopolis, a district of Tentyra,[4] net the crocodiles
hange them up on persea trees, flog them severely, mangling them with all
the blows in the world, while the creatures whimper and shed tears;
finally they cut them up and eat them . . ."!

Other writers, particularly Juvenal[5] (Satire 15), told how the citizens
of these two towns delighted in upsetting each other's religious ceremonies. The feud was so serious that it sometimes resulted in deaths and
vindictive cannibalism (see p. 88).
Few Ancient Egyptians, however, would regularly eat crocodile
flesh except during religious rituals or at the conclusion of "revenge-
hunts." Herodotus (II, 69) implied that the custom was not restricted to
Ks, or to the region of Dendera, but that it extended to Elephantine. The
majority of positive reports, however, localized it to the north of Thebes.
Plutarch (*I. and O.*, 371, 50, D) was most positive in his assertion

". . . in the town of Apollonopolis it is an established custom for every
person without exception to eat of a crocodile . . ."

Diodorus (1, 35, 6) did not admit that this was really practiced

". . . they are seldom slain by the inhabitants; for it is the custom of most of
the natives of Egypt to worship the crocodile as a god, while for foreigners
there is no profit whatsoever in the hunting of them since their flesh is not
edible . . ."

The techniques by which the inhabitants of Dendera and *Ks* subdued
the scaly saurians were described, much embellished, by the Greeks and
Romans. Diodorus (1, 35, 5) even offered a "small history" of Egyptian
hunting techniques

". . . [the earliest Egyptians] used to catch these beasts with hooks baited
with the flesh of pigs[6] . . . [while in later periods] . . . they hunted them
sometimes with heavy nets and sometimes from their boats with iron
spears[7] which they strike repeatedly into the head[8] . . ."

Once landed, the thrashing crocodiles were still dangerous and Herodotus (II, 70) reported that they were subdued by smearing their eyes with mud, after which the quarry was very easily mastered.

Other writers offered more spectacular descriptions

". . . [men] actually dive into the river and mounting on their back as if riding a horse, when they yawn the head thrown backward to bite [they] insert a staff into the mouth, and holding the staff at both ends with their right and left hands, drive their prisoners to land as if with bridles . . ." (*N.H.*, 8, 38, 93)

This description might be regarded as "literary licence" were it not still to be seen among the tribesmen of southern Sudan who ride crocodiles to show their bravery, exactly as the Seminole Indians do with alligators in Florida. Even today the old men in Upper Egypt tell tall stories of leading the ferocious crocodile with sticks inserted into its mouth in the precise manner depicted by Pliny!

The crocodile was worshipped at several localities, two renowned sites being Kom Ombo and *Shdt*. The god Sebek (Fig. 8.1), personified by a crocodile, was known by the Greeks as Suchos. The site of *Shdt* was even renamed by the Greeks and Romans after the sacred animal and appears in their texts as Crocodilopolis, later called Arsinoe, a major town of Fayoum during the Greek and Roman Periods.

Suchos crocodile worship in the Fayoum has been discussed by more than one ancient writer, and Strabo (17, 1, 38) remarked, after he viewed the feeding of this sacred beast, that it led a remarkably easy life feeding on grain, meat and wine!

The temple dedicated to Sebek at Kom-Ombo (Fig. 8.1) represents an unusual contradiction in Egyptian religion for, although the crocodile was a Sethan animal, there was, at this site, parallel worship of the god Horus (Khons-Hor), paradoxically considered to be the *son* of Sebek.

Deification of the crocodile puzzled the Greek and Roman visitors who offered varied explanations for this unusual aspect of Egyptian religion. Diodorus (1, 89, 2–3) mentioned two possible reasons. The first was the legend of King Mena, who, when he wished to cross Lake Moeris, was helped by a crocodile that offered him a ride upon its back. The second reason postulated by Diodorus was one of security for, he said

". . . the robbers that infest both Arabia and Libya do not dare to swim across the Nile because they fear the beasts whose number is very great . . ."

Plutarch (*I. and O*, 381, 75B) offered a more imaginative explanation

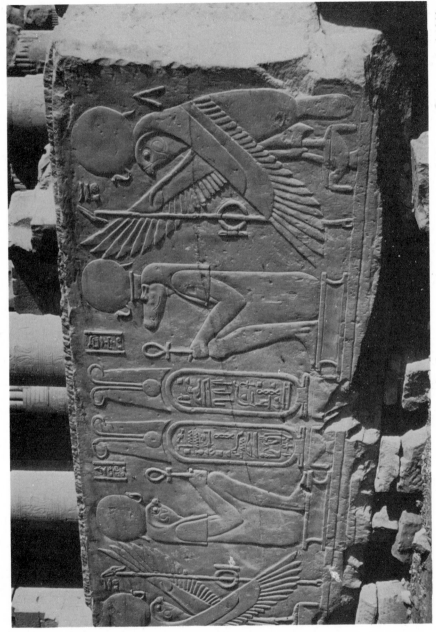

Fig. 8.1. The crocodile god Sebek between Horus gods. Temple of Kom-Ombo. Ptolemaic-Roman. Photographed 1969.

". . . he is declared to be a living representation of God, since he is the only creature without a tongue; for the Divine Word has no need of a voice . . .!"

A common peasant belief credited this reptile with unusual instincts

". . . it lays as many eggs as a goose and, by a kind of prophetic instinct, incubates them always outside the line to which the Nile in that year is going to rise at full flood . . ." (Pliny, *N.H.*, 8, 37, 89)

Aelian (8, 4) reported another ominous augury of a sacred crocodile (possibly Suchos?)

". . . Ptolemy was calling to the tamest of the crocodiles, but it paid no attention and would not accept the food he offered. And the priests realized that the crocodile knew that Ptolemy's end was approaching and consequently declined to take food from him . . ."

The same parallel, using the prophetic instincts of the Apis bull, was told of Germanicus Caesar (Chapter 3, p. 133 and note 40).

Egyptian herdsmen, however, knew the dangers they ran from crocodiles, and one wonders at the nature of their worship that perhaps fluctuated between dread and awe. Artists commonly portrayed the beast lying in wait beneath the unruffled water of the canals (Fig. 3.24). and Aelian (5, 23) aptly described the dangers from its presence

". . . this is the way in which crocodiles lie in wait for those who draw water from the Nile: they cover themselves with driftwood and, spying through it, swim up beneath it. And the people come bringing earthen vessels or pitchers, or jugs. Then, as men draw water, the creatures emerge from the driftwood, leap against the bank, and seizing them with overpowering force make a meal of them. So much for the innate wickedness and villainy of crocodiles . . ."!

Elsewhere, he enlarged on these dangers

". . . it is not easy even to wash one's feet nor can one draw water in security; why, one cannot even walk along the river banks freely and off one's guard . . ." (Aelian, 10, 24)

Though such a description mainly applied to village women, Aelian (6, 53) also described the plight of thirsty dogs

". . . [they] do not put their heads down and drink for fear some creature from below may creep up and seize them; and so they run along the brink, lapping with their tongue and snatching or, one might say, positively stealing their drink . . ."

However, a resigned fatalistic attitude seemed to permeate the character and beliefs of most Egyptians regarding the daily danger presented by the crocodile. Some uneducated peasants held that by shouting at a retreating crocodile, the animal would disgorge the body of anyone recently eaten, whereupon the corpse could receive a more proper "burial" (Pliny, *N.H.*, 8, 38, 93). It remained, however, for the people of Dendera and *Ks* to fight efficiently against this reptilian threat, and the deeds of these citizens received a passing compliment from Pliny

> ". . . the creature in question is terrible against those who run away but runs away from those who pursue it . . ." (8, 38, 92–93)

Today, the crocodile is no longer a threat in Egypt. The construction of dams and the increase in population produced restrictive barriers and more "hunters." In time crocodiles were exterminated and the "face of the crocodile" so feared by Ancient Egyptians has disappeared from the Egyptian landscape.

The Crocodile in Egyptian Medicine

Physicians were concerned not only with cures and prescriptions that utilized crocodile fat and dung, but with treating severe lacerations caused by this beast. The Ebers Medical Papyrus lists "what is done for bites by a crocodile"

> ". . . if thou examinest a crocodile-bite, and thou findest that its flesh has been thrown aside and its two sides are separated, then thou shalt bandage it with fresh meat the first day . . ." (*Eb.*, LXIV, 436)

One prescription, of questionable flavour, utilized the dung of a crocodile and was ingested

> "*To eradicate asthma* (?): dung of crocodile, *sb* ᶺ of dates, sweet beer, are ground, mixed together and eaten in 1 day . . ." (*Eb.*, LV, 333)

The majority of prescriptions which used the dung of crocodiles were related, however, to eye disorders or scalp diseases (*Eb.*, LVII, 344; LX, 379, LXIV, 437)

The rationale of these prescriptions is unclear, even if one assumes them to be based on the principles of homeopathy. In any case, the Greeks took up this disreputable medication and called it "crocodilea" (*N.H.*, XXVIII, 108)

Lizard

We know of no reference to the consumption of lizards but parts or the whole of this animal were used, together with other ingredients, in external applications

"*To expel pterygium*(?): lizard's dung" (*Eb.*, LIX, 371)
"*To expel bending of the hairs into the eyes* (trichiasis?): lizard's blood" (*Eb.*, LXIII, 424)
"*To make the hair grow*: a pounded black lizard" (*Eb.*, LXVI, 469)

Pliny (8, 38, 91) recommended the use of a specific lizard, native of the Nile, the *skink*, as an aphrodisiac and antidote. The first of these indications occurs also in Dioscorides (2, 71), and in Arab writings (Abdul Latif al-Baghdady 1965, p. 97). Today, in rural Egypt, its fat is massaged into the limbs to alleviate rheumatism and to enhance virility, and a gecko, in a home, is an omen of good luck.

Snakes

Neither is there evidence of snake eating, although Aelian (11, 34) reports one instance of eating "snake-eggs"

". . . one, Cissus by name, was the victim of a plot on the part of a woman whom he had once loved and later married; he ate some eggs of a snake, which caused him pain; he was in a grievous state and in danger of death. But he prayed to the god [Sarapis], who bade him buy a live moray and thrust his hand into the creature's tank. Cissus obeyed and the moray fastened on and clung to him but when it was pulled off it pulled away the sickness at the same time . . ." (Aelian, 11, 34)

Snake-fat was used medicinally to

"make the hair of a baldheaded person grow" (*Eb.*, LXVI, 465),

which recalls the English traditional names of hair tonics sold to anxious settlers in the western parts of the United States during the last century.

An unusual external application to remove a thorn included ground sloughs of snakes, with oil, and a boiled unidentified animal (*Eb.*, LXXXVIII, 727).

Apart from the occasional eating of a live snake by snake-charmers during their festivals, a practice that cannot be considered as a regular food habit, snake consumption is unknown today in Egypt. It seems unlikely that it was any more common in Ancient Egypt.

Turtles

Shells and bones of turtles have been reported from refuse deposits dated to the Sebilian horizon (*MAE*, p. 67). It is not possible to determine the extent of the use of this animal in the diet of early man, but it may be presumed that it was of but minor significance. Artistically, a unique example of a marine Turtle can be seen in the temple of Hatshepsut at Deir el Bahari (Fig. 8.2).

There is no report dated to either Dynastic, Greek or Roman Periods that specifically mentions the turtle as a source of food. The medical papyri do prescribe, however, their shell and bile for external use. *To cause the hair to fall out*, one could use burnt shell of tortoise with hippopotamus fat (*Eb.*, LXVII, 476). *If (the ear) grew fatty*, it was used as a dusting powder with the head of a shrewmouse, the *mndr*(?) of a goat, and thyme (?), (*Eb.*, XCI, 766). *To loosen a child in the belly of a woman*, a dressing of *nys* (?) of tortoise, *hkwn* (?), turpentine, *dsrt*-beer (?), and oil was available (*Eb.*, XCIV, 807). Shell of tortoise was also included in salves *to expel a hoof-like excrescence in the mouth of a wound* (*Eb.*, LXXI, 539), and *to prevent stinging in the summer* (*Eb.*, LXXXVI, 710).

Retrospectively, the most interesting prescription is the application of gall of tortoise to the eyes to expel "white spots" (leucoma) (*Eb.*, LVII, 347). In another prescription (*Eb.*, LXII, 405), fish bile (Dawson, 1933) was used. These compare with the Biblical story of Tobias who was directed by an angel to cure his father's leucoma with fish bile (11, 13–15). A relation between the Egyptian and Biblical prescriptions is suggested further along the story, when the demon Asmodaeus, who had previously killed all the precedent matches of Tobias's bride, was expelled with a preparation of the same fish and took refuge in Egypt (see also p. 379).

In the early thirteenth century A.D., Abd al Latif al Baghadadi (1965, p. 105) mentioned a variety of marine turtle that was used for food along the coast at Alexandria

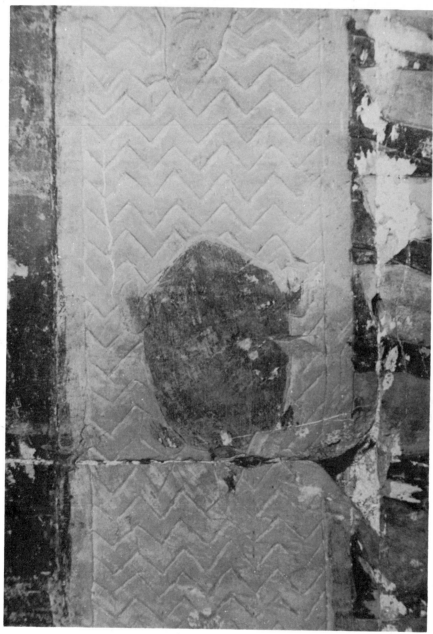

Fig. 8.2. Turtle. Temple of Queen Hatshepsut Deir el-Bahari, Thebes, New Kingdom. Photographed 1969.

". . . the Tarseh . . . is a large turtle which weighs nearly 400 weights . . . I have seen this at Alexandria. They cut it in portions, and it is sold as they sell beef. Its flesh is shaded with green, red, yellow, black, and other colours. There come from its body nearly 400 eggs, all alike hen's eggs, except that their shell is more soft. They make of these eggs a kind of confection which, being congealed, is shaded with green, red, and yellow like the flesh . . ."

Despite such notice, it must be concluded that the turtle was not an important food.

Shellfish

The word "shellfish" recurs in ancient texts as an all inclusive term embracing both marine and freshwater creatures possessing a hard external protective shell as their sole unifying feature. This broad categorization would place in the same group some molluscs (snails and clams), arthropods (lobsters, crabs, crayfish and barnacles), and even the spiney sea-urchin (an Echinoderm). The latter is eagerly sought today as an appetizer in the eastern Mediterranean. It would also seem to exclude the squid and octopus, molluscs that superficially bear little resemblance to the clam or snail, and the lethargic sea-cucumber, another Echinoderm quite distinct from the sea-urchin.

Taxonomically, such ambiguous terms as "shellfish" and "seafood" should be discarded. But as, throughout ancient texts, both terms are frequently used, we have tried to place these interesting animals into more logical groupings, keeping in mind the differences between "literary" and "scientific" classifications.

As we shall see, there is little evidence of consumption of marine shells and other seafood in Pre-Dynastic times; but one should bear in mind the near total destruction of Ancient Egyptian vestiges along the northern coast, and the sparseness of population along the Red Sea, which probably also explain, at least partly, the absence of saltwater fish in ancient artifacts.

A general pattern seen in modern Egypt concerns the avoidance of all molluscs in months without the letter "R" principally as a protection typhoid fever. These are, of course, the hottest months of the year and the link to the foreign names of the months point to the foreign origin of this tradition.

Molluscs

Clams (Various Freshwater and Marine Species)

Deposits of human refuse dating to the Sebilian type horizon indicate that early man in the Nile Valley consumed great quantities of freshwater clams. Hayes (*MAE*, p. 68) reports the identification of the following species from the upper Paleolithic-Mesolithic Sebilian zone: *Aetheria elliptica, Cleopatra bulimoides, Corbicula consobrina arlini, Viviparus unicolor, Nodularia (Caelatura) nilotica, Unio (Caelatura) nilotica,* and *Unio willcocksi.* Many of the shells were utilized as utensils and ornaments, but their abundance is consistent with the concept that their primary use was alimentary. This conclusion is substantiated as the Post-Sebilian sequences are examined. The Fayoum "A" peoples were fond of *Spatha cailliaudi,* the common Nile freshwater mussel, as were members of the Merimdian and Omarian groups (Hayes, *MAE*, 95, 112, 119).

Dawson (1932) translated as "freshwater mussel"(?) the word *wd ꜥy.t,* the interior of which was utilized in Egyptian medicine: (*Eb.*, XXVII, 119; XXXIV, 165, XXXV, 182; XLV, 225), but there are no records known to us to indicate that freshwater or marine mussels were eaten during the 3000 years of the Dynastic Period. The first such record is a statement from the Ptolemaic Period by Athenaeus (*Deipnos.*, 3, 87, F)

". . . but ear-mussels[9] found on the island called Pharos,[10] opposite Alexandria, are more nourishing than all the aforesaid kinds, though, they are not so digestible . . ."

He also discussed another edible clam

". . . *Tellinae* are found at Canobus[11] in large numbers and are abundant about the time when the Nile is rising. Of these the regal are more tender and light, and promote digestion; moreover they are nourishing . . ." (*Deipnos.*, 3, 90, C–D)

There is some confusion among ancient writers as to the *Tellis.* Athenaeus recorded two identifications, either ". . . what the Romans call *Mitulus* ("Mussell") . . ." (*Deipnos.*, 3, 85, E–F) or a type of "seasnail," or more specifically, a kind of limpet (*Patella* sp.) (*Deipnos.*, 3, 85F–86, A).

Snails (Various Freshwater, Marine and Land Species)

There is less evidence for the consumption of snails by the Pre-Dynastic Nilot than for clams. Snail-shells were found at the Omarian type horizon (*MAE*, p. 119), but whether they were a freshwater, marine or land species was not indicated. Hayes (*MAE*, p. 129) records also the finding of "conch"[12] shells in the Maadian type horizon; evidence that would apparently indicate trade with the Red Sea.

Not until Post-Dynastic times is there definite record of snail consumption in Egypt. The first reference is ambiguous in terms of the variety involved

". . . 10 choinikes[13] of snails as [partial payment for rent] . . ." (Lindsay, p. 298)

But there is in Egypt an interesting land snail commonly found in the western desert. This hardy mollusc estivates (the invertebrate equivalent of hibernation) through the harsh burning summers by secreting a thick membrane over the opercular opening of the shell. When the rare curiosity of desert rains occurs, the snail dissolves the membrane, after which it forages about, reproduces, and either re-estivates or dies. Finds of these snails provide a life-sustaining food for persons lost, stranded, or held prisoner while in the desert (Belgrave, 1923, p. 123); and the modern Awlad Ali bedouins occasionally roast this snail over an open fire and take delight in eating them. Such concentrations of snails could have provided Ancient man, dynastic desert explorers, and the unfortunate army of Cambyses that perished on its way to Siwa, with emergency "rations."

Squid and Octopus

Squid and octopus were carved in the reliefs of Queen Hatshepsut's funerary temple at Deir el Bahari, but, as we have already said, these merely illustrate a South Red Sea or even an Indian Ocean fauna.

During the eighteenth dynasty trade was established between the Egyptians and the Minoan inhabitants of the Island of Crete, and there are many proofs of cross-cultural contacts. If by this time the Egyptians were not fully aware of the potential of cephalopods as food, they certainly would have learned it from the Minoans, as an examination of the interesting and naturalistic Minoan pottery would indicate (Fig. 8.3).

No text has come to our attention that indicates that squid or octopus were eaten in Egypt prior to the Arabic Period. On the other hand, present day visitors to the eastern Mediterranean commonly encounter both on the menu. It is tempting to assume that Ancient Egyptians, or the Ptolemaic Greeks in Alexandria were, likewise, connoisseurs of this fare, for there is evidence that both Greek and Roman banquets, at least in coastal cities, included squid and octopus. However, one must guard against the temptation to make assumptions concerning behavioural patterns through broad expanses of time, or to assume that the firmly ingrained food habits of modern man indicate historical precedents of great antiquity. It is recorded (*Eb.*, LXXXVIII, 732) that, medically, cuttlefish *ns-s*, literally "the tongue of the pond," was part of an application to remove splinters, and of other local remedies. It was one of the species illustrated in the above mentioned relief of Deir el Bahari.

Arthropods I: Crustaceans

Barnacles (Balanus spp.)

From a modern western viewpoint, these sessile crustaceans, usually considered by sailors and mariners to be major pests, could scarcely appeal to anyone's appetite. Athenaeus (*Deipnos.*, 3, 91, A), however, appreciated their role in the epicurean banquets of his time

"... and the barnacles, which take their name from their likeness to the acorn on oaks, differ according to locality. For the Egyptian are sweet, tender, well-flavoured, nourishing, have abundant liquor, and are diuretic and good for the bowels . . ."

Despite this reference that dates to Ptolemaic times, there is no evidence that barnacles were consumed by the Dynastic Egyptians.

Crayfish (Palinurus vulgaris)

Athenaeus (*Deipnos.*1 6, 244, B) quotes from Machon (p. 399) regarding a banquet given by Ptolemy Soter, where "genuine crayfish" were

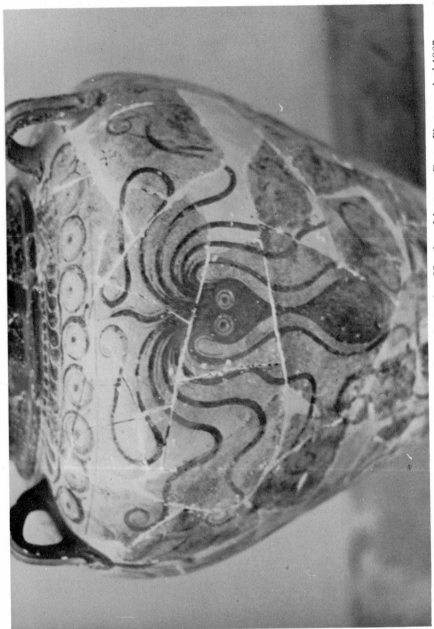

Fig. 8.3. Minoan pottery showing a cephalopod as a decoration. Heacleon Museum, Crete. Photographed 1967.

offered to the guests. The specification, "genuine crayfish" may imply a distinction between the marine lobster and the freshwater crayfish which superficially resemble one another. But it seems doubtful that crayfish were eaten during the Dynastic Period.

Lobster *(Hommarus gammarus)*

Biblical and religious scholars have joined with the archaeologist and zoologist in an attempt to ascertain a "just cause" for the religious exclusion of arthropods among foods. One hypothetic explanation of avoidance is the rapid spoilage of such forms, whereas salted fish presented no such danger.

Lobsters are not mentioned in Ancient Egyptian texts. Even though one is depicted in the eighteenth dynasty "Queen-of-Punt" reliefs (Fig. 8.4) of Deir el Bahari; this illustrated Red Sea fauna from the extreme south of the Red Sea and does not necessarily indicate use made of the examples depicted.

These were obviously eaten during the Greek Period, for Athenaeus praised the fine quality of the lobsters from Alexandria and the Libyan coastline (*Deipnos*, 1, 2, B). Indeed, his reference to "genuine crayfish" (*loc. cit.*) implies that they were consumed, at least by the wealthy, along the Egyptian sea coasts.

Arthropods II: Insects

Locusts *(Acrydium peregrinum)* znḥm *(F., 233)*, or ʿapšyt (? beetle)

". . . even these of them ye may eat; the locust after his kind, and the bald locust after his kind . . . and the grasshopper after his kind . . ." (*Leviticus*, 11, 22)

In marsh scenes of the Old Kingdom, particularly at Saqqara, locusts form a part of the habitual scenic background (Fig. 8.5). They (ʿpsyt) are listed in the Berlin papyrus (no. 59) as a fumigation; and in

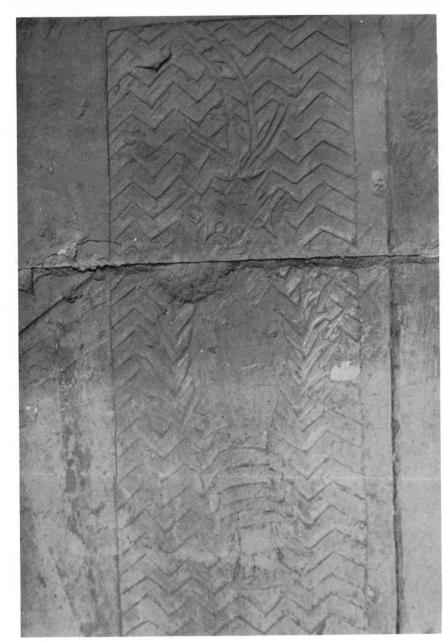

Fig. 8.4. Lobster. Funerary temple of Queen Hatshepsut. Deir el Bahari. New Kingdom. Photographed 1969.

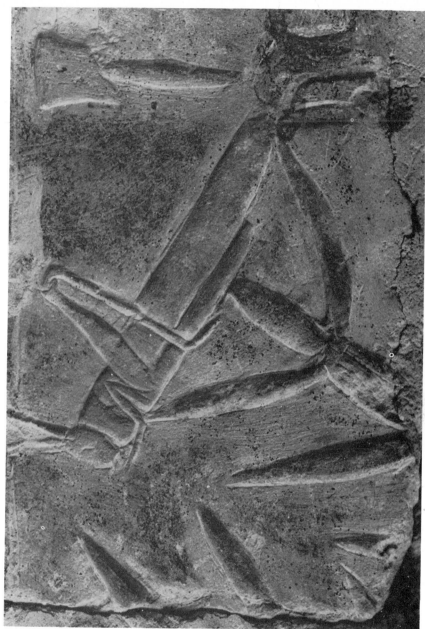

Fig. 8.5. Locust. Mereruka's Tomb. Saqqara. Old Kingdom. Photographed 1969.

the London papyrus (*L.*, 11) in an incantation, not as a drug in the proper sense.

A point upon which there is agreement among certain authors is that the Mosaic dietetic laws were meant clearly to distinguish between the Children of Israel and their former masters. So viewed, Biblical permission may be construed as a means of accentuating a cultural difference between the two, since the lack of evidence of consumption in Ancient Egypt may reflect a conjectural abhorrence or taboo.

Information available on peoples elsewhere indicates that locusts were acceptable to Parthians (Pliny, *N.H.*, XI, XXXV, 106); and Strabo (*Geo.*, 16, 4, 12) described an Asiatic people

> ". . . who are blacker than the rest and shorter in stature and the shortest-lived; for they rarely live beyond forty years, since their flesh is infested with parasites. They live on locusts. . . they cast smoking timber in the ravines, lighting it slightly and thus easily catch the locusts for when they fly above the smoke they are blinded and fall. The people pound them with salt, make them into cakes, and use them for food."

By Arabs, locusts have always been considered a delicacy, from the Arabian peninsula to Morocco.

Miscellaneous Insects

Hayes (*MAE*, p. 48), as well as others, stated that larvae and grubs formed part of the diet of the earliest Nilots. This, of course, is pure speculation based in large measure on present-day food-gathering techniques of primitive peoples, particularly in Australia and south-western Africa. A full account of such practices as known today is given by Bodenheimer (1951), whose work should be consulted for more details concerning entomophagy in the modern world. It may be mentioned, in concluding this chapter, that ant oil is widely used in southern Sudan, but there is no evidence that it was known or used in Ancient Egypt.

Notes: *Chapter 8*

1. During that period, Edfu was called Apollonopolis Magna.
2. Sometimes called "Ombos-of-the-North" to differentiate it from the "southern" Ombos, the modern Kom Ombo.

3. Aelian's informants here certainly exaggerated the feelings of the children's parents! This should be compared, however, with the Aztec and Babylonian offerings to the gods, and possibly, with the old legend of the bride of the Nile, until lately commemorated yearly, by ceremonially throwing into the Nile, on the day of the flood, a statuette of a girl.

4. Tentyra, site of the village of Dendera, gave its name also to the inhabitants of *Ks*, who were thus called Tentyritae. Such was their reputation that some appeared in Rome as crocodile-wrestlers and trainers for the amusement of the populus (Strabo, 17, 1, 44).

5. Juvenalis was exiled to Egypt during the reign of the Emperor Domitian (A.D. 81–96), and some believe he was garrisoned at Aswan. His feelings towards the citizens of the country of his exile were, in general, bitter.

6. First mention of this technique described by Diodorus is in Herodotus (II, 70) ". . . the hunter baits a hook with a chine of pork, and lets it float into the midst of the river; he himself stays on the bank with a young live pig, which he beats. Hearing the cries of the pig, the crocodile goes after the sound, and meets the chine, which then the hunters pull the line . . ."

7. Abd al-Latif al Baghadadi, reputedly knowledgeable in regard to Arabic science, foods and natural history, reported that iron would not pierce the skin of crocodiles (1965, p. 93). This error can be attributed, perhaps, to his informants, and one would suspect he did not himself witness such a hunt during his visit to Egypt in the early thirteenth century A.D.

8. Aelian (10, 24) offered a credible description of the Egyptian hunting technique ". . . now the people of Egypt called Tentyritae know the best way to master the beast: the most effective way of wounding it is to strike it in the eyes or armpits and even in the belly. . ."

9. Probably *Mitulus* sp.

10. The island of Pharos at Alexandria was the site of the lighthouse, one of the seven wonders of the Ancient World.

11. Mis-spelling of Canopus.

12. An ambiguous term applied to any large marine snail.

13. Sometimes spelled *Choenix*, approximately one litre.

Chapter 9   *Sweetening Agents*

The desire for sweet-tasting nutrients is inborn in most animals, and has been cleverly exploited in their training and taming. In humans, it is detectable at birth and cannot, therefore, be attributable to the mere "learning" of the rapid satiation effect of sugars, or of the sweetness of reward. In adults, this craving has been so strong throughout history that kings and the wealthy reserved sweets for their own tables, or offered them to their gods; and that, once the cheap production of sugar made it available to the masses, the enormous demands for it inspired political moves and the unspeakable cruelties of slavery in sugar plantations (Aykroyd, 1967).

Various factors that control this fondness for sugars have been recently discussed in a symposium edited by Kare and Maller (1967). The contributors showed that, basically, it is instinctive; but that it is modulated by deficit or satiation (Jacobs, 1967, pp. 187–200), by homoeostatic and endocrine mechanisms (enhanced by hypoadrenocorticism, corrected by gluco-corticoids, not by DOCA) (Henkin, 1967, pp. 95–103), or by early conditioning. Experiments have further shown that, in animals, needs and dietary habits may override palatability; that motivational changes tend to be relatively short-lived, whereas the effects of learning last longer (de Ruiter, 1967, pp. 83–88), and that the calorie intake is less influenced by palatability in wild species (rats) than in their domesticated brethren (Maller, 1967, pp. 201–202). Man's taste for sweetness is present at birth, hence his historical quest to satiate it.

Several sweet substances are naturally found in food, and they vary in the intensity of the sensations they elicit in the same or in different species. In man, the sweetness of the principal of these diminishes in the following order: fructose, sucrose, glucose, lactose. These are found in different proportions in various foods.

According to Winton and Winton (1935, 1945) raw sugar cane juice contains, on the average, sucrose 12% and levulose and invert sugar 1·7%; and beet juice, sucrose 18·5%. By USA standards, white sugar, whether from cane or from beet, contains at least 99·5% sucrose (Winton and Winton, 1945). Sucrose is the principal sugar in dates, but inversion before picking causes the transformation of as much as 20–25% of it

(Winton and Winton, 1935, Vol. II, p. 486). Lactose is the sugar in milk. Honey contains from 67–75% of invert sugars and from 2–3% sucrose. The sugar content of several fruits is shown in Table 1.

Accordingly, the proportion in which the different sugars occur in the human diet varies with the type of food consumed. Before the discovery, development and world-wide distribution of cane sugar, relatively little sucrose was ingested. But, nowadays, according to calculations made by Page and Friend (1974), of the total of 200 g of sugars daily consumed per person in the United States, two-thirds are made of sugar and syrups, one-eighth comes from dairy products, one-eighth from fruits and the remainder from other foods.

Reckoned as individual sugars, in the United States in 1972, sucrose accounted for 61·8% of the total; lactose, for 12·5%; glucose, for 6·4%; maltose, for 2·7%; levulose, for 1·7%; other sugars, for 3·2%; and the rest was undetermined. Honey accounted for less than 2%.

Sugar (Sucrose)

Cane Sugar

Sugar (from Sanskrit *Karkara*, meaning sand) is a relatively recent addition to diet. Its history has been extensively studied by Deerr (1949–50) and by Aykroyd (1967). Until the beginning of the nineteenth century, it was obtained exclusively from the sugar cane (*Saccharum officinale*), a grass apparently first cultivated in Southeast Asia, and of which no wild ancestors are known for certain. From India, where crude sugar was probably manufactured around 500 B.C., it spread eastwards to China, *c.* 100 B.C. But the Chinese, who had learnt from India in A.D. 640 how to prepare a crude form of molasses, used only to boil and skim the juice which, when cold, left a black paste. Around the thirteenth century, according to Marco Polo (1929, p. 240), some Egyptians

> ". . . who happened to be at the Court (of the Great Khan) taught the people to refine the sugar with the ashes of certain trees."

Westward, production of sugar slowly spread to the Mesopotamian valley, probably in the sixth century B.C. As Aykroyd pointed out (1967,

Table 1

Sugars content of fruits and honey

	Total solids	Glucose	Fructose	Invert sugar	Sucrose	Maltose
Apricot	14·44	1·73	1·28	—	5·84	—
Carob, cured	88·50	—	—	11·24	23·17	—
Date, cured	84·60	—	—	—	—	—
Fig	14·98	—	—	——10·80——	—	—
Grape, v. labruscana	19·13	6·86	7·84	—	2·25	1·58
Grape, v. vinifera	17·97	5·35	5·33	—	1·32	2·19
Pomegranate	21·73	—	—	11·61	1·09	—
Honey	82·00	33·7	37·1	—	—	1·1

Data from Winton and Winton (1945) and Sipple and McNutt (1974).

p. 11), the land of Canaan was flowing with milk and honey (Exodus, 33, 3), not with milk and sugar. The Jews heard of it much later.

> "Thou hast bought me no sweet cane with money . . ." Isaiah (43, 24)

and Jeremiah asked,

> "To what purpose cometh there to me incense from Sheba and the sweet cane from a far country?" (6, 20)

This must have happened around the end of the Babylonian exile for, although Isaiah lived long before, it is currently accepted by Biblical scholars that the book called by his name was put together by many hands over a long period of time.

Strabo (XV, I, 20) quoted Nearchos, Alexander's admiral, as having seen in the Punjab reeds that yielded honey although there were no bees, and a tree

> ". . . from the fruit of which honey is compounded . . ."

His following remarks, however, make it difficult to identify this fruit with the sugar cane, for he added that those who ate the fruit raw became intoxicated.

Dioscorides described sugar thus

> "And there is a kinde of concrete Hony, called sugar (sakcharon), found in reeds in India and in Arabia ye Happy, like in consistence to salt, and brittle to be broken between the teeth, as salt is. It is good for the belly and stomach being dissoluted in water, and soe dranck . . ." (II, 104)

Pliny (*N.H.*, XII, XVII) mentioned it as a medicine

> "Arabia also produces cane sugar [saccharon] but that grown in India is more esteemed. It is a kind of honey that collects in reeds, white like gum, and brittle to the teeth . . . it is only employed as a medicine."

At the same period

> ". . . honey from the reed called sacchari . . ."

was shipped from India to the Somali coast (Schoff 1912, pp. 27, 90, 285). This does not necessarily indicate Arabia as its source, for it is known that Arabian seamen and traders kept the sources of their goods closely guarded secrets, and acted only as middle men to many a commodity which they led their clients to believe that they produced.

Although remnants of a wild kind of sugar cane were found in Omarian deposits in Egypt (*MAE*, p. 119), it is only in the seventh century, A.D., that the developed cane was brought by the Arab invaders to Egypt, where conditions were most favourable to its production, and whose sugar was long considered the best. It later spread west—and northwards, helped by the Crusaders and by Venetian merchants, and its subsequent widespread cultivation, first in West Africa, then in the New World, has been ably told by Deerr and by Aykroyd.

Beet Sugar

It was in 1740 that Marggraf in Germany demonstrated that sugar could be crystallized from beets. The industrial development of the process enabled Napoleon to combat the monopoly of the sugar trade closely held by the British. Within two years 334 factories of beet sugar were functioning, and all import was forbidden in France. According to a doubtful story, that nevertheless reflects political mores at that time, the widespread destruction of French beet-sugar factories by the allied troops after Waterloo was ordered by the Duke of Wellington to stifle the danger to English industry.

A development similar to that which happened in France occurred during the American Revolution when the Patriots, cut off from their West Indies supplies, produced sugar from maize stalks (Winton and Winton, 1945, p. 607). Nowadays, the world production of sugar is in the ratio of 60 from cane, 40 from beet.

This historical schedule of appearance of sugar from cane in the Mediterranean area only from the sixth century A.D. indicates that despite Egypt's important role in sugar production in modern times, sugar *per se* was not a food of the Ancient Egyptian.

Sugar is a ready source of energy and quickly produces satiety. Early after its introduction only the wealthy could afford it, and the consumption of it was quite limited in contrast to use levels today. One of the complications that may follow retention of sweet foods in the interdental spaces and around the teeth is caries due to plaque formation and fermentation in the presence of appropriate microorganisms. As early a writer as Aristotle noted that soft sweet figs could harm teeth, and he attributed the harm either to the viscous pulp of the fig adhering to the gums and insinuating itself into the dental interstices causing decomposition, or to friction of the small hard grains during mastication (*Problems*, XXII, 14). Aykroyd (1967, p. 117) cited the historically bad state of Queen Elizabeth's teeth that was ascribed to her undue fondness for sweetmeats. In Ancient Egypt an increasing intake of honey, fruit and pastries might have been one of the reasons for the rising incidence of caries with luxury reported by Ruffer (1921), and by Elliot-Smith and Dawson (1924), although these authors considered only the softness or hardness of foods as possible factors.

The consumption of sugar *per se* could not have been a factor in this rise. In recent times the infectious nature of caries has been stressed and the opportunities for the more affluent members of ancient society to acquire such flora has been noted in Chapter 2. The modern role of sugars in nutrition is well covered in the recent monograph edited by Sipple and McNutt (1974).

Honey (byty)

"Thy lips, O my spouse, drop as the honey-comb; honey and milk are under thy tongue." (Song of Solomon, 4, 11)

As told in an ancient legend, one day, long ago, the god Ra wept, and the tears that dropped from his eyes turned into a bee that, forthwith, made its honeycomb and busied itself with flowers (Derchain, 1965). For millenia, this miraculous honey provided sweetness to mankind, and apiculture was one of the most important and most protected industries, since it took the place of modern sugar production (though it hardly equalled it in extent), and provided beeswax, that was needed for worship, fighting, cosmetics and a variety of other purposes.

But, like sugar in the first centuries of its appearance in Europe, honey was a highly expensive commodity that only the wealthy could afford. This industry of luxury, at first restricted to honey gathering from wild bees, thrived especially well in the Delta, where the wide spreads of cultivated land suited its industrious producer. Thus did the bees deserve to be a symbol of the North and to appear in the royal protocols. One of the earliest designations of Kings was their *nisw* and *byty* name (Fig. 6.45), where *byty*, meaning "The One of the Bee" was their title of rulers of the North, and *nisw*, "The One of the Reed," their title of rulers of the South.

At least in the early periods, honey must have been a royal prerogative. It was mentioned exclusively in religious texts, not in any known secular document or private tomb (Kueny, 1950). In the Old Kingdom, it was mentioned among the presents sent by Pepi II (sixth dynasty), with the Count, Bearer of the Royal Seal, Governor of the South, Sole Companion, and Ritual Priest, Sebni, to the "countries of the negroes" (*A.R.*, I, 366).

In the Middle Kingdom, deposits were made in private tombs (Maspero, 1885–1886) but, although apparently in common usage, as an offering it was presented only to gods.

From that dynasty on, honey is seen listed among funerary and temple offerings (*A.R.*, II, 571; IV, 770), and in rations issued to important officials, like the "King's messenger and standard bearer" (*A.R.*, III, 208); during the eighteenth dynasty, Ineni, who enjoyed great favour with Thutmose II, could boast of having been supplied with honey from the royal table (*A.R.*, II, 117).

From the number and quantities of donations to temples, it is clear that honey played an important role in temple rituals, and local supplies, that could hardly satisfy the demands, had to be supplemented by tribute exacted from vassal countries like Palestine and Syria (*A.R.*, II, 462, 472, 518).

Honey was especially agreeable to the god Min. Montet (1950) could identify the titles of two high officials involved in the provision of honey in Min's rituals: the *ȝfty*, who probably kept bees, and the *bity*, who was more concerned with the gathering of honey and, possibly, took part in desert expeditions to collect wild honey. One of the high officials of Rameses IV, *Ouser-mare-nakhty* bore the titles, among others, of "Purveyor of honey to Min, Who is in the laboratory at Coptos (Min's domain), and Messenger to the Mysterious District." Montet concluded that the Coptos laboratory was the place where secret preparations were made, such as the "divine matter" prepared by the *smȝty*, another priest of Min, an ointment destined to anoint the divine members of the statue of Min.[1]

The temples, indeed, made a great consumption of this delicacy. Special gatherers were appointed to that effect (*A.R.*, IV, 206) and armed aids accompanied them to enforce the impositions

> ". . . I made for thee archers and collectors of honey . . . I established for them tax officials to conduct them and to collect their annual impost for thy august storehouse." (*A.R.*, IV, 324)

Rameses III included it in practically every one of his offerings (*A.R.*, IV, 151–412), and among "the things exacted, the impost of all the people and serf-labourers" of the temple.

Under the twenty-first dynasty, the "great chief" Namlot is recorded as having made a payment for honey, payable to the treasury of Osiris in bas-relief in the Chamber of Seasons of Ne-Woser-Re's solar temple at Abusir (von Bissing, 1905). The scene (Fig. 9.1) clearly shows, at the extreme left, a man kneeling in front of a pile of jars, and holding before his mouth an elongated vessel.

Apiculture in Egyptian Iconography

> *He who desires honey must suffer the bee stings.*
> (Popular saying)

As early as the fifth dynasty, apiculture, as a profession, was illustrated in a bas-relief in the Chamber of Seasons of Ne-Woser-Re's solar temple at Abusir (von Bissing, 1905). The scene (Fig. 9.1) clearly shows, at the extreme left, a man kneeling in front of a pile of jars, and holding before his mouth an elongated vessel.

Above his head, the word *nft*, "to breathe" or "to exhale," is clearly written. This has been variously interpreted as "blowing" smoke, or any other bee-repellent, or as imitating the call of an old "queen," as do bee-keepers today in Egypt (Kueny, 1950). The latter possibility seems confirmed by a sentence of the Leyden papyrus

> ". . . they [the bees] are called with a flute . . ." (Spiegelberg, W., quoted by Kueny, 1950)

and by a passage from Isaiah (VI, 18)

> "And it shall come to pass in that day that the Lord shall hiss for the fly that is in the uttermost of the rivers of Egypt, and for the bee that is in the land of Assyria."

To the right of the kneeling man, another worker is pouring the contents of a jar into a long, wide-mouthed vessel; two groups of men (the second very deteriorated) pour something from a low rounded vessel into high narrow jars. To the extreme right, a spherical pot is being sealed; two already sealed pots are stored on a shelf, and a bee is very obviously displayed, giving the clue to the whole scene.

The most important series of such scenes, however, are certainly the ones in Rekhmire's tomb at Thebes (eighteenth dynasty), where this important vizier presides a function called

> "Reception of grain, honey, and all precious things in the White House [Treasury] of the Temple; sealing of all Treasures . . . by virtue of his office as the Master of Secret Things, the Hereditary Prince, the Vizier."

Dressed in state robes and holding a scepter, Rekhmire receives officials from various districts, advancing in four rows to bring their dues. Of the thirty-one still preserved, ten bring in honey (*A.R.*, II, 717). In the remaining scenes (Davies, 1943), Rekhmire ceremoniously watches over the manipulation of the precious liquid. From right to left, there are displayed extraction from the hives, no doubt after smoking out the bees with the lamps held by the standing man, filling three different kinds of jars, and sealing in flat containers (Fig. 9.2).

Other illustrations are found in a badly preserved eighteenth dynasty tomb (Save-Soderbergh, 1957), and the tomb of Pabes (twenty-fifth dynasty) (Fig. 9.3). They show an arrangement quite similar to the more traditional bee-hives still seen today in the Egyptian countryside, where claypipes are piled up in rows and stoppered with mud (Fig. 9.4).

Kueny (1950), reviewing present-day apicultural practices in Egypt, finds several other features similar to those shown in the above illustration He noted that present-day honey producers prepare three "grades": "virgin" honey, which is the first honey expressed from the combs, and is usually kept for the personal consumption of the producer; "second grade," obtained by pressing the combs with 6–12% water, destined to the market; and a "third," obtained by further crushing the residue. He makes the interesting suggestion that the three kinds of jars, in both Ne-Woser-Re's and Rekhmire's illustrations, in each of which a distinct operation seems to be carried out, might likewise represent the production of correspondingly different "grades" of honey. If this hypothesis be verified, these might correspond to the varieties called light-coloured *stf*, red *dsrt* (Hayes, 1951), *pw-g'*, *mḥ-tt*, and honey for cakes of Ramses III's records (*A.R.*, 4, 300, 350).

Finds of Honey

Apart from the finds described by Maspero there have been, according to Kueny (1950), many specimens of honey discovered in tombs from

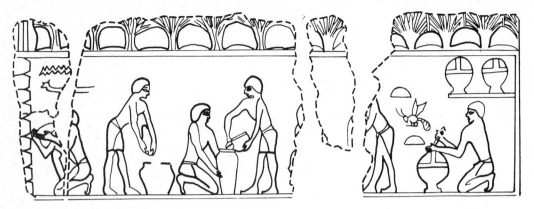

Fig. 9.1. Honey production. Ne-Woser-Re's Solar Temple. Old Kingdom. Redrawn from Kueny (1950).

the Middle Kingdom onwards. Two small jars from Tut-ankh-Amon's tomb, labelled "honey of good quality," were examined by Lucas (1962, p. 26) who could not identify their contents although, in one, when treated with hot water, an indication was a slight smell suggestive of caramel. Another material from the same tomb was black and resinous-looking, and covered with the kitinous remains of beetles and innumerable crystals of some sugar, suggesting that the material had been either honey or a fruit juice.

Zander (1941, p. 180) described a honeycomb found at Deir el-Medineh in a tomb dating to the nineteenth dynasty, *c.* 1350 B.C. The typical hexagonal design (Fig. 9.5) indicated its source to be an Apis bee, and the small size of the cells, when compared to present-day honey-combs suggested *Apis mellifica unicolor fasciata*. When the hard, dark brown, glistening contents were dissolved in water, he identified a predominance of pollen of *Mimusops schimperi* and *Balanites aegyptiaca* with scant specimens of *Graminae*, *Caryophyllaceae*, *Trifolium*, *Melilotus*, *Vicia*, *Cruciferae*, *Rosaceae*, *Thymelaceae*, and *Polygalaceae*. Although he advised caution in interpreting his results, he concluded, from the completely different pollen composition of present day Egyptian honey, that the flora from which bees gathered their honey has suffered considerable change since Pharaonic times, and has shifted from garden and wild trees to clover-like herbs (*op. cit.*, pp. 216–218).

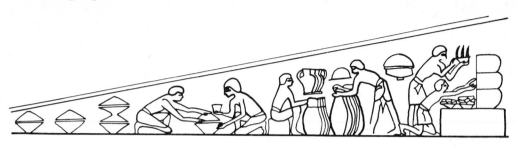

Fig. 9.2. Tomb of Rekh-mi-Re at Thebes. New Kingdom. Handling of honey. Redrawn from Davies (1943).

Uses of Honey

Apart from its utilization in the pure state, honey was incorporated in cakes and pastries, and was used to prime beer and wine (see Chapters 13 and 14).

It was one of the components of *Kyphi* of the enigmatic composition which so much has been written and so little is known, and which was variously said to be made of sixteen (Plutarch, *I. and O.*, 80), or of ten ingredients (Dioscorides, 1, 24).[2]

In the field of Ancient Egyptian medicine we have seen honey in remedies for *polyuria*. But it was extensively used for other conditions, principally as a flavouring agent or as a vehicle. Lefebvre (1956, p. 196) quotes about 60 prescriptions that included it. Its wide indications may be judged from the following examples:

Local applications:

In ointments—to expel the rose (? erysipelas), with myrrh (*Eb.*, XXIV, 95)
to treat headache, with tamarix, natron, burnt bones of various fish, ladanum (*Eb.*, XLVIII, 248)
to soften the knees, with fat meat, and flour (*Eb.*, LXXVI, 603)

Eye remedies—with human (? pork) bile (*Eb.*, LXI, 392)
with tortoise bile (*Eb.*, LVIII, 360)
with galena (*Eb.*, LXI, 395)
with malachite for pterygium (*Eb.*, LIX, 373)
for pterygium (*Eb.*, LIX, 369)

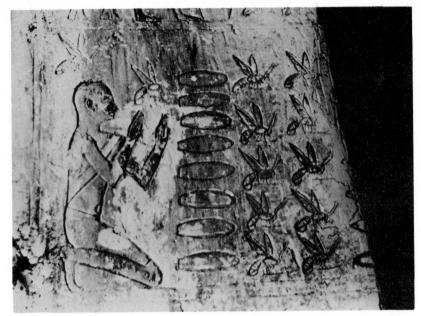

Fig. 9.3.

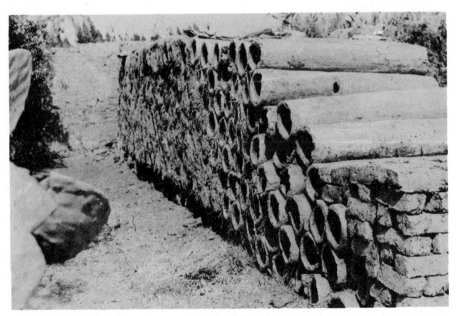

Fig. 9.4.

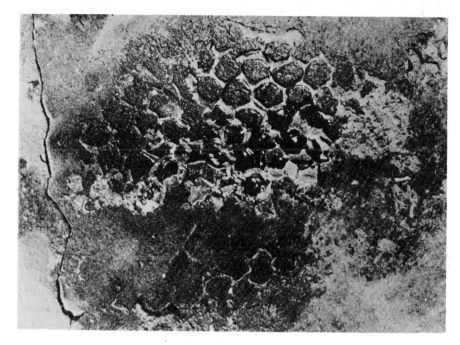

Fig. 9.5.

Fig. 9.3. Collecting honey from cylindrical hives. Tomb of Pabes. Thebes. New Kingdom. Photographed 1969.

Fig. 9.4. Traditional bee-hive, made of clay pipes, still in use in rural Egypt side by side with more modern models. Qaliub, just north of Cairo. Photograph taken in August 1974. This kind of bee-hive is gradually being replaced by modern types.

Fig. 9.5. Honey cake. Deir el-Medineh. Nineteenth dynasty. Reproduced from Zander (1941).

As wound dressings—*Eb.*, LXIV, 435; *Ber.*, 52, Sm. Nos. 10, 15, 18, 26 with Nubian earth and oil (*Eb.*, LXXVIII, 619)

Local applications—to the leg, with brain of silurus (*Eb.*, XXX, 128) for an ailing toe, with bone-marrow ?, fat, and oil (*Eb.*, LXXVIII, 620)
for a toe nail that is falling; with natron, terebinth, resin, oil, and Nubian earth (*H.*, 179)
for trembling of fingers, with terebinth, cummin, yellow ochre, natron, figs, Nubian earth (*Eb.*, LXXIX, 624)

As a mouth wash—for ulceration of gums, with sycamore, frankincense, and water (*Eb.*, LXXII, 554)

In a suppository—to cool the anus, with pignon, juniper, frankincense, cuttlebone, yellow ochre, cummin, myrrh, and cinnamon (*Eb.*, XXI, 140)

Internally—as an aperient, boiled with ʿ ꜣ t, mustard, oil (*Eb.*, XLI, 203); with manna, gum, yellow ochre, oil (*Eb.*, XLI, 205)
to expel "death" in the belly of man (*Eb.*, XXXV, 182)
to treat cough, honey is included in twelve prescriptions, e.g. with cream and cummin (*Ber.*, 31)[3]
with cream and beer (*Eb.*, LIV; 315, *Ber.*, 29, 31, 34, 37)

In other cases, "fermented" honey was specified—against "rising of water in the eyes" (cataract ?) with goose fat (*Eb.*, LX, 379)
against blindness, with colocynth (*Eb.*, LXIII, 420) or with colocynth and galena (*Eb.*, LXII, 399)
with humours of pig's eye, galena, yellow ochre, to be injected in the ear (*Eb.*, LVII, 356); this was to be accompanied by a magic spell (see below).

Honey was a useful adjunct in magic therapy. While administering the last prescription (*Eb.*, 356) the physician had to say,

"I have brought this which was applied to the seat of yonder and replaces a redoubtable, redoubtable suffering."

The following spell had to accompany the application of tortoise bile and honey on the lids

"It is thundering in the southern sky since the evening, there is rough weather in the northern sky, as corpses fell into the water, and Re's crew were landing at their shore, because the heads fell into the water. Who shall bring them?

. . . I shall bring them. I have brought your heads, I have attached them to your necks . . . I have fastened your cut-off heads in their place . . . I have brought you to expel affliction caused by a god, by dead man or woman . . ." (*Eb.*, LVIII, 360)

Another prescription (*Eb.*, LX, 385) is a spell to be recited while anointing the eye with fermented honey and rush-nut

"Come, Chrysocoll (Malachite?); Come, thou green one: Come, discharge from Horus's eye. Come, secretion from Atum's eye. Come, fluid that has come out of Osiris! Come to him and expel from him water, matter, blood, dim sight, blindness, afflictions caused by dead man or woman . . ."[4]

Finally, the "Incantations for Child and Mother" (*Zaub.*, 2, 4) contain the following poetic spell

"Disappear, you who come in the dark with his nose behind him; his face turned; but from whom that for which he came will flee . . .
Did you come to kiss that child, I shall not allow you to kiss it
Did you come to appease it, I shall not allow you to appease it
Did you come to harm it, I shall not allow you to harm it
Did you come to take it away, I shall not allow you to take it away
I made a charm for him against you, of melilotus that harms you, of onions that destroy you; of honey, sweet to man, bitter to the dead.[4]

Honey in Greece

The Greeks, too, made a great use of honey. Pythagoras who led a very frugal life, lived principally on it

"He led his whole life through with very little expense, often he was satisfied with honey only." (Athenaeus, *Deipnos.*, X, 418)

On the opposite end of the scale of extravagance, a man, complained of his son's spending on a dinner

"Four flute girls have to be paid, and a dozen cooks, and artisans who demand honey by the bowlful." (Athenaeus, *Deipnos.*, IV, 172)

At the very extreme of hedonism, a Cyrenaic philosopher, Aristoxenus,

"in his excess of luxury, used to water the lettuce in his garden with wine and honey!" (Athenaeus, *Deipnos.*, 1, 7)

Beeswax

Beeswax was an extremely useful by-product of apiculture. It was used medicinally as a vehicle for external applications: (*Eb.*, XLVIII, 252; LXXVIII, 613; LXVIII, 484; LXIV, 435; LXXXVIII, 731). Another prescription, presumably to be given orally, merely said

". . . to be taken for four days."

It was a remedy against burning of the anus and pain in the feet, and it included colocynth, fresh dough, goose fat, and water (*Eb.*, XXXII, 153).

The embalmers utilized it to pack mummies and to plug the eyes, ears, nose, mouth and embalming incisions (Elliot Smith and Dawson, 1924, pp. 113, 117, and 124). During the twenty-first dynasty, the figures of the four sons of Horus, that were placed in Canopic vessels, were sometimes made of beeswax (Lucas, 1962, p. 303). But there is no truth in statements that honey was used in Egyptian embalming (Lucas, p. 27), as it was by the Greeks (Posener, 1962, p. 127).

Fruit Juices

The proletariate, unable to obtain, or to afford honey, sweetened their food with fruit juices, probably evaporated to a syrupy consistency. In a picture of a twelfth dynasty tomb at Beni Hassan, a liquid is being stirred over a fire and strained through a cloth (Fig. 9.6). As this scene adjoins one of vintage, it may be illustrating the production of grape syrup. In Tut-ankh-Amon's tomb, a jar was found labelled "unfermented grape juice of good quality from the temple of Aten" (Cairo Museum, No. J. 62324). Lucas (1962, p. 27), who examined two specimens from Deir-el-Medineh, found them to contain 17% and 24·4% respectively of glucose, and concluded that they were the remains of either honey or grape sugar. Of a much later date, the Zenon papyri (Edgar, 1931) mention grape syrup. These preparations were presumably similar to the "debach" of the Bible (Exodus, III, 8), a word that was translated "honey", and to the thickened concentrated fruit extracts called "debs" in Syria and Lebanon.

Date juice, and possibly other fruit juices were added to sweeten or "to prime" beer (discussed in Volume 2).

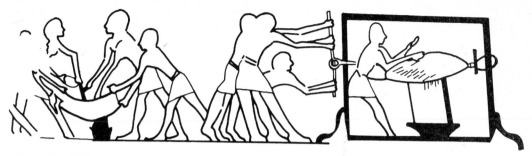

Fig. 9.6. Beni Hassan (Tomb no. 15). Pressing grapes. Left: Straining the juice through a cloth. Redrawn from Newberry and Fraser (1833–94).

In *medicine*, fruits found ready applications as taste correctives in addition to their possible pharmacodynamic properties. Their list, after Lefebvre's translation (1956), covers practically all the varieties known at the time: *calamus aromaticus* (*Eb.*, XCVIII, 853); *caroub* in a mouth rinse (*Eb.*, LXXXIX, 746), or in oral mixtures (*K.*, 3; *Eb.*, LIV, 314; *Eb.*, VII, 22); *cyperus esculentus* (*Eb.*, IX, 28; XI, 34; LV, 334); *cyperus rotundus* "rush nut" (*Eb.*, LXI, 385); *dates*, in mouth rinses (*Eb.*, LXXXIX, 746), or in oral mixtures (*Eb.*, VII, 22; *Eb.*, LV, 333; LXXXIX, 745); *figs*, (*Eb.*, LI, 291; LV, 334; LXVII, 477); *grapes* (*Eb.*, LI, 291; *Eb.*, LV, 334); *juniper* (*Eb.*, 334, LV); *melilotus officinalis* (*Eb.*, XX, 64; *Zaub.* 1, 9–26); *melon* (*Eb.*, XCVIII, 852); *pomegranates* (*Eb.*, XVI, 50); *sycamore*, in a mouth rinse (*Eb.*, LXII, 554), and in mixtures (*Eb.*, XX, 65; XLII, 207); *watermelon* (*Ber.*, 193).

This, in addition to *sweet beer*, that was probably beer sweetened with a fruit juice or syrup (*Eb.*, LI, 291; LV, 333); and to unidentified fruits *iaou* (*Eb.*, LVI, 337), *iched* (? Sebesten), *Eb.*, XXXIX, 198), *kesbet* (*Eb.*, LVI, 342), and *semet* (*Eb.*, LXVII, 477).

Notes: Chapter 9

1. Honey, however, is not mentioned among the components of this particular preparation.
2. Dioscorides wrote that *Kyphi* was welcome to the gods and that the Egyptian priests used it abundantly. He added that there were many ways of making it, of which one used cyperius, juniper berries, plum raisins, resinae

repurgatae, calamus aromaticus, aspalathus, juncus odoratus, myrrh, old wine, honey (I, 24).

3. Dioscorides also believed that honey was good for cough (II, 82) and prescribed it with cummin (II, 33), as did the Berlin papyrus (*Ber.*, 31).

4. The "dead", i.e. evil souls, enemy spirits and demons.

Chapter 10   *Salt*

Salt in Antiquity

No animal organism can function or survive without adequate provision of minerals, of which—as a relic of the marine origin of all animal life—common salt (sodium chloride) is most abundant in the body. As a result, this mineral, of all others, was singled out by man to be added in its crystalline state to his diet.

However, that people may live in total ignorance of salt was known, ever since Homer related that Odysseus was advised to look for a people who ate no salt. These were, according to Pausanias (I, XII), the *Epeirotes*, the majority of whom, even after the capture of Troy, knew nothing of the sea, nor even as yet how to use salt, witness the words of Homer in the Odyssey

> "That done, a people far from sea explore
> Who ne'er knew salt, or heard the billows roar
> Or saw gay vessel stem the wat'ry plain
> A painted wonder flying on the main" (Odyssey, XI, 121–3, *The Poems of Alexander Pope*, 1967)

In Greece, itself, the use of salt appears to have been a late development. The Homeric poems nowhere mention the addition of salt to sacrifices. Athenaeus explained why

> ". . . But mindful to this day of the earlier customs, they roast in the flame the entrails in honour of the gods without adding salt. For they had not as yet discovered its application to that use. But since it pleased them later to do so, they added salt from that time on, although when holy rites are performed they still observe the ancestral custom." (*Deipnos.*, XIV, 23, 661)

In a note to that passage, the author of one translation, C. B. Gulick (1941, p. 43), remarked that there is no reason to doubt that the Ancient Egyptian prohibition to use sea-salt, that we shall discuss later, was also the rule in Greece; although salt was permitted in the cult of Aphrodite.

Schleiden (1875, p. 4) quoted many travellers who explored areas where salt was never used. It was unknown in several central American countries before the Spanish conquest and, before the European explorations the same was true in central Africa, where the saying, "he adds salt to his food" meant "this is a wealthy man." In Pre-Columbian North America salt was used south of a well-defined line of demarcation, while it was not all utilized to the north of it (Kroeber, 1941–42). Whether this had any relation to the dominant diet remains to be shown.

When man first learnt the use of salt is enshrouded in the mists of the remotest past. Parallel to the Ancient Greeks' ignorance of this seasoning, the original Indo-Europeans and the Sanskrit speaking peoples had no word for it. This apparent lack of salt-craving in early people could have been a result of their reliance on raw or roasted meat. Later, when with the invention of boiling the sodium content of meat was reduced, and when the shift to an agricultural economy introduced vegetables in increasing amounts, sodium chloride became a basic need to provide an adequate sodium intake and, more important still, to counterbalance the high potassium content of plants.

Thus, whereas most languages use the expression "bread and salt" as a general metaphor for food, none speaks of "meat and salt." In many countries, to share bread and salt is to establish the most sacred ties of loyalty that it would be sacrilegious to break. One of the most solemn oaths in the East is to swear by them. To place salt on the table is an expression of the utmost trust. To spill it is to break the trust and is still considered an omen of evil that can be dispelled only by appropriate gestures, like picking it up with the fingers and casting it over one's left shoulder (the side of the devil).

Either from the belief that men were mutually bound when they ate salt together, or from the idea that salt was a preservative and thus a sign of perpetuity, the binding by salt as a sign of inviolability is attested in the Bible

". . . neither shalt thou suffer the salt of the covenant of thy god to be lacking from thy meat offering; with all thine offerings thou shalt offer salt." (Leviticus, 2, 13)

This is stressed again and again in the Scriptures

"And thou shalt offer them before the Lord, and the priests shall cast salt upon them, and they shall offer them up for a burnt offering unto the Lord." (Ezekiel, 43, 24)

Salt was specifically mentioned in the donations to rebuild the Temple of Jerusalem

"And that which they have need of, young bullocks, and rams, and lambs, for the burnt offerings of the God of Heaven, wheat, salt, wine . . ." (Ezra, 6, 9)

And Artaxerxes ordered that unlimited quantities be made available without prescribing how much

". . . And I, even I, Artaxerxes the King, do make a decree to all treasurers which are beyond the river, that whatsoever Ezra the priest . . . shall require of you, it be done speedily, unto an hundred talents of silver . . . and salt." (Ezra, 6, 21—22)

But some of the Jews who were antagonistic to the promoters of the project wrote to Artaxerxes to warn him against the people of Jerusalem, asserting their loyalty since, they said

"We have been salted with the salt of the palace and it was not meet for us to see the king's dishonour." (Ezra, 4, 14)

It is tempting to see in the emphasis on adding salt to oblations a gesture of gratitude that manifests itself by giving back to God part of his bounties, in the same way as

". . . setting apart uont the Lord all that openeth the matrix and every firstling that comes of a beast." (Exodus, 13, 12)

The addition of salt in that context would be a reflection of a prized culinary habit.

It is, therefore, surprising to find that the Scriptures specifically cite salt only with meat offerings, not with offerings of wheat and oil, although they recommend adding it to all offerings

"With all thy offerings thou shalt offer salt." (Leviticus, 2, 13)

This distinction certainly contradicts the previously stated thesis that, at the origin, salt was not added to meat, but that it became necessary when cereals became important dietary constituents.

In the New Testament, salt is called "a good thing". Salt is good

". . . but if the salt shall have lost his savour, wherewith shall it be seasoned." (Luke, 14, 34; Mark, 9, 49)

"Ye are the salt of the earth: but if the salt have lost his savour, wherewith shall it be salted." (Matthew, 5, 13)

The hedonic Romans had the same high regard for this commodity.

"Heaven knows a civilized life is impossible without salt and so necessary is this basic substance that its name is applied metaphorically even to intense mental pleasures. We call them *sales* [wit] . . . But the clearest proof of its importance is that no sacrifice is carried out without the *mola salsa*." (Pliny, *H.N.*, XXXI, XLI)

Plutarch's guests were of the same opinion

"First there is salt, without which practically nothing is eatable. Salt is added even to bread and enriches its flavours; this explains why Poseidon shares a temple with Demeter. Salt is also the best relish to season other relishes . . . all meat is either a dead body or part of one. But the effect of salt upon meat, like the addition of a veritable soul, is to lend flavour and an agreeable quality to it." (*Moralia, Table Talk*, IV, 4, 668)

To explain the origin of salt, the Greeks had many theories, all set in the same poetic vein. The physics of evaporation being still unknown to them, they regarded salt as the fruit of an interaction between fire and water, two of the four Cosmic elements. Pythagoras was credited with saying that

"it should be brought to table to remind us of what is right; for salt preserves whatever it finds, and it arises from the purest sources, sun and sea." (Diogenes Laertus, VIII, 35)

Salt sources were holy in some countries. Tacitus (*The Annals*, XIII, 57) in his relation of the war between the Hermunduri and the Chatti over a river that produced plenty of salt, wrote

"They have not only a passion for settling every question by arms, but also a deep-rooted superstition that such localities are specially near to heaven . . . It is they think through the bounty of divine power, that in that river and in these forests salt is produced not as in other countries by the drying up of an overflow of the sea . . . but by a combination of two opposite elements, fire and water . . ."

The human appetite for salt as for many commodities is now divorced, however, from the need for it; and the amount used is almost wholly governed by culture and early habits. Among possible factors, the continuing habit of using salted foods, that allowed early man to survive from season to season, may have encouraged excessive use. But, though so much attention has been paid to the provision of salt, less concern was shown until recently to its excess in the diet, or to factors that favour its retention in the body. These, at least in animals, cause renal lesions and hypertension even independently of adjuvents like adrenal steroids, and it is certain that, in man and animals, restriction of excessive intake or the addition of potassium lower blood-pressure and, in animals, prolong survival (Meneely *et al.*, 1957).

Salt in Egypt

According to Plutarch, the Egyptian priests shunned salt because, like anything connected with the sea, they associated it with Typhon (Seth)

"The Nile, therefore, which runs from the south and is swallowed up by the sea in the north . . . For this reason, the priests keep themselves aloof from the sea, and call salt the 'spume of Typhon', and one of the things forbidden to them is to set salt upon a table; also they do not speak to pilots; because these men make use of the sea, and gain their livelihood from the sea . . . This is the reason why they escew fish . . ." (*I. and O.*, 363, 32)

Elsewhere, he said

"[They] make it a point of religion to abstain completely from salt, even eating their bread unsalted"

and he explained that they abstained from it because of the aphrodisiac properties sometimes attributed to it (*Table Talk*, IV, 10, 684, 685).

In partial contradiction to the above, he also suggested that abstinence was kept only on certain religious occasions

"[They] use no salt with their food during their periods of holy living, [because salt] by sharpening their appetite, makes them more inclined to drinking and eating." (*I. and O.*, 352, 5)

It is certain, however, that salt was not regarded in Egypt as impure in an absolute sense; or, else, this might have been thus construed only in Plutarch's days, which is unlikely. On some occasions, it was used in religious ceremonies. According to Herodotus

"At Sais when the assembly at the Isis Festival lamented over the death of Osiris, they all lit lamps filled with a mixture of oil and salt." (II, 62)

These contradictions may be reconciled in the light of Arrian's account of the oasis of Amon (Siwa)

"There are natural salts in this district, to be obtained by digging; some of these salts are taken by the priests of Amon going to Egypt. For whenever they are going towards Egypt, they pack the salt into baskets woven of palm leaves and take them as present to the King or someone else. Both Egyptians and others who are particular about religious observance, use this salt in their sacrifices as being purer than the sea-salts" (*Anabasis Alexandri*, III, 4, 3–4).

Thus, whereas sea-salt might have been considered impure, salt quarried in the oasis of Amon or, in fact, any salt other than sea-salt, was not. It was an offering acceptable to Kings and gods. According to Dawson, salt, with natron and wine, being all excellent preservatives, were probably first employed in mummification because they were credited with life-giving or life-preserving properties (1929, pp. 29–30). That such ideas were current among the Ancients is confirmed by the above quoted citation of Pythagoras "For salt preserves whatever it finds," a concept on which Plutarch expanded.

"Consider also whether this other property of salt is not divine too . . . As the soul, our most divine element, preserves life by preventing dissolution of the body, just so salt, controls and checks the process of decay. This is why some of the Stoics say that the sow at birth is dead flesh, but that the soul is implanted in it later, like salt, to preserve it . . . Ships carrying salt breed an infinite number of rats because, according to some authorities, the female conceives without coition by licking salt.[1] But it is more likely that the saltiness imparts a sting to the sexual members, . . . for this reason perhaps, womanly beauty is called 'salty' and 'piquant' when it is not passive, nor unyielding, but has charm and provocativeness. I imagine that the poets called Aphrodite 'born of the brine' . . . by way of alluding to the generative property of salt . . ." (*Table Talk*, V, 10, 685)

We find in the literature many examples accrediting the acceptance of this commodity. Khounanoup the "Eloquent Peasant" or "Oasian" as he is sometimes called, hero of a twelfth dynasty popular tale, left his home in the "Oasis of Salt" (Wadi Natroun),[2] loaded with his products, that included salt, to sell them in Egypt (Lefebvre, 1949). Rameses III donated to temples large quantities of common salt (*A.R.*, IV, 299–348).

Khounanoup presumably traded his salt for other products, since minted money was as yet unknown. Salt has always been a readily bartering commodity, highly prized for its dietetic, taxable, or trade value.

In the days of Marco Polo (1929, p. 175), Tibetan Tartars used it instead of paper money; and Schleiden (1875, p. 70) quoted the price of a picture of Christ by Holbein, sold for 2,000 tons of salt. So great was the value of salt that wars were waged over its sources, like the war related by Tacitus, between the Hermunduri and the Chatti (Chapter

10, p. 446). Strabo (*Geo.*,XV, 1, 30, 700) thought worthy of record that Alexander the Great's armies were accompanied by a mining engineer who found, near the present site of Lahore, a mountain of salt sufficient for the whole of India. Pliny told of another mountain of salt in Oromenus of India, that brought to the Rajah greater revenues than those from gold or pearls (*N.H.*, XXXI, 7).

This was a legacy of old ways. In Rome, salt found its place even in military payments; hence the word "salarium" or salt-money (Pliny, *H.N.*, XXXI, 88, 89), from which came "salary" and its deratives. Selling it to enemies, like selling weapons or wheat, was punishable by death according to the Codex Justiniani

> "*Cotem ferro subigendo necessariam hostibus quoque uenundari, ut ferrum et frumentum et sales, non sine periculo capitis licet*" (lib., XXXIX, IV, 11). (It is not licit, under capital penalty, to sell to the enemy the whetstone to sharpen iron; as well as iron, wheat or salt.)

Sources and Varieties of Salt in Egypt

Although Herodotus obviously exaggerated when he stated that all the soil of Egypt exudes salt to the extent that the Pyramids were injured by it (II, 12), salt was easily obtained from many sources. Herodotus specifically mentioned the Pelusiac salt pans where salting factories cured fish for export (II, 15), an aspect of salt use that we have discussed in previous chapters.

Pliny (*N.H.*, XXXI, XXXIV–XLII) divided salt into two kinds: one, natural, made by condensation; the other, artificial, by drying. It was made around Egypt, he added, by the sea itself which permeates the soil, soaked by the Nile. He mentioned artificial salines on the coast and natural sources in Pelusium as well as beneath the sand in the desert between Egypt and Arabia, and in the Western Desert. The latter source still provides the oasians of Kharga, Dakhla and Farafra, with a very impure kind. Pliny also described a lake near Memphis that yielded a "blushing red" salt; a well-known phenomenon in the Mariut salines where brine waters and salt are at times coloured red under the action of various microorganisms.

But we do not know which methods of purification the Ancients utilized to obtain the pure salt they used, that was quite free from natron and sulphate, as shown by analysis of specimens from the sixth dynasty found in Gebelein, and of undated salt bricks from Deir el-Medineh (Lucas, 1962, p. 269).

Several varieties are mentioned in the texts: just "salt," "northern" salt, and an unidentified "*spr*" salt. But the differences between them are unknown. Herodotus, who stated that salt quarried in Libya was of two colours, white and purple (III, 186), is no more informative on this point. But, at least in Greek times, gourmets put different kinds of salt to different uses

> "To season meats and foods, the most useful one melts easily and is rather moist, for it is less bitter. For preserved meat the more suitable salt is sharp and dry." (Pliny, *H.N.*, XXXI, 86, 87)

Elsewhere Pliny talks of "spiced" salts (XXXI, XLI), a variety also mentioned by Athenaeus (*Deipnos.*, IX, 336b), and Plutarch (*Table Talk*, V, II, 812). But these were probably later ameliorations introduced by Greek epicureans.

A natural variation, difficult to identify, is the fragrant salt of Arabia, reported according to Strabo (16, 4, 20) by Poseidonus.

Salt and the Authorities

The production, sale and distribution of salt were considered of sufficient importance to the national economy to justify the affectation of special salt-gatherers to the temples. Rameses III gave a preferential status to those he appointed to Khnum's temple at Elephantine, by issuing a decree protecting them against exactions, appropriations, or any adverse (legal) procedures (*A.R.*, IV, 148); but there is no indication that it was subject to any impost or that it constituted a Royal or governmental monopoly.

In Rome, salt was the object of a State Monopoly first in the sixth century B.C. In the beginning of the Second Punic War a salt tax, imposed by Livius to cover war expenses, gained him the hatred of the people, and the nickname "Salinator." Thereby began the long story of salt taxing in Europe that was, in subsequent history, at the root of many uprisings and revolutions.

During Ptolemaic and Roman times, and in Egypt conforming to the policy of all Hellenistic states, salt was taxed at every stage of its handling. The State became the sole supplier to dealers and brokers; and these had to pay for their licences. The retail price was fixed; and all subjects, except a few privileged, were subjected to a very unpopular salt tax.

Medical Uses of Salt

Salt entered in the composition of a large number of recipes administered through all possible routes.

Orally, a mixture to open the bowels, contained "northern" salt, senna and fresh dates (*Eb.*, IV, 13). Another, for anal conditions, combined "northern" salt with balanites oil, honey, sweet beer and fermented mucilage (*Ber.*, 16, 5–17, 1).

Through an undetermined route, probably orally, "fresh salt" and honey (*Eb.*, XCIV, 801) or "northern" salt, dates, wine and oil (*Eb.*, XCIV, 799), were thought to speed delivery.

Anal applications and suppositories were made with "salt", water melon, honey, and *?ibw* (*Eb.*, XXXI, 139); or "salt", myrrh (or ? olibanum), frankincense (? terebinth), rush nut, celery, coriander, oil, *?mehtet* (*Eb.*, XXXII, 145); or "northern" salt, bran, oil, honey (*Ch. B.*, 5, 7–8).

In enemas, "northern" salt was mixed with balanites oil, honey, sweet beer and *?mhwy* (*Eb.*, XLIX, 265).

To treat gynaecological conditions, "fresh" salt, terebinth (?frankincense), *bsbs* (? fennel), onion, *djsrt* (beer or a milk preparation?), and fly droppings (*Eb.*, XCIV, 802), were injected *per vaginam*.

With other ingredients, it was also applied to burns (*Eb.*, LXVIII, 484), and to the eyes to treat pterygium (?) (*Eb.*, LIX, 365).

Other Uses of Salt

The non-dietary and non-medicinal uses of salt were many: metal smelting, gold refining, and the manufacture of glass (Forbes, 1955, p. 162 f). But its main applications were in relation to food, as a seasoning or to cure meats (see chapters on beef, fowl and fish). There is no mention that it was used in sacrifices.

Notes: Chapter 10

1. A statement repeated by Aristotle "Some people say, indeed stoutly maintain, that if they merely lick salt, mice become pregnant, without copulation (*Historia Animalium*, VI, XXVII).
2. *Natroun* [or natron], a natural mixture of sodium carbonate and bicarbonate that must not be confused with nitre (potassium nitrate, saltpetre).

Index of Popular Sayings

Sayings are listed in the order in which they appear

I

Index to Volumes 1 and 2

The subentries have been arranged in order of reference, rather than in alphabetical order.

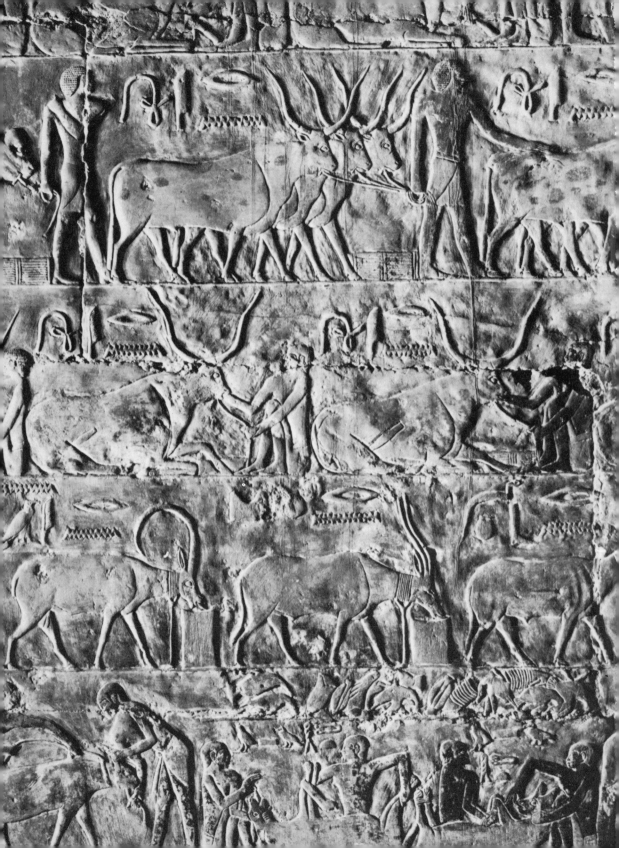